Praise for *Take Care of Yourself*

"Take charge of your health! If you don't, who will? There is no better guide to the path and no more honest assessment of medical ills than you will find in this book. It not only covers maintaining your health but also prepares you for managing new problems that come along. *Take Care of Yourself* leaves you well prepared to 'take charge!'"
— C. Everett Koop, MD, Former Surgeon General, U.S.

"Since its initial publication, *Take Care of Yourself* has probably done more for the health and peace of mind of Americans than any other book. As a bonus, it helps to curb rising health care expenditures."
— Victor R. Fuchs, Henry J. Kaiser Jr., Professor Emeritus, Stanford University; author of *Who Shall Live? Health, Economics and Social Choice*

"*Take Care of Yourself* is a book of pure genius: clear, concise, authoritative, trustworthy. It provides the foundation of our new consumer-driven health care system."
— Regina E. Herzlinger, Professor, Harvard Business School; author, *Consumer-Driven Health Care*

"*Take Care of Yourself* is a must for every person with a new symptom who wonders, 'What do I do now?' The advice is clear and sensible. This book helps me to self-manage my health conditions and assures me that I am making the right decisions. It is a must-have book for my health care bookshelf."
— Kate Lorig, RN, Dr. PH, Professor, Stanford Patient Education Research Center

"There are a remarkable number of award-winning wellness programs that use *Take Care of Yourself* to improve employee health and reduce the need for medical care. It's no wonder: the book is a lifesaver. It tells you so much you can do to address your own health problems immediately, effectively, and efficiently."
— Carson E. Beadle, Chairman, The Health Project

Important Addresses and Telephone Numbers

Please take a moment to put these numbers together here so that you can find them fast when you need them.

Emergency Room _____

_____

Poison Control Center _____

_____

911/Ambulance _____

_____

Family Physician _____

_____

Pediatrician _____

_____

Specialist (specify) _____

_____

Dentist (office) _____

_____

Dentist Emergency Number _____

_____

Hospital (main number) _____

_____

Take Care of Yourself

BOOKS BY THESE AUTHORS

The Arthritis Helpbook
by Kate Lorig and James F. Fries

Taking Care of Your Child
by Robert H. Pantell, James F. Fries, and Donald M. Vickery

Take Care of
YOURSELF

The Complete Illustrated Guide to Medical Self-Care

TENTH EDITION

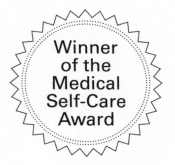

Winner
of the
Medical
Self-Care
Award

James F. Fries, MD and Donald M. Vickery, MD

Da Capo
LIFE
LONG

Many of the designations used by manufacturers and sellers to distinguish their products are claimed as trade-marks. Where those designations appear in this book and Da Capo Press is aware of a trademark claim, the designations have been printed in initial capital letters (e.g., Excedrin).

Instructions on the abdominal-thrust maneuver for choking (pages 82–85) have been adapted from the National Safety Council publication *Family Safety and Health*, Winter 1986–1987.

The drawing on fishhook removal from the foot (page 118) is adapted from George Hill, *Outpatient Surgery* (Philadelphia: Saunders, 1973).

The decision chart on alcoholism (page 305) has been adapted from J. A. Ewing, "Detecting Alcoholism: The CAGE Questionnaire," *Journal of the American Medical Association* 252 (1984): 1905.

Information on substance abuse (pages 307–309) has been adapted from Donald M. Vickery, *Lifeplan: Your Personal Guide to Maintaining Health and Preventing Illness* (Reston, VA: Vicktor, 1990).

The table on pages 324–325 has been adapted with permission from G. J. Pfeiffer, *Taking Care of Today and Tomorrow* (Reston, VA: The Center for Corporate Health Promotion, 1989).

The table on page 332 has been adapted from Howard W. Ory, "Mortality Associated with Fertility and Fertility Control: 1983," *Family Planning Perspectives* 15, no. 2 (March/April 1983).

Design and production by Eclipse Publishing Services
Set in 10.5 point New Baskerville

Cataloging-in-Publication data for this book is available from the Library of Congress.

First Da Capo Press edition 2017
ISBN: 978-0-7382-1973-8 (paperback)
ISBN: 978-0-7382-1974-5 (e-book)
LCCN: 2017946578

Published by Da Capo Press
www.dacapopress.com
@DaCapoPress

Note: The information in this book is true and complete to the best of our knowledge. This book is intended only as an informative guide for those wishing to know more about health issues. In no way is this book intended to replace, countermand, or conflict with the advice given to you by your own physician. The ultimate decision concerning care should be made between you and your doctor. We strongly recommend you follow his or her advice. Information in this book is general and is offered with no guarantees on the part of the authors or Da Capo Press. The authors and publisher disclaim all liability in connection with the use of this book.

LSC-C

10 9 8 7 6 5 4 3 2

To Our Readers

This book is strong medicine. It can be of great help to you. The medical advice is as sound as we can make it, but it will not always work. Like advice from your doctor, it won't always be right for you. This is our problem: if we don't give you direct advice, we can't help you. If we do, we'll sometimes be wrong. So here are some qualifications:

▲ If you're under the care of a doctor and receive advice contrary to this book, follow the doctor's advice; the individual characteristics of your problem can then be taken into account. This is especially important if you have been diagnosed with a chronic condition.

▲ If you have an allergy or a suspected allergy to a recommended medication, check with your doctor, at least by phone, before following the advice in this book.

▲ Read medicine label directions carefully; instructions vary from year to year, and you should follow the most recent.

▲ If your problem continues to concern you beyond a reasonable period, you should see a doctor. We suggest for most problems what a reasonable period might be.

Contents

List of Tables

Preface

"Take Care!" With this traditional parting phrase, we express our feelings for our friends and show our priorities. When I see you again, be healthy. Keep your health. Not "Be rich!" or "Be famous!" but "Take care of yourself!"

This book is about how to take care of yourself. For us, this phrase has four meanings:

First, "take care of yourself" means maintaining the habits that lead to vigor and health and that postpone aging. Your lifestyle is your most important guarantee of lifelong vigor, and you can postpone most serious chronic diseases by making the right choices about how to live. You can prevent most bad health.

Second, "take care of yourself" means periodic monitoring for those few diseases that can sneak up on you without clear warning, such as high blood pressure, cancer of the breast or cervix, glaucoma, or dental decay. In such cases, taking care of yourself may mean going to a health professional for assistance.

Third, "take care of yourself" means to respond decisively to new medical problems. Most often, your response should be self-care, and you can act as your own doctor. At other times, however, you need professional help. Responding decisively means that you pay particular attention to the decision about going, or not going, to see the doctor. This book, more than any other, helps you make that decision.

Many people think that all illness must be treated at the doctor's office. In fact, most new problems already are treated at home, and a much larger number could be. The public has not had guidelines to determine when the doctor is needed and when not. In the United States, the average person sees a doctor slightly more than five times a year. Over 3 billion prescriptions are written each year, about eight for each man, woman, and child. Medical costs now average over $8,000 per person per year—over 18% of our gross national product. In total, over $3 trillion each year. Among the billions of different medical services used each year, some are lifesaving, some result in great health improvement, and some give great comfort. But some are totally unnecessary, and some are even harmful.

In our national quest for a symptom-free existence, we make millions of unnecessary visits to doctors—as many as 70% of all visits for new problems. For example, 11% of such visits are for uncomplicated colds. Many others are for minor cuts that do not require stitches, for tetanus shots despite current immunizations, for minor ankle sprains, and for the other problems discussed in this book. But while you don't need a doctor to treat most coughs, you do for some. For every ten or so cuts that don't require stitches, there is one that does. For every type of problem, there are some instances in which you should decide to see the doctor and some in which you should not.

These are critically important decisions. If you delay a visit to the doctor when you really need medical attention, you may suffer unnecessary discomfort or leave a serious illness untreated. On the other hand, if you go to the doctor when you don't need to, you waste time, and you may lose money or dignity. You may lose confidence in your own ability to judge your health and in the healing power of your own body. You can even suffer unnecessary physical harm if you receive a drug that you don't need or have a test that you don't require. Your doctor is in an uncomfortable position when you come in unnecessarily and may feel obligated to practice "defensive medicine" just in case you have a bad result and a good lawyer.

This book, above all else, is intended to help you with the decision of when to see your doctor. It gives you a "second opinion" within easy reach on your bookshelf. It helps you make sound judgments about your own health.

The fourth meaning of our title is this: your health is your responsibility; it depends on your decisions. There is no other way to be healthy than to "take care of yourself." You have to decide how to live, what to do to age more slowly, whether to see a doctor, which doctor to see, how soon to go, whether to take the advice offered. No one else can make these decisions, and they profoundly affect your future health. To be healthy, you have to be in charge.

Take care of yourself!

James F. Fries, MD
Stanford, California

Donald M. Vickery, MD
Evergreen, Colorado

Acknowledgments

We are grateful to many people for their help with this tenth edition, including the thousands of readers who have written with suggestions and encouragement and the hundreds of health workers, corporations, and health plans that have used previous editions in their programs and practices.

We particularly thank Dr. Stuart Altman, Carson Beadle, Dr. Karen Bolenhorn, Dr. William Bremer, Dr. Grace Chickadonz, Dr. Peter Collis, Charlotte Crenson, Ann Dilworth, Dr. Edgar Engleman, Dr. Jack Farquhar, Dr. Jonathan Fielding, William Fisher, Sarah Tilton Fries, the late Elizabeth Fries, Victor Fuchs, Dr. Ron Goetzel, Regina Herzlinger, Jo Ann Gibely, Dr. Robert Harmon, Dr. Halsted Holman, J. W. Hornsby, Dr. Robert Huntley, Dr. Donald Iverson, the late Dr. C. Everett Koop, Dr. Julius Krevans, Dr. Kenneth Larsen, Dr. Kate Lorig, Florence Mahoney, Michael Manley, Dr. Larry Matson, Lawrence McPhee, Dr. Dennis McShane, Dr. Eugene Overton, Dr. Robert H. Pantell, Charles L. Parcell, Christian Paul, Clarence Pearson, William Peterson, George Pfeiffer, Dr. Robert Quinnell, Nancy Richardson, Dr. Robert Rosenberg, Dr. Ralph Rosenthal, Craig Russell, Dr. David Satcher, Dr. Douglas Solomon, Dr. Michael Soper, Warren Stone, Dr. Richard Tompkins, the late Dr. Donald Vickery, Dr. William Watson, and Dr. Craig Wright for their advice and support.

How to Use This Book

Welcome to *Take Care of Yourself*. We've tried to make this book very easy for you to use. We want you to be able to quickly find the information you want, from emergency advice to preventive measures that will help you stay healthy for a long time.

To get the most from this book, here's a good way to read it:

Today

▲ Read the introduction that follows and Chapter 3, "Emergencies," so that you can develop a plan for dealing with a medical problem or emergency before one happens.

▲ Write the telephone numbers of your Emergency Room, Poison Control Center, and other resources on page ii.

▲ Read about what you need in your "Home Medicine Chest" in Chapter 2.

▲ Leaf through the rest of the book and read what interests you.

Today or Over the Next Month

▲ Read Part I carefully. Consider the six keys to health and the preventive steps you can take to keep yourself and your family healthy.

▲ Read Part III and consider your medical coverage. Review any questions about your health insurance with your coverage provider.

▲ Once again, leaf through the whole book and read what interests you.

When a new medical problem arises, you'll quickly be able to find advice and suggestions in Part II, "Common Problems." Then you can perform home treatment or contact your doctor, whichever the book advises.

With *Take Care of Yourself,* you'll handle common medical problems effectively and confidently. You'll save money by not going to the doctor when you don't have to, and you'll save yourself grief by recognizing problems before they grow. By living a healthier life, you can live a happier life.

When you face a medical problem, consider these six steps:

1. *Is emergency action necessary?*

   Usually the answer is obvious. The most common emergency signs are listed and described in Chapter 3, "Emergencies," on pages 78–87. It's a good idea to read the chapter now so that you're prepared. Fortunately, the great majority of complaints don't require emergency treatment.

2. *Look up your chief complaint or symptom.*

   Part II contains information on more than 175 common medical problems; these make up over 98% of new problems. Determine your chief complaint or symptom—a cough, an earache, dizziness—and look up that problem. Don't jump to conclusions about the cause of the problem: chest pain, for instance, may indicate indigestion rather than a heart attack. (Look that problem up under Chest Pain, page 260.) Each problem discussion contains a decision chart to help you choose between home treatment and a call or visit to the doctor.

   Use the chart on page xxv to find the appropriate problem section. The chapters in Part II are organized by type of complaint and by area of the body: skin problems; bones, muscles, and joints; and so on. You can also look up a symptom in the contents or the index.

3. *If you have more than one problem, turn to the section for your worst problem first.*

   You may have more than one problem, such as abdominal pain, nausea, and diarrhea. In such cases, look up the most serious complaint first, then the next most serious, and so on. If you use more than one chart, play it safe: if one chart recommends home treatment and the other advises a call to the doctor, call the doctor.

4. *Read all of the general information for the problem.*

   The general information describes possible causes of each problem, methods for treating it at home, and what to expect at a doctor's office, if you need to go. This material gives you important information about interpreting the decision chart. If you ignore it, you may inadvertently choose the wrong action.

5. *Go through the decision chart.*

   Start at the top. Answer every question, following the arrows indicated by your answers. Don't skip around: that may result in errors. Each question assumes that you've answered the previous question.

6. *Follow the treatment indicated by the decision chart.*

   Sometimes the decision chart will instruct you to go to another section. More often you'll find one of the instruction icons shown below and on the next page. Sometimes you'll find an illustration showing you how to carry out the home treatment for the best results.

   Don't assume that an instruction to use home treatment guarantees that your problem is trivial and may be ignored. Home treatment must be used carefully if it is to work. As with all treatment, home treatment may not be effective in a particular case, so don't hesitate to visit a doctor if the problem doesn't improve.

   If the chart indicates that you should consult a doctor, it doesn't necessarily mean that the illness is serious or dangerous. Many less serious problems require a physical examination to diagnose the cause, and facilities at the doctor's office can make accurate diagnosis possible.

The charts usually recommend one of the following actions, noted by the symbol to the left.

▲ **Seek Medical Care Now**

Go to your doctor or health care facility right away. In the general information, we try to give you the medical terminology related to each problem so that you can anticipate some words your doctor may use during your conversation.

▲ **Seek Medical Care Today**

Call your doctor's office and say that you're coming in. Describe your problem over the phone as clearly as you can. Review Chapter 13 about communicating with your doctor so that you can get the most from your visit.

▲ **Make Medical Appointment**

Schedule a visit to your doctor's office anytime during the next few days. Before the appointment, review Chapter 13 about communicating with your doctor.

▲ **Call Medical Advisor**

Often a phone conversation with your doctor or physician assistant will enable you to avoid an unnecessary visit, which is one way of using medical care more wisely. Remember that most practices don't charge for telephone advice; they regard it as part of their service to regular patients. Please don't abuse this service in an attempt to avoid paying for medical care.

If your every call results in a recommendation for a visit, the doctor is probably sending you a message: come in and don't call. This is unfortunate, and you may want to look for a doctor willing to put the telephone to better use.

▲ **Use Home Treatment**

Follow the instructions for home treatment closely. These steps are what most doctors recommend as a first approach to these problems.

There are times when home treatment is not effective, even though you do it conscientiously. Think the problem through again, using the decision chart. The length of time you should wait before calling your doctor can be found in the general information in most sections. If you become seriously worried about your condition, call the doctor.

For quick access to your chapter, open to the appropriate tab.

Emergencies (Chapter 3)

Does the person show any of these emergency signs?
▲ Major injury
▲ No pulse or breath
▲ Unconsciousness
▲ Active bleeding
▲ Stupor or drowsiness
▲ Disorientation
▲ Shortness of breath while resting
▲ Cold sweats
▲ Severe pain

Yes

Emergency
Go to the emergency room or call 911 for help immediately. Turn to page 79, in the black-edged pages, for more instructions.

No

Is the person choking and unable to speak or cry out?

Yes

Emergency
Turn to page 82.

No

Has the person swallowed poison?

Yes

Emergency
Turn to page 86.

No

NONEMERGENCY
Identify the type of problem and turn to the beginning of the chapter with the corresponding blue tab on the edge of the book. Or look up the problem in the index or the table of contents.

For recommendations on a healthy lifestyle for you, Chapter 1

For advice on your Home Medicine Chest, Chapter 2

Common Injuries, Chapter 4

Ear, Nose, Throat, Eye, and Mouth Problems, Chapter 5

Skin Problems, Chapter 6

Childhood Diseases, Chapter 7

Bones, Muscles, and Joints, Chapter 8

Chest, Abdominal, and Urinary Problems, Chapter 9

Generalized Problems, such as fever, stress, or addiction, Chapter 10

Women's Health, Chapter 11

Sexual Problems and Questions, Chapter 12

Introduction

You can do more for your health than your doctor can.

We introduced the first edition of *Take Care of Yourself* in 1976 with this phrase. The concept that health is more a personal responsibility than a professional one was controversial at that time, although it can be found in the earlier writings of René Dubois, Victor Fuchs, and John Knowles, among others. But the idea was still foreign to a society heavily dependent on experts of every kind and seemingly addicted to ever more complex gadgetry and medications.

What a difference forty years can make! The report of the Surgeon General of the United States, *Health Promotion and Disease Prevention,* contains this statement, once considered a radical phrase: "You, the individual, can do more for your own health and well-being than any doctor, any hospital, any drugs, any exotic medical devices." The report goes on to detail a strategy for improved national health based on personal effort. The strategy of *Take Care of Yourself* is now a nationally accepted one. Your health depends on you. We are proud that this book has played a role in the changing national perception of health.

In 1991, the Department of Health and Human Services released an important document called *Healthy People 2000: National Health Promotion and Disease Prevention Objectives.* It laid out health goals for the nation for the year 2000; they had long been the goals of *Take Care of Yourself.* Some were met, more were not.

In 2000, the *Healthy People 2010* goals were set. Some of the 2010 targets:

▲ Increase the number of people participating in moderate daily physical activity to at least 30% of people (currently 21%)
▲ Reduce overweight problems to no more than 20% of people (currently 35%)
▲ Reduce dietary fat intake to an average of less than 30% of calories (currently 36%)

▲ Reduce cigarette smoking to less than 15% of adults (currently 24%)

▲ Reduce alcohol intake by 20% (from 2.54 to 2.0 gallons, or 7.5 liters, per person per year)

▲ Increase fiber intake to five servings a day on average (currently two a day)

We are pleased to support these national goals, and you will find many specific suggestions in *Take Care of Yourself* for how to reduce your personal health risks in the direction of the national goals.

The first nine editions of *Take Care of Yourself* included more than 200 printings totaling over 17 million copies in North America alone. This book has been translated into over 25 languages. It has been the central feature of many health promotion programs sponsored by corporations, health insurance plans, and other institutions. Acceptance by professional review panels is testimony to the soundness of the medical advice provided here. It is also a testament to visionary health directors who see the need for new approaches to health improvement.

Evidence That This Book Works

Does *Take Care of Yourself* work? Can you improve your health with the aid of a book? Can you use the doctor less, use services more wisely, save money? Absolutely. *Take Care of Yourself* has been more carefully evaluated by critical scientists than any health book ever written, and the evaluations have been published in major medical journals. These studies involved an aggregate of many thousands of individuals and cost nearly $4 million to perform. The results of all of these studies have been positive.

▲ A report in the *Journal of the American Medical Association* described a randomized study in Woodland, California. As determined by lot, 460 families were given *Take Care of Yourself,* and 239 were not. Visits to doctors by those who were given *Take Care of Yourself* were reduced by 7.5% compared with those not given the book. Visits to doctors for colds decreased by 14%.

▲ A report in the *Journal of the American Medical Association* compared the use of *Take Care of Yourself* in a health maintenance organization with a random control group. Medical visits were reduced 17%, and visits for minor illnesses were reduced 35%. This large study of 3,700 subjects over five years obtained its data directly from medical records, had a rigorous experimental design, and found statistically significant reductions in medical visits in both Medicare and general populations.

▲ A major study reported in the journal *Medical Care* detailed an experiment at 29 work sites that reduced visitation rates for households of 5,200 employees by 14%—1.5 doctor visits per household per year—after distribution of *Take Care of Yourself*.

▲ A report in the *American Journal of Health Promotion* analyzed health risks in over 250,000 people given *Take Care of Yourself* and Healthtrac materials and followed for up to 30 months. The decrease in health risks was consistent at about 10% per year, and applied equally to young and old ages and to those with less or more education.

▲ The *American Journal of Medicine* reported a randomized two-year controlled trial of nearly 6,000 Bank of America retirees. The people who received *Take Care of Yourself* and the Senior Healthtrac program reduced health risks by 15% compared with control groups. Furthermore, they saved about $300 per person.

▲ A randomized trial of 59,000 people reported in the *American Journal of Health Promotion* showed that these same materials improved health and saved over $8 million for the California Public Employees Retirement System.

▲ The *American Journal of Health Promotion* reported a study of over 8,000 employees of a large bank, with major improvements in health status and reductions in medical costs.

▲ In 2002, RAND released a report to Medicare recommending evaluation of health education programs involving *Take Care of Yourself* as a Medicare benefit.

▲ In 2004, MEDSTAT submitted its evaluation design report to Medicare with the same conclusions and recommended immediate implementation of a demonstration project. Then Secretary of Health and Human Services Tommy Thompson agreed.

Why does *Take Care of Yourself* "work," while other resources do not appear to work as well? We think it may be because of:

▲ **Medical Quality.** We are doctors ourselves, and we get a lot of help from our friends.

▲ **Medical Currency.** We make revisions every printing, almost once a month, to keep up with new knowledge.

▲ **Branching Logic.** Our decision guidelines are branching algorithms, which are more accurate and easier to use than linear lists.

▲ **Health Confidence Improvement.** You have to be confident to use recommendations. We work hard to help you build up your confidence so you can control your own health.

We, as a nation, are in the midst of a health care cost crisis. Costs now average over $8,000 per person per year—more than double those of many countries. Many people can no longer afford insurance. The *Take Care of Yourself* solution is simple: stay healthy, and when you do need to make a medical decision, make it wisely. Healthier people need less medical care.

For every heart attack prevented, the health care system saves over $200,000, and you may save your own life. By preparing a living will, you may save your family thousands of dollars, and you can increase the dignity of your care if you develop a terminal illness. Even the common cold that you treat at home may save $300 or more in doctor bills, laboratory tests, X-rays, and medication.

Some ask why you should work to reduce medical care costs when you have insurance? You paid for it; why not use it?

We are reminded of the "tragedy of the commons." In a small mountainous village in Spain, each family had one goat, which represented their total wealth. The village goats grazed on the common land inside the circle of huts and provided milk and cheese. One man reasoned that if he had two goats, he would be twice as wealthy, and the commons could surely support one more goat, so he raised two goats. Then another man did the same. And another. And another. Eventually the grass was all eaten up, the goats died, and the villagers starved.

The health care crisis can be controlled if we all work to decrease our need for and use of medical services. Now is a time to work for the common good: to preserve common resources. Your good health is its own reward. It feels better to be healthy than not. A vigorous lifestyle, a continuing sense of adventure and excitement, the exercise of personal will, and the acceptance of individual responsibility are essential to—and benefits of—the healthy life. Take care of yourself. You will help the broader society. And your loved ones will thank you for it.

PART I

The Habit of Health

CHAPTER 1

A Pound of Prevention:
Your Health Is in Your Hands

When we wrote *Take Care of Yourself* (TCOY) in the 1970s, it was quickly recognized as a self-care book that could help you solve your medical problems. You can make your own health decisions following reasonable and well-studied guidelines. You can save money and prolong your good health. TCOY works because the science is sound, factual, and clearly stated. It has helped many millions of people.

This tenth edition extends these approaches and algorithms as they have evolved. Even more importantly, it develops the emerging science of postponing aging and the processes by which you plan in advance to achieve a healthy long life for yourself and your family.

The truth is that you can do much more than any doctor to maintain your health and well-being. But first you have to get into the habit of health. And you have to have a plan. At the age of 50, individuals with good health habits can be physically 30 years younger than those with poor health habits. In other words, at age 50 you can feel as if you're 65 years old or 35 years old. Your health is in your hands.

The major health problems in the developed world are chronic long-term illnesses in middle age and beyond, and trauma at young ages. These illnesses, which include heart disease, cancer, emphysema, and liver cirrhosis, cause nearly 85% of all deaths. They also account for about 80% of all sickness in the United States. Over two-thirds of cases of these illnesses can be postponed, and most of these can be prevented.

You can greatly reduce the infirmities and pain associated with disease, as well as the deaths, by having a good plan for health. For example, only two years after your last cigarette, you return to the normal risk level for heart attacks. After ten years, you're back to nearly normal risk for lung cancer. In only a few weeks, exercise programs begin to contribute to your health and well-being. For many chronic diseases, not only can you slow the rate of progression, but you can also reverse part of the damage.

In this book, we emphasize the importance of making a life plan for prolonging youth and postponing aging. You can reduce damage to your future health by avoiding health risks in the first place.

If you want to achieve the healthiest life, you need to plan ahead. This is "the power of prevention."

Your plan for good health can prevent many nagging, nonfatal health problems such as hernias, back pain, varicose veins, and osteoporosis. And it can prevent the development of serious medical issues such as cancer, heart disease, and stroke; it is far better to prevent these diseases than to diagnose and treat them. By developing the habit of health, you can reduce the number of illnesses you'll have in your lifetime. As an even bigger bonus, you'll feel much better and have more energy. Good health is its own reward. An ounce of prevention is better than a pound of cure. Think of what a pound of prevention can do! Prevention is the most effective way to reduce lifetime illness, to retain vigor, and to postpone aging and death.

Postponing Aging

What is the greatest health challenge of our time? The answer may surprise you: aging. Aging affects the most people, results in the most deaths, and causes the most infirmities and misery. A cure for human aging is not on the horizon, but *postponing* the aging processes is practical already. We discuss the science and the data of human aging in this chapter.

You are likely to want to start postponing your aging earlier in your life than you had thought, set higher expectations for yourself, work at it harder, and keep it up longer than you had previously planned. You are much less likely to postpone your aging if you do not have a plan, or if you fail to carry out the plan you already have. This book is meant to guide you on your path toward lifelong health.

There are no magic elixirs, no new and improved diets, no fountains of youth, no miracle drugs. Any new health fad may have its moment, but there is little prospect of a cure for aging or a major reversal of established aging processes. However, if you are willing to put in a bit of careful work, there is likely to be very good news for you in your effort to prolong your health and delay your death.

Aging begins early in life and, in most cases, progresses slowly for decades before death. Aging begins in childhood, not in retirement. Aging has much to do with accumulated damage, the "death by a thousand cuts." It has relatively little to do with diseases directly, although diseases, often themselves caused by ignoring health risks, may hasten the damage. What does this mean for you? You can best achieve improvement in your future health by reducing your personal health risks, sustained over time.

The slow development of the infirmities, disabilities, and malfunctions of advancing age mostly result from overlooked health risks that gradually damage the body. The cause of the damage usually precedes the damage by quite a long time. Sun exposure comes decades before melanoma; the first cigarette, decades before lung cancer; the too-high lipid intake, years before the earliest fatty streak in the artery and decades before the heart attack or congestive heart failure. Alcohol comes before the car crashes, the cirrhosis, and the liver failure. Obesity precedes hernias and diabetes. The joint injury precedes osteoarthritis.

We introduced the term "Compression of Morbidity" in 1980 to point out that we can improve health and extend life by decreasing health risks and delaying morbidity (the occurrence of disease). Simply put, it means postponing the age of onset of chronic illness, thus reducing the time at the end of life when a person is sick or disabled. If the onset of the first chronic illness is postponed, the burden of lifetime illness may be compressed into a shorter period before the time of death.

Gompertz Law, first described in 1825 by British actuary Benjamin Gompertz, observed that mortality rates double in humans every eight years of life. No exceptions to Gompertz Law have been found after nearly two centuries. Other mammalian species also exhibit a doubling of mortality rates with increasing age. Compressing the infirm period of life between a postponed onset and exponentially increasing mortality will reduce lifetime morbidity. Many geriatricians and gerontologists are now converging toward the view that the limit to human life is fixed at about 115 years. A Frenchwoman, who died in 1997, was said to be 122 years old; no new such claims have been made in the last twenty years. While the exact number of supercentenarians (persons 110 years of age and older) is difficult to determine, recorded cases indicate that the majority are women. The oldest living person at the time of this writing was 116. The average age at death in developed countries is projected to continue to rise over at least the next century. But the age of the oldest among us will not.

We now have a clearer understanding of aging and illness than we did in 1980. Aging processes can be detected early in life, often before age 20 or so. For the sprinter, it may be "losing a step." For the chess master, it may be losing matches more frequently. Later effects of aging are more obvious. Perhaps the hair is grayer and the stairs are more difficult. The first losses in function are inconveniences; later they become impairments.

Our own aging becomes apparent to all of us at some point, usually in our forties, fifties, or later. This does not mean that we are "old," and decreases in certain abilities may be more than compensated for by increased experience and accumulated knowledge. Many of those aging today will find it easier to add life to their years than years to their life.

The Six Keys to Health

Good news! There are only six major keys for good future health:

1. Vigorous, regular, serious, lifelong exercise
2. Not smoking
3. Moderate use of alcohol and other intoxicants
4. Maintenance of a moderate weight
5. Reduction of accidental injuries
6. Wise use of professional prevention

Here's more good news: most individuals don't even need to worry about all six keys. You're probably already a nonsmoker. Quite possibly your body weight isn't too far from where it needs to be. If you drink alcohol at all, your alcohol intake is probably already moderate. Maybe you already do some exercise, and you have some good dietary practices. Most likely you take some measures, such as using your automobile seat belts, to reduce your chances of serious injury. And you probably work with your doctor to have some of the periodic screening tests that you need. You may well have only two or three areas that need additional serious work. Focus on these.

Vigorous, Regular, Serious, Lifelong Exercise

Physical and mental exercise is the single most important key to lifetime health. It prevents obesity. It tones the muscles, strengthens the bones, and makes the heart and lungs work better. It increases your physical reserve and your vitality. Exercise eases depression, assists the function of the bowels, leads to sound sleep, and aids in every activity of daily life. Exercise helps prevent heart disease, high blood pressure, stroke, and many other diseases.

Physical exercise means aerobic conditioning that results in an increase in pulse rate and sweating while exercising 90 minutes a week, maintained over a lifetime. One hundred eighty minutes a week—or more—is even better. This commitment is more serious and aggressive than most recommendations you may have seen, particularly the lifelong aspect. You have to mean it to achieve it.

People who do not seriously persist with lifetime exercise are unlikely to maintain the full benefits. Changing from one exercise regimen to another of equal intensity is fine. Your resting pulse rate should decrease, preferably to 60 beats per minute or slower. Some people find that having a dog helps motivate them to exercise. Make exercise fun, exercise with others, and vary the specific exercises over time to decrease the effects of any injuries.

Mental exercise is, of course, in many ways the equal of physical exercise but defies description because of its great variability. Its attributes vary across individuals and across activities, and maintaining strong mental health requires different kinds of mental activity.

One of the authors has found physical satisfaction in climbing the seven continental summits and running the Boston Marathon, and mental satisfaction in writing 450 scientific articles, or having a beer with friends or a quiet evening in family conversations. Other people have different lists of preferred activities and get there by different paths. Have fun doing something you like to do, every day if possible.

The Three Types of Exercise

Exercise comes in three different types: aerobic (endurance, cardiovascular) exercises, strengthening exercises, and stretching exercises. There are advantages and limits to each type.

Aerobic (endurance, cardiovascular) exercise is a requirement for fitness and vitality. This exercise is the most important kind. The word "aerobic" means that during the exercise period, the oxygen (air) that you breathe in balances the oxygen that you use up. During aerobic exercise, a number of good things happen. Your heart speeds up to pump larger amounts of blood. You breathe more frequently and more deeply to increase the oxygen transfer from the lungs to the blood. Your body develops increased heat and compensates by sweating to keep your temperature normal. You build endurance.

As a result of aerobic exercise, the cells of the body develop the ability to extract a larger amount of oxygen from the blood. This improves the function of all of the cells of the body. As you become more fit, these effects increase. The heart becomes larger and stronger and can pump more blood with each stroke. The cells can take up oxygen more readily. As a result, your heart rate when you're resting doesn't need to be as rapid. This allows more time for the heart to repair itself between beats.

Strengthening exercises are the traditional "body-building" exercises that build stronger muscles. Squeezing balls, lifting weights, and doing push-ups or pull-ups are examples. These exercises can be very helpful in improving function in a particular body part after surgery (for example, knee surgery) where it's necessary to rebuild strength. They also help to strengthen your bones, since bones react to stress by becoming stronger; they can help strengthen bones even at advanced ages.

You should never use anabolic steroids or any other drugs as part of a strengthening program. By so doing, you may damage your future health.

Stretching exercises are designed to help keep your body loose. Everyone should do some of these exercises, but they don't have many direct effects on health. Be careful not to overdo these exercises. Toe-touching, for example, should be done gently, without bouncing. Stretch relatively slowly, to the point of discomfort and just a little bit beyond.

Stretching exercises can be of great benefit in these situations:

▲ If you have a joint that's stiff because of arthritis or injury
▲ If you've just had surgery on a joint
▲ If you have a disease condition that results in stiffness

There's nothing mysterious about the stretching process. Any body part that you can't straighten or bend completely needs to be frequently and repeatedly stretched; a good rule is twice daily. Over weeks or months, you can often regain motion of that body part.

For most people, however, stretching exercises are useful mainly as part of the warm-up for aerobic (cardiovascular) exercise activity. Gently stretching before you begin aerobic exercise is important for three reasons:

▲ It helps to warms up the muscles.
▲ It makes the muscles looser.
▲ It may decrease the chances of injury.

Stretching again after you complete aerobic exercise can help prevent stiffness.

Your Aerobic Program

Aerobic exercise is important for all ages. It's never too soon to develop the habit of lifetime exercise. It's never too late to begin an aerobic exercise program and to experience the often dramatic benefits. There are, of course, a few difficulties in beginning a new exercise program. If you've lost fitness by avoiding exercise for some time, start at a lower level of physical activity than a more active person would. You may have an underlying medical condition that limits your choice of exercises; if so, ask your doctor for advice about exactly how to proceed.

Some people worry that (1) exercise will increase their heart rates; (2) they have only so many heartbeats in a lifetime; so (3) they may be using them up. But our hearts are not preprogrammed to run out after a certain number of beats. In addition, because of the decrease in their resting heart rates, fit individuals actually have 10% to 25% fewer heartbeats in the course of a day, even after allowing for the increase during exercise periods. Aerobic training also builds good muscle tone, improves reflexes, improves balance, burns fat, aids the bowels, and makes the bones stronger.

Other people worry about destroying their joints with too much exercise or about sudden death while exercising. The truth is the opposite. Those who exercise have much less disability than those who don't, and the ligaments that support their joints actually become stronger. And while very occasionally a person does have a heart attack during exercise, the overall chances of a heart attack are very greatly decreased by aerobic exercise. Total knee replacements are needed *less* frequently in persons who exercise regularly.

Heart Rate. Much has been made of reaching a particular heart rate during exercise, a rate that avoids too much stress on the heart and yet provides the desired training effect. Cardiologists (heart specialists) often suggest that a desirable heart rate during exercise is 220 minus your age times 75%. For example, at age forty, your target exercise heart rate is 180 x .75 = 135 beats per minute. It can be difficult to count your pulse while you're exercising, but you can check it by counting the pulse in your wrist for 15 seconds immediately after you stop and then multiplying by 4.

As your training progresses, you may wish to count your resting pulse, perhaps in bed in the morning before you get up. The goal here (if you don't have an underlying heart problem and aren't taking a medication such as propranolol, which decreases the heart rate) is a resting heart rate of about 60 beats per minute. An individual who isn't fit will typically have a resting heart rate of 75 or so.

We generally find this whole heart-rate business a bit of a bother. There really are no good medical data to justify particular target heart rates. You may wish to check your pulse rate a few times just to get a feel for it, but it doesn't have to be something you watch extremely carefully. Aerobic exercise shouldn't be "all out." If you can't talk to a companion while you're exercising, you're probably working too hard; on the other hand, if you don't work up a sweat in a 70°F environment, you may not be exercising hard enough.

Aerobic Choices. Your choice of a particular aerobic activity depends on your own desires and your present level of fitness. You should be able to grade the activity; that is, you should be able to easily and gradually increase both the effort and the duration of the exercise over time.

Walking slowly isn't a true aerobic exercise, but it provides important health benefits. If you haven't been exercising at all, start by walking. A gradual increase in walking activity, up to a level of 100 to 200 minutes per week, usually should precede attempting a more aerobic program. First get in the habit of putting in the exercise time, then increase the effort. Walking briskly can be aerobic, but you need to push up the pace quite a bit to break a sweat and increase your heart rate. Walking uphill can quite quickly become aerobic.

Jogging, swimming, and brisk walking are appropriate for all ages. At home, stationary bicycles or cross-country ski machines are also helpful. We have seen people confined to bed using a specially designed stationary bicycle. Some individuals like to use earbuds or wireless headphones while they exercise; others exercise indoors while watching the evening news. Remember that aerobic exercise can't be "start and stop." Aerobic activity can't come in bursts; it must be sustained for at least 10 to 12 minutes during each exercise period. The most recent recommendations are for 15- to 30-minute exercise periods three to seven days a week. We suggest working toward 30 minutes, six or seven days a week, as a minimum goal.

Cautions. If you have a serious underlying illness, particularly one involving the heart or the joints, or if you're over age 70, ask your doctor for specific advice. Advice from your doctor should always take precedence over recommendations in this book. For most people, however, a doctor's permission to start exercising is not needed. We recommend mentioning your exercise program to your doctor while on a visit for some other reason. A good doctor will encourage your exercise program and perhaps assist you in choosing goals and activities.

Some doctors recommend that you have an electrocardiogram (ECG), an exercise electrocardiogram, or even a coronary arteriogram before you start exercising, particularly if you're over 50. We have difficulty seeing what this accomplishes because (1) gentle, gradual exercise is a treatment for heart problems anyway, and

(2) the tests produce up to 80% "false-positive" results, suggesting that you have problems when you don't. Many doctors (including us) don't think these tests are necessary, regardless of age, unless you (the patient) have specific, known problems. If a doctor recommends a coronary arteriogram (X-ray study of the arteries of the heart after injecting a dye into the arteries) before you begin an exercise program, you should seek a second opinion to see if you actually need this test

"Crash" exercise programs are always ill advised. You have to start gently and go slowly. There's no hurry, and there's a slight hazard in pushing yourself too far too fast. Age alone is not a deterrent to exercise. Many seniors who have achieved record levels of fitness, as indicated by world-class marathon times for their age, started exercising only in their 60s, 70s, or even 80s. A man over 100 years old has climbed Mount Fuji. One of the authors of this book (JFF) climbed nearly to the summit of Mount Everest in Asia and successfully climbed the highest peaks of the other six continents in his 50s.

Getting Started. Assess your present level of activity to determine where to start. Set goals for the level of fitness you want to achieve. Your final goal should be at least one year away, but you may want to develop in-between goals for one, three, and six months. Select the aerobic activity you want to pursue. Choose a time of day for your exercise. Develop exercise as a routine part of your day. We recommend that exercise be regularly performed for at least five or six days of the week; if you exercise all seven days, take it easy one or two days each week. Younger individuals can frequently become fit with exercise periods three or four times a week. For seniors, gentler activities performed daily are more beneficial and less likely to result in injury. You can make ordinary activities like walking or mowing the lawn aerobic by doing them at a faster and constant pace.

Start slowly and gently. Your total exercise activity shouldn't increase by more than about 10% each week. Each exercise period should be reasonably constant in effort. When you're walking, jogging, or whatever, you can use both distance and time to keep track of your progression. When starting out, keep a brief diary of what you do each day to stay on track. Slowly increase your exercise *time* to at least 90 to 100 minutes per week before you work to increase the *effort* level of the exercise. Get accustomed to the activity first and then begin to push it a bit. Again, progress slowly. The bottom line is patience and common sense.

Each exercise period should start with warming up by doing your intended activity at about 50% of normal intensity. This is one of the most important ways of avoiding muscle and joint problems during exercise.

Be sure to loosen up with stretching exercises after warming up and after exercise periods, and to wear clothing warm enough to keep your muscles from getting cold and cramping.

Handling Setbacks. No exercise program ever progresses without problems. After all, you're asking your body to do something it hasn't done for a while. It will occasionally complain. Even after you have a well-established exercise program, there will be interruptions. You may be ill, go on a trip where it's difficult to exercise, or sustain an injury. But the inevitable setbacks shouldn't change your overall plan.

Common sense is the key to handling setbacks. Often you can substitute another activity for the one you're having trouble with and thus maintain your fitness program. Sometimes you just have to stop for a while.

When you begin again, don't immediately start at your previous level of activity; losing fitness is a surprisingly rapid process. On the other hand, you don't have to start again at the beginning. The general rule is to take as long to get back to your previous level of activity as you were not exercising. If you can't exercise for two weeks, gradually increase your activity over a two-week period to get back to your previous level.

Topping Out. After your exercise program is well established, make sure that it becomes a habit you want to continue for a long time. Two hundred minutes of aerobic exercise a week (about half an hour a day) or more seems to give the best results. There is no medical evidence that more than that is of additional value. Many people won't want to exercise this much, and that's perfectly fine. You can get most of the benefits with less activity. At 100 minutes a week, you get almost 90% of the gain that comes with 200 minutes. At 60 minutes a week, a total of one hour, you get about 75% of the benefits that you get with 200 minutes.

Exercise should be fun. Often it doesn't seem so at first, but after your exercise habits are well developed, you'll wonder how you ever got along without them. Once you're fit, you can take advantage of your body's increased reserve to vary your activity more than you did during the early months. You can change exercise activities or alternate days of hard exercise and easy exercise. At that point, we hope you're a convert to exercise programs. You then can work to introduce others to the same benefits.

Not Smoking

Avoiding cigarette smoking is the second major key to future good health. Smoking causes over 300,000 deaths per year in the United States and has adverse effects on many physical functions and diseases.

Think of that as two fully loaded 747s crashing every single day. Lung cancer and emphysema (chronic lung disease) are the best-known and among the most miserable outcomes. However, smoking causes atherosclerosis to develop faster, and that problem affects smokers whether or not other diseases occur. Atherosclerosis results in heart attacks and strokes, angina pectoris (heart pains), intermittent claudication (leg pains), and many other problems. Pipe and cigar smoking don't have the pulmonary (lung) consequences that cigarette smoking does, but they can lead to cancer of the lips, tongue, and esophagus. Nicotine in any form has bad effects on the small blood vessels and thus increases your chance of heart attack. E-cigarettes perpetuate the tobacco habit and may encourage children to start smoking.

Think also about how ugly this habit is, the physical (second-hand smoke) and psychological effects on your kids, the dirty looks from strangers, the accelerated aging, the financial and other costs (such as forest fires and house fires), and other consequences. It's time to stop this foolish habit completely. Life is already too short.

It's never too late to quit. Only two years after your last cigarette, your risk of heart attack returns to average. It actually decreases substantially the very next week after quitting! After only two years, there's a decrease in lung cancer risk by perhaps one-third, and after ten years, the risk is back to nearly normal. The development of emphysema is stopped for many people when they quit smoking, although this condition doesn't actually reverse. But most people who quit smoking will enjoy major health benefits the rest of their lives.

Moreover, you'll notice at once that your environment becomes friendlier when you're not a smoker. A lot of the daily hassles that impair the quality of your life go away when you stop offending others with your habit.

Here are some tips for quitting:

▲ Decide firmly that you really want to quit. You need to believe that you can. Set a date on which you will stop smoking. Announce this date to your friends. When the day comes, stop.

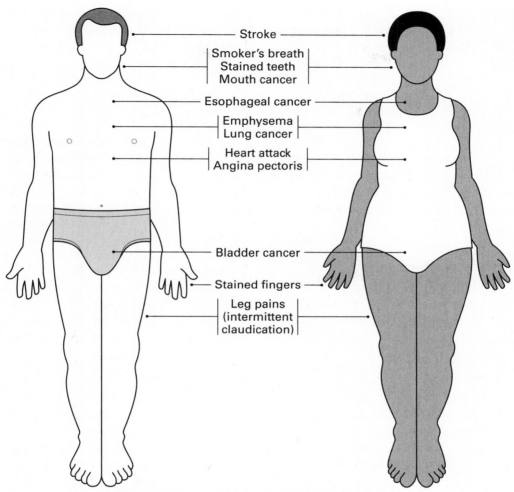

- Stroke
- Smoker's breath
- Stained teeth
- Mouth cancer
- Esophageal cancer
- Emphysema
- Lung cancer
- Heart attack
- Angina pectoris
- Bladder cancer
- Stained fingers
- Leg pains (intermittent claudication)

Smoking. The damage occurs at many sites throughout the body.

▲ You can expect that the withdrawal from nicotine may make you nervous and irritable for about 48 hours. After that, there's no further physical addiction. The psychological craving can sometimes last a very long time; often, however, this craving is quite short.

▲ Reward yourself every week or so by buying something nice with what would have been cigarette money.

▲ Combine your stop-smoking program with an increase in your exercise program. The two changes fit together naturally. Exercise will take your mind off smoking and decrease your tendency to gain weight in the early weeks after you stop smoking; this weight gain is the only negative consequence of quitting smoking.

The immediate rewards of not smoking include better-tasting food, happier friends, less coughing, increased stamina, more money, fewer holes in your clothes, and membership in a larger world. If you have children, you become a better role model for them.

Many health educators are skeptical about a slow reduction of smoking; they stress that you need to stop completely on a "quit date." We don't think this is always true. For some people, rationing is a good way to get their smoking down to a much lower level, at which point it may be easier to stop entirely. For example, the simple decision not to smoke in public can help your health and decrease your daily hassles. To cut down, keep in your cigarette pack only those cigarettes that you'll allow yourself that day. Smoke the cigarettes only halfway down before extinguishing them. Then, set a quit date.

Many good stop-smoking courses are offered by the American Cancer Society, the American Lung Association, and your local hospital. Most people don't need these, but if you do, they can help you be successful. Try to quit by yourself first. Then, if you still need help, there's a lot of help available.

Nicotine chewing gum or nicotine patches may help some people quit; your doctor can give you a prescription and advice.

Your decision to stop smoking is one example of your ability to make your own choices. If you're trapped by your addictions, you can't make those choices. Victory over smoking improves your mental health, in part, because quitting is difficult. Winning this fight can open the door to success in other areas.

Twenty-two percent of U.S. adults smoke cigarettes; in 1964, it was 54%. A hundred million Americans have successfully quit; you can too.

Moderate Use of Alcohol and Other Intoxicants

Avoiding binge encounters with alcohol, other acute intoxicants, or chronic substance abuse is the third key to better health. Alcohol can be good for you, in moderation; two drinks a day actually decrease heart disease and overall death rates below the level of nondrinkers. Red wine, in moderation, appears to be the healthiest form of alcohol. But excessive alcohol intake is a serious problem for some people in every age group.

Intoxications are mostly due to alcohol, and more alcohol problems come from abuse rather than use. Substance abuse causes far too many suicides, homicides, depressions, liver transplants, and auto crashes, in addition to the known physical and mental effects of overuse of prescription pain medications.

Among the potentially fatal complications are:

▲ Damage to the liver
▲ Delirium tremens (the DTs) from alcohol withdrawal
▲ Car, motorcycle, and private plane accidents, and domestic violence in which alcohol plays a role

There are many other complications that aren't fatal but that decrease the quality of your life. A drinking problem makes a person dependent on the next drink, interferes with emotions and thinking, and burdens loved ones, diminishing everyone's quality of life.

Fortunately, alcoholism is a disease from which many people recover, although recovery is a lifelong process. There are about a million recovered alcoholics in the United States; between half and three-quarters of the people who attempt rehabilitation succeed. Among some highly motivated groups, the success rate is much higher. For example, more than 90% of physicians and airline pilots who participate in highly structured, monitored programs stay in recovery. Success depends on personal characteristics, early treatment, the quality of the counselors or support program, access to the right medical services, and the strong support of family, friends, and coworkers.

We discuss the warning signs and treatment of alcoholism on page 304. Refer to this section if you have any questions about your drinking. Usually this problem gets too little attention too late. Be alert for alcohol-related problems in family and friends, express your concerns to them, and cooperate in helping them establish a program for alcohol control or elimination. You can save their lives and perhaps even save your own.

Maintenance of a Moderate Weight

Controlling obesity and its complications is the fourth key to better health. Obesity, increasing rapidly, has greatly reduced the health gains people otherwise achieved from reductions in smoking and increases in exercise activity. Heart disease, stroke, falls, liver disease, and a general increase of problems in every other category accompany obesity. People who drink diet soft drinks often seem to be fat. Fast food appears to have addictive qualities. Look in your mirror, look at the scale, look around you; get the weight off and keep it off.

Weight Control

Excessive body weight compounds many health problems. It stresses the heart, the muscles, and the joints. It increases the likelihood of hernias, hemorrhoids, gallbladder disease, varicose veins, and many other problems. Excess weight makes breathing more difficult. It slows you down, makes you less effective in personal encounters, and lowers your self-image. You snore more if you're overweight. Fat people are hospitalized more frequently than people with normal weight; they have more heartburn, more surgical complications, more cases of breast cancer, more high blood pressure, more heart attacks, and more strokes.

Weight control is a difficult task. Think of "weight control" as "fat control," and it will fit in well with your other good health habits. For most of us, the problem and the solution are personal, not medical. (Excess weight is very seldom due to thyroid disease or other specific illness.) Like the other habits that change your health, management of this problem begins with recognizing that it is a problem. Weight control requires your continued attention. There are genetic factors that act to make weight control very difficult for some. For those of us with a potential problem, we must have lifelong vigilance.

Increasingly, exercise is recognized as an important key to weight control. Part of every weight-control program should be an exercise program. Obesity isn't just the result of overeating; obese people, when studied carefully, are found to move around less and therefore to burn too few calories. There's nothing very mysterious about calories. Thirty-five hundred calories equals about one pound (450 g) of fat. If you take in 3,500 calories fewer than you burn, you lose a pound. If you take in 3,500 calories more than you burn, you gain a pound.

There are two important phases to weight control: the **weight-reduction phase** and the weight-maintenance phase. Surprisingly, the weight-reduction phase is easier to manage. Here, the method you use to lose weight doesn't matter too much, although you should check with your doctor if you plan to lose a large amount of weight unusually quickly. You want to be sure that the diet you intend to follow is sound. (We discuss diet in more detail later in this section.) Complex carbohydrates are important to most sound diets. During the weight-loss stage, many of your calories are provided by your own body fat and protein as they're being broken down and burned as fuel; thus, you need less fat and less protein in your diet during this period. Weight-loss diets usually have a gimmick of some kind that encourages you and helps you

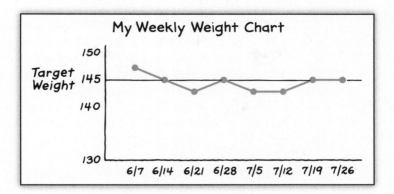

remember the diet, and there are dozens of books available with "secret" tips.

Recently, the gimmicks have been of the "Atkins" or "low-carb" variety. Before that there were low-protein, low-fat, liquid-protein, the "drinking man's" diet, and many others. Note that the various gimmicks contradict each other. The new fads, like the others, can result in some weight loss at first, but after a year, little weight has been lost. Over the long term, there are concerns about deficiencies of calcium, fiber, and other nutrients, and about elevation of LDL (bad) cholesterol with the low-carb diets, but few problems have been found in the first 6 to 12 months.

Remember that weight loss is naturally slow; even a total fast will cause weight loss of less than one pound a day. More rapid changes in weight are generally due to loss of fluid. The first few days of a diet often give you a false sense of accomplishment as you lose fluid. Then, when the rate of weight loss slows, you may think that the diet has failed. You have to be patient with this weight-loss phase.

Most people have some success in losing weight. If you set a target, tell people what you're trying to do and stick with the effort for a while. You can probably lose weight. One pound a week is a reasonable goal. This requires elimination of the equivalent of one day's food each week.

The **weight-maintenance phase** involves staying at the desirable weight you've achieved. This is more difficult, and it requires continual attention. Weigh yourself regularly (perhaps weekly) and record the weight on a chart. Draw a line at your desired weight and maintain your weight below the line, using whatever method works best for you. Keep exercising. Accept no excuses for increasing weight; it's easier and healthier to make frequent small adjustments in what you eat than to try to counteract binges of overeating with crash diets. Keep yourself off the dietary roller coaster. Failure at weight maintenance accounts for most diet failures.

If you can't lose weight, make yourself physically fit—**the fit but fat solution.** Recent scientific studies show that "fit but fat" people do a lot better than those who are sedentary and obese. Becoming aerobically conditioned returns heart disease and other risks for obese persons to nearly normal. Starting to exercise is easier for many obese people than losing weight and can be nearly as helpful for your heart.

We have not, in previous writings and here, been very enthusiastic about diet and nutrition as promoted in the lay press. We have never seen either health improvement nor even lifetime weight control with fad diets. In contrast, we think that a diet with reduced caloric intake and an exercise program, continued for many years, can show positive results and can even save money.

We present new data later in this chapter strongly indicating that exercise, lean body mass, and cigarette avoidance have impressive benefits for your long-term health.

There is always a new diet in the news, often with words like "easy" and "fast," claims of weight loss, and images of young slender actresses, while the people on the street seem to be fatter every year. Somebody is getting conned.

The exception to these "beware of the hype" cautions is the "Mediterranean diet." This exists in a number of variations and emphasizes low saturated fats, little sugar, and lots of fruits and vegetables. Studies have shown this diet works pretty well, and people also tend to stay on Mediterranean-type diets for a lot longer.

Most people can't easily make sudden, radical changes in diet, so they may not maintain them. In general, you should move slowly in making changes to your current diet. Develop good dietary habits slowly over a long time span. The more changes you make, the greater the benefits. Table 1 provides guidelines for a healthy diet.

At the same time, don't forget to exercise; diet is not the best way to deal with obesity. Exercise is.

Fat Intake

Excessive total fat and saturated fat are the worst aspects of the typical American diet. Excessive fat intake is the major cause of atherosclerosis (hardening of the arteries' inner lining), which leads to heart attacks and strokes. The U.S. government's *Healthy People 2010* goals call for people to reduce their total fat intake to less than 30% of the total calories they consume and their saturated fat intake to

Table 1: Your Diet for Health	
Protein	Reduce protein intake from red meat; increase protein from whole-grain foods, vegetables, poultry, and fish.
Fat and Cholesterol	Decrease total fat intake to less than 30% of total calories. Greatly decrease the saturated fats found in whole milk, most cheeses, and red meat. Switch to vegetable oils, canola oil, soybean oil, corn oil, peanut oil, or olive oil.
Carbohydrates	Increase total carbohydrates, emphasizing whole-grain foods, vegetables, cereals, fruit, pasta, and rice; these contain "complex" carbohydrates.
Alcohol	Moderate use or less; "moderate" is approximately two drinks daily.
Fiber	Increase fiber intake, with emphasis on fresh fruits and vegetables and whole-grain foods.
Salt	Decrease to about 4 grams per day (average intake in the United States is 12 grams per day). Avoid added salt in cooking or at the table and avoid heavily salted foods, such as most snack foods. Further decrease salt intake if medically recommended.
Calcium	Standard recommendations are for at least 1,000 mg per day for men after age 65 and 1,500 mg per day for women after menopause. For reference, nonfat milk has 250 mg per glass. Use powdered nonfat milk in foods such as soup. If necessary, use calcium supplements.

less than 10%. The current U.S. average is 37% of calories as total fat and nearly 20% as saturated fat.

We think that you should try for 30% of calories as total fat but only 7% as saturated fat. Stricter diets have been shown to actually *reverse* some early artery hardening. In some cases, patches on the artery walls nearly disappear. Such improvements have been seen both in monkeys given high-fat diets and then normal diets and exercise, and in X-ray studies of human hearts.

Cholesterol

An elevated serum cholesterol level is one sign warning you to reduce dietary fat. A good level is "200 or less"—that's 200 milligrams (mg) of cholesterol per deciliter (dl) of blood. Some advocate even stricter standards, particularly in persons with known heart disease. Measurement of cholesterol is only a very rough guide to your dietary needs, however, and everyone will benefit from decreasing fat intake. The actual chemistry of fats in the body is very complicated. The waxy white cholesterol not only comes from your diet but is also manufactured in your liver. This cholesterol production in turn is related to the various other fats in your diet. Attached to the cholesterol itself are high-density lipoproteins (HDL), which actually help prevent atherosclerosis, and low-density lipoproteins (LDL), which make heart problems much more likely. The LDL (bad cholesterol) travels "outbound" from the liver and can deposit on the inside walls of blood vessels. The HDL (good cholesterol) takes cholesterol "inbound" back to the liver for removal and can help remove plaque from arterial walls.

You can simplify this whole complicated business by simply cutting down on the largest sources of saturated fat in your diet. Fortunately, there are easy approaches to reducing saturated fat intake.

- ▲ Instead of butter, use soft or liquid **margarine.** Some evidence suggests that solid margarines are no better for you than butter. Avoid "trans fats," which are hazardous and are found in many margarines and many foods. Check the label for "trans fats." If there are any, don't buy.
- ▲ Use **low-fat** or **nonfat milk** instead of whole milk. The calcium and other nutrients in milk are very good for you, but the saturated fat is bad.
- ▲ Cut down the number of **eggs** per week; two eggs a week or fewer is a good ration.
- ▲ To reduce fat intake from **meats,** don't eat meat often. A good rule for many people is to avoid having red meat two days in a row. This easy rule brings variety to your diet. Remember, the white fat in red meat is really the problem. Pork, bacon, hot dogs, and sausage are not red but usually contain a great deal of saturated animal fat. When you do have meat, trim the fat extensively before cooking, broil so that some fat burns or runs off, and cook the meat longer so it's well done. For meat lovers, a good (and economical) practice is to buy small cuts of meat; surround a four- or five-ounce steak with large portions of vegetables.
- ▲ **Don't fry foods,** which usually adds saturated fat. If you do fry, avoid saturated fats such as palm oil and coconut oil; although these are vegetable oils, they're saturated fats that are bad for your arteries. Monounsaturated fats—such as olive oil, peanut oil, and canola oil—may actually be good for you.

What about other ways to lower your serum cholesterol and other fats (lipids) in the bloodstream? As we discuss in the following sections, fish is excellent food, and fiber (in vegetables, celery, apples, beans, and whole-grain breads and cereals) actually acts to lower serum cholesterol by binding some cholesterol in the bowel before the cholesterol can be absorbed. Adequate calcium intake, needed for strong bones, also lowers blood pressure and probably the blood lipids. Your exercise program lowers your total cholesterol and also increases the good HDL in your blood. When you stop smoking, your HDL cholesterol goes up. Good health habits all seem to fit together.

Protein

What's the best protein for your diet? Probably that from whole-grain foods. The official national nutritional guidelines recommend that you substitute complex carbohydrates (such as whole-grain foods and cereals) for some of the fat and some of the protein in your diet. The complex carbohydrates are more slowly digested and provide a more even source of energy.

Fish is extremely good for you; you should plan at least two fish meals a week. Interestingly, the best fish for you are the high-fat kinds that live in cold water, such as salmon or mackerel. These contain a kind of fish oil that is good for your heart and actually lowers your serum cholesterol level. Do not be overly concerned about the mercury that is in some fish and has resulted in adverse publicity. The good health that comes from fish usually outweighs any problems; moderation is suggested for pregnant or nursing mothers.

Chicken and other poultry are good neutral foods. They contain less fat than red meat, though still some cholesterol; they have much less fat if you remove the skin.

Salt Intake

Having too much sodium (salt) in your system tends to retain fluid in your body, increasing your blood pressure and predisposing you to such problems as swollen legs. Your heart has to work harder with the increased amount of fluid volume. Thus, it's good to decrease your salt intake.

The average person in the United States takes in about 12 grams of sodium each day, one of the highest levels in the world. Our convenience foods and fast foods are usually loaded with salt. Salt is in ketchup, in most sauces, and in hidden form in many foods. You need to read the labels to find it: look for "sodium," not "salt."

The recommended amount of salt is four grams (about two grams sodium) per day. You'll get plenty of salt in your food without adding more. People with high blood pressure, heart failure, or some other problems may need to reduce salt much more radically and should discuss desirable levels with their doctor.

Do you have a craving for junk foods? Don't despair—there are healthy snacks! One of our favorites: popcorn, air-cooked, sprayed with butter-flavored PAM instead of butter, and sprinkled with a little Parmesan cheese. Even better, try popcorn with olive oil instead of butter, unsalted peanuts in the shell, or French bread basted with olive oil and toasted with oregano or garlic. Try low-salt whole-grain pretzels. To add flavor to foods, use lemon juice, pepper, or herbs rather than salt.

Fiber

Adequate fiber is important to your future health. Fiber is the indigestible residue of food that passes through the entire bowel and is then eliminated in the stool. It's found in unrefined grains, cereals, vegetables (particularly celery), and most fruits.

The beneficial effects of fiber come from its actions as it passes through the bowel. Fiber attracts water and provides consistency to the stool so that it may pass easily. The increased regularity of bowel action that results turns out to be very important; it decreases the chances of diverticulitis, an inflammation of the colon wall. Fiber also acts to decrease problems with constipation, hemorrhoids, tears in the rectal wall, and other minor problems. Finally, fiber binds cholesterol and helps eliminate it from the body.

We must emphasize that the natural-fiber approach to maintaining regular bowel movements is much better than using laxatives and bowel stimulants, which have none of the advantages of fiber. You need to get the fiber habit and to avoid the stimulant and laxative habit.

Calcium

Everybody needs enough calcium. Sufficient calcium is particularly important for senior men and even more important for senior women. Our national trend toward better health habits has decreased our intake of calcium-containing milk and cheese. Hence, calcium levels for many people have dropped below what is desirable, and calcium supplements are often needed.

Women over age 50 should have at least 1,500 mg of calcium each day, and men over age 65 at least 1,000 mg. A glass of non-fat milk contains about 250 mg of calcium. Add in the odds and ends of calcium in various foods and a typical daily intake is usually around 500 mg. Therefore, many people need some sort of calcium supplement. The most popular forms are Tums and Os-Cal; each tablet contains 500 mg of calcium. One or two tablets a day will usually do it.

It's important for you to remember the "calcium paradox." Just having enough calcium in your diet doesn't really help because the extra calcium is not, for the most part, absorbed by the body. You need both to take in enough calcium and to give your body a stimulus to absorb it. Weight-bearing exercise is a strong stimulus for your body to absorb more calcium and to develop stronger bones. Exercise is for everyone. For women after menopause, estrogen supplementation also can provide a strong stimulus for absorption of calcium. This possible treatment should be discussed with your doctor since it is not always recommended.

Diet Supplements

What about fish oil capsules? These contain the good fish oils, such as those found in salmon and mackerel, which lower the serum cholesterol level. Five capsules are about equivalent to one serving of salmon, but they cost less than salmon. Many experts believe that fish oil is the only supplement, other than a multivitamin, that most Americans should consider.

The good effects of some vitamin supplements, particularly vitamin E, have been supported by some, but not all, research. We discuss these in detail on pages 74–75.

Aspirin Treatment

What about taking a tablet of low-dose aspirin (81 mg) every day to thin the blood? This regimen has shown major benefits for those at increased risk for heart attacks. Take it in addition to making your dietary changes. Even very small doses of aspirin thin the blood and prevent clots in the arteries and veins, but these same doses can result in excessive bleeding. Studies of regular aspirin use have shown a major decrease in the number of heart attacks, but this was partly compensated for by increases in other diseases, including gastrointestinal bleeding and hemorrhagic strokes. We believe that aspirin treatment should be undertaken after discussion with your doctor, and generally not by those below age 40 or 50. The U.S. Preventive Services Task Force recommends 81 mg of aspirin daily for persons with a 3% or greater chance of a heart attack in the next five years; this generally means men over 50 and women over 65 years of age.

Drugs to Lower Cholesterol

Cholesterol-lowering drugs such as the "statins" (atorvastatin, lovastatin, pravastatin, etc.) and some other drugs are powerful and very important, helpful drugs. But we recommend that you discuss such medications with your doctor. They will usually be recommended if you are at higher risk for heart disease because of one or more of the following risk factors:

▲ You have had a heart attack.
▲ A parent or a sibling had a heart attack before age 40.
▲ You have elevated cholesterol levels, diabetes, high blood pressure, or smoke cigarettes.
▲ Your doctor has diagnosed the metabolic syndrome (obesity, insulin resistance, high triglycerides, and low HDL "good" cholesterol).
▲ Your cholesterol or other lipids remain above a desirable range after you have made appropriate modifications to your diet.

Your goal for cholesterol and triglyceride levels will depend on which risk factors you have. Particularly nasty combinations of risk factors may result in a goal as low as 70 for LDL cholesterol, a level so low that it will necessarily require drugs in addition to lifestyle changes.

Note also that the statins appear to reduce the risk of heart disease beyond their effect on cholesterol, a benefit that may be related to reduction of inflammation.

The "statins" do cause muscle and tendon aches and pains quite frequently and serious muscle or liver disease rarely.

Reduction of Accidental Injuries

Accidents, considered broadly, are a major cause of injuries and deaths. Minimizing them is the fifth key to future good health. Car crashes are the biggest cause of injuries and deaths, but fires, airplane accidents, floods, earthquakes, drownings, and many other causes also contribute. Many of these events are readily preventable. Prevention includes proper use of seat belts and child seats and abiding by speed limits. Now we have to add the dangers and distractions of talking and texting while driving, and multitasking as a distracting cause of death and injury. We are too often our own worst enemies.

Seat Belts and Helmets

Automobile seat belts reduce death and injury by 75%—but only when people wear them! Wear seat belts all of the time, whether you're a driver or a passenger. Strap little kids into a secure car seat. Air bags are great, but you still need to buckle the belt. All the time. And, thousands of people, mostly children and young adults, die or suffer severe head injuries because they neglected to wear a helmet while bicycling, motorcycling, skiing, or skating. Wear one!

Seat belt and helmet use symbolizes the other healthy actions you can take to avoid injury. This simple and easy-to-achieve habit greatly reduces health risks, and adopting the habit means that you've thought ahead, considered the probabilities and the risks, and taken action to preserve your future health. The same kind of thinking will help you reduce other risks. Studies show that people who always use their seat belts have also lowered their risks in other ways. They're less likely to be smokers, for example, and they're less likely to drink and drive.

Impairment

The other extremely important, preventable contribution to auto-motive injury is alcohol or, less frequently, impairment by other drugs. Often it seems the intoxicated driver survives intact, while passengers in the other car suffer. Your primary responsibility to yourself and those around you is not to drive when under the influence. You can wreck your life, not just your car. We believe, however, that responsibility extends to passengers as well. Don't ride with an impaired driver under any circumstances. Walk, call a cab, or go with someone else. Before a party, appoint a "designated driver" who is responsible for staying sober. Hide the car keys from someone who has had too much to drink.

The new kind of impaired driver is one who is distracted by cell-phones, email, and social media. We've all noticed these people suddenly swerving into the next lane repeatedly, usually in broad daylight. This is a risk to life and limb, of a similar magnitude to alcohol intoxication. Don't drive while texting, reading, arguing with a passenger, or distracted in any way.

Water

Drownings are also usually preventable. Watch children whether they are in a pool, lake, or ocean. Wear life preservers on small boats. Don't go boating with an impaired captain, and don't be one yourself. Don't dive into hard objects or shallow depths. Watch out for the undertow. Use common sense.

Fire

Fires are usually preventable tragedies. They're started by overloaded electrical systems, faulty heaters, smoking in bed, hot ashes in garbage cans, careless use of fireworks, playing with matches, inadequate fireplace screening—all avoidable hazards. Fires are even more likely to hurt people when there are no smoke detectors or no fire extinguishers. Having well-placed and functioning smoke detectors in your home is another proof that you're thinking ahead, considering probabilities and risks, and taking action to protect your future.

Falls

Most broken bones are caused by falls, and most falls are preventable. Clutter in the home, no grab bars in the bathroom, poor lighting, the wrong shoes, careless use of ladders, unsteady walking because of alcohol or other drugs—all are causes.

Firearms

Gunshot wounds are a major cause of death in our society, especially among young people. Adolescents with thoughts of suicide are much more likely to succeed in killing themselves if they have a gun available. Criminals, especially in the illegal drug trade, often use guns without regard for whom they injure. Use common sense to protect yourself from crime. Take extreme care in using and storing firearms. Lock ammunition securely away from the firearm.

Wise Use of Professional Prevention

Professional prevention refers to assistance needed from doctors, nurses, other health professionals, medical institutions, pharmacists, self-care books, and other sources. We list it as the sixth key, and it is a pervasive need. In this book, professional prevention is appropriate wherever a diagram says "Seek Medical Care Today," "Seek Medical Care Now," or "Call Medical Advisor." Professional prevention includes vaccinations, baby care, periodic checkups (only if strongly suggested by your doctor), emergency room visits (when the problem discussion ends with "Seek Medical Care Now!"), dental care, and many others.

Sometimes, we have to admit, a health professional may suggest unnecessary services. You will need to be ready, politely but firmly, to seek a second opinion when a medical suggestion doesn't seem right for you.

The most important part of prevention, developing good health habits, has been discussed above. This is your personal responsibility. But the idea of preventive medicine also includes five other strategies that involve health professionals, and it's important to understand both the strengths and the limitations of these strategies:

▲ The checkup or periodic health examination
▲ Screening for early problems

▲ Early treatment for problems
▲ Immunizations and other public health measures
▲ Health risk appraisal

Periodic Checkups

An annual checkup is still recommended by some schools, camps, employers, and the army. However, doctors seldom go to each other for routine checkups. Checkups don't detect treatable diseases early with any regularity, and they may raise false confidence; that is, they may encourage the false belief that if you're regularly checked, you don't need to concern yourself as much about developing good health habits.

Your primary interest is in finding conditions about which something can be done, and for this, the checkup is unfortunately not very useful. If you use the techniques described above to reduce your health risks, and if you attend to new symptoms as discussed in Part II of this book, you'll gain few advantages from an annual "complete checkup."

Are complete checkups ever worthwhile? Yes. The first examination by a new doctor allows you to establish a relationship with him or her. Increasingly, the periodic checkup is not as much for the detection of disease as for the opportunity to counsel the patient about poor health habits, so that patients can do a better job of personal disease prevention. We applaud this change and look to doctors to further refine their skills at influencing their patients to take care of themselves.

Screening for Early Problems

Although complete checkups may offer limited benefits, periodic screening tests in several specific areas are important. Try to arrange these tests when you visit your doctor for another reason so as not to require a special trip.

Blood pressure test. High blood pressure is a significant medical condition that gives little warning of its presence. During adult life, it's advisable to have your blood pressure checked at least every year or so. This measurement can easily be done by a nurse, physician's assistant, or nurse's aide; a doctor's visit isn't required. If high blood pressure is found, a doctor should confirm it, you should confirm it again by taking your blood pressure a number of times while you are relaxed at home, and you should carefully attend to the measures needed to keep it under control (see High Blood Pressure, page 294).

Pap smear. If you're a woman over age 20, you should have a Pap smear taken every year or so. Some authorities now recommend beginning annual Pap smear testing at the age of first sexual activity, decreasing its frequency to every three to five years after the first three tests are negative, and again increasing the frequency to every one or two years after age 40. This test detects cancer of the cervix, the portion of the womb (uterus) that protrudes into the vagina. In early stages, this cancer is almost always curable. See Chapter 11, "Women's Health," page 310, for more information.

Breast examination. Women over age 25 should practice breast self-examination (BSE) monthly. Any suspicious changes should be checked by a doctor. While the effectiveness of BSE in the detection of cancer is arguable, we believe that knowing whether a lump is new or old, getting larger or smaller or varying in size, can be helpful. Women with large breasts can't practice self-examination with as much reliability as other women and may wish to discuss other screening procedures with their doctors. We recommend mammography as a yearly screening procedure for women after age 50, and others believe screening should start at age 40. Women who have already had a breast tumor should follow their doctors' recommendations. Women with a strong history of breast cancer in their family should begin mammography screening by age 40. See pages 310–311.

The importance of these few examinations is underscored by their availability as a public service, free of charge, at many city and county clinics. The U.S. Preventive Services Task Force consists of the leading experts on the science of screening procedures. Its recommendations are summarized in Table 2 and closely parallel our views about screening.

The value of other screening tests is more dubious. Some doctors believe that routine glaucoma tests and tests for blood in the stool after age 30 are worthwhile, and others don't.

Many news stories have suggested that screening with prostate-specific antigen (PSA) determinations, with or without digital rectal examination, revolutionizes the outlook for prostate cancer and promises to save many men's lives. Unfortunately, there's no convincing evidence yet that this screening improves the outlook for avoiding prostate cancer.

Early Treatment
In several areas, treatment before symptoms occur can be very important. These treatments include statins for cholesterol reduction,

Table 2: Recommended Adult Screening Procedures

Procedure	Recommendation
Pap smear for cervical cancer (women)	Annually for 3 years starting at age 21, or when sexual activity begins, whichever is earlier. If these first 3 tests are negative, every 3 years from then on.
Fecal occult blood tests for colorectal cancer	Annually after age 50.
Colonoscopy for colorectal cancer	Every 3 to 5 years after age 50; every 10 years if last screening negative If a parent or sibling has had colon cancer, colonoscopy every 3 to 5 years after age 40.
Breast cancer screening (women)	Monthly self-examination. Yearly physician examination after age 40. Annual mammogram after age 50, or after age 40 if mother or a sister has had breast cancer.
Lipid screening	Lipid profile measured at intervals of 5 or more years up to age 70.
High blood pressure screening	Recommended, incidental to other health care services (no special visit is needed).
Diabetes screening	Glucose tolerance test or glycosalated hemoglobin test recommended for pregnant women between the 24th and 28th week of gestation, or women with diabetes in their family who are planning to become pregnant. Otherwise not recommended.
Asymptomatic coronary artery disease screening	Screening with exercise stress testing *not recommended.*
Lung cancer screening	Screening *not recommended.*
Osteoporosis screening	Screening *not recommended.*
Prostate screening	PSA test *not recommended.*

multidrug control of high blood pressure, and tight control of blood glucose in early diabetes.

An effective health maintenance strategy includes seeking medical care promptly whenever an important new problem or finding appears.

The guidelines in Part II of this book can help you select those instances in which you should seek medical care. In most cases, you can take care of yourself with home treatment. However, you must respond appropriately when professional care is needed.

To ensure timely treatment, you need to make a plan ahead of time.

▲ Do you have a doctor? Do you discuss prevention with your doctor?

▲ If you need emergency care, where will you go? To an emergency hospital? To the emergency room of a general hospital? To the on-call physician of a local medical group?

▲ If you're not sure what to do after consulting this book, whom can you call for further advice?

▲ Have you written down the phone numbers you need or stored them in your cellphone?

Only rarely will you need emergency services. But the time that you need them is not the time to begin wondering what to do. If you have a routine problem that requires medical care, where will you go? Is there a nearby doctor? Who has your medical records? Chapter 13, "Working with Your Doctor and Your Health Care System," will help you answer these questions. Plan ahead.

Immunizations

Immunizations have had far greater impact on health in the developed nations than all of the other health services combined. Only a few years ago, smallpox, cholera, paralytic polio, diphtheria, whooping cough, and tetanus killed large numbers of people. These diseases have been effectively controlled by immunization in the United States and in most other developed nations. Smallpox has been eradicated from the entire world, and there's no longer any need for smallpox immunization. An incredible success story!

Unfortunately, many Americans have become lax or skeptical concerning the need for or safety of childhood immunizations. As a result, there has been a resurgence of measles, mumps, and rubella. You and your children can reap the benefits of immunizations while minimizing their risk by following the recommendations in Table 3a on page 31. The measles vaccine has been proven NOT to cause autism!

Keep a record of your immunizations on the form on page 352. Don't allow yourself to be reinoculated just because you've lost records of previous immunizations. If you haven't had a tetanus shot for 10 years or so, ask for a booster shot while visiting the doctor for another reason. You can eliminate future trips to the doctor by being protected for the next 10 years.

In general, don't seek out the optional immunizations. Flu shots, for example, are only partially effective and often cause a degree of

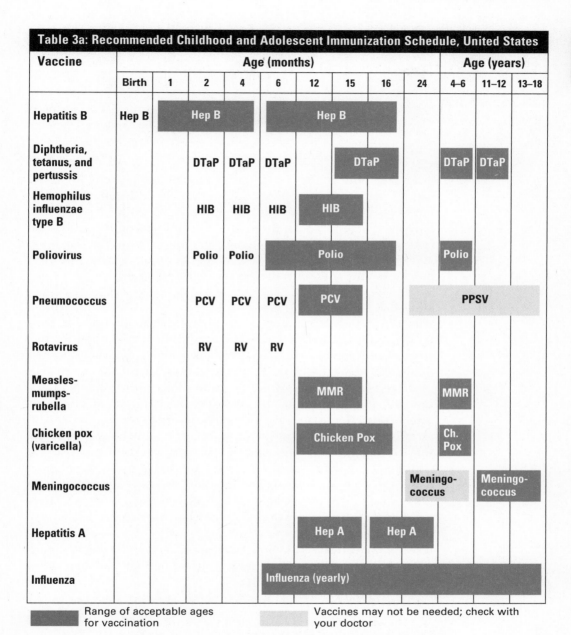

Table 3a: Recommended Childhood and Adolescent Immunization Schedule, United States

Vaccine	Age (months)									Age (years)		
	Birth	1	2	4	6	12	15	16	24	4–6	11–12	13–18
Hepatitis B	Hep B	Hep B			Hep B							
Diphtheria, tetanus, and pertussis			DTaP	DTaP	DTaP		DTaP			DTaP	DTaP	
Hemophilus influenzae type B			HIB	HIB	HIB	HIB						
Poliovirus			Polio	Polio	Polio					Polio		
Pneumococcus			PCV	PCV	PCV	PCV			PPSV			
Rotavirus			RV	RV	RV							
Measles-mumps-rubella						MMR				MMR		
Chicken pox (varicella)						Chicken Pox				Ch. Pox		
Meningococcus									Meningo-coccus		Meningo-coccus	
Hepatitis A						Hep A	Hep A					
Influenza					Influenza (yearly)							

Range of acceptable ages for vaccination

Vaccines may not be needed; check with your doctor

Adapted from the Centers for Disease Control, United States Public Health Service

Table 3b: Recommended Adult Immunization Schedule	
Schedule/Frequency	**Vaccine**
Every 10 years	T(d) adult tetanus, diphtheria
Over age 65/once	Pneumococcal
Over age 65, or with chronic illness such as lung disease/yearly	Influenza (flu)

fever and aching; they're generally recommended only for those over 65 and for those with severe major diseases. Recent studies do, however, suggest that adults over 40 who get a flu vaccine yearly have fewer sick days than those who don't. We recommend that the optional immunizations (including pneumonia and flu, Table 3b above) be taken only on the recommendation of your doctor. They have a definite role for some people, but not for all.

Health Risk Appraisal

Your future health is largely determined by what you do now. Your lifestyle and your habits have a dominant influence on how healthy you are, how healthy you'll be, how much time you'll spend in hospitals, and how rapidly you'll "physiologically" age.

Recently, techniques have been developed for mathematically estimating your future health risks. These techniques are variously termed "health risk appraisal," "health hazard appraisal," or "health assessment." You complete a questionnaire or otherwise provide information about your lifestyle and health habits. Your responses are mathematically combined to estimate your likelihood of developing major medical problems such as heart disease and cancer. Other estimates such as your "physiologic" age also may be calculated. These techniques form an increasingly important part of comprehensive health education programs such as those with which we have been involved: Healthtrac, Senior Healthtrac, and Informed Choice. They also have a potentially large role in helping you shape your own personal health program.

You should know several things about health risk appraisals:

▲ The results are only estimates. Even though they're based on the best medical studies, data are incomplete and may not apply equally to all populations. In general, the estimates may be accurate to within 10% to 20%. Think of health risk scores as similar to IQ or achievement test scores; they're approximately correct but not exact.

▲ The predictions are only averages. Some people will do better than the tests predict and others worse.

▲ Any single assessment represents you at one point in time, but your actual risks depend on the changes you make and your average lifetime health habits as well. Regular repeated assessments can reveal your current status and the benefits you've achieved through lifestyle changes.

▲ A good health risk appraisal should be based only on those relatively few risk factors that are scientifically well established and associated with major health factors. These include cigarette smoking, exercise, automobile seat belt use, helmet use, alcohol intake, obesity, dietary fiber, salt, fat intake, blood pressure, cholesterol levels, and stress level.

▲ The health risk assessment itself provides no health benefits unless it results in you changing your health-related behaviors, and the risk assessment might even frighten you unnecessarily. Therefore, these assessments are best used as part of a program that not only identifies risk but also educates you, motivates you to change, provides suggestions and recommendations, and reinforces positive changes.

▲ Such programs, termed "tailored print interventions," have been proven effective. They are increasingly used by corporations, health plans, and government. More and more of these programs now include use of the Internet. Medicare now has completed a major demonstration project over the past ten years, the Senior Risk Reduction Program. This study of tailored interventions involved 85,000 Medicare beneficiaries and used this book.

We're enthusiastic about the growing role of health promotion programs that focus attention on prevention of disease and the use of good health assessment tools. Well-designed programs are already having a large effect in decreasing human illness. As a bonus, they also reduce medical care costs.

Much of what's written about healthy behaviors makes the whole process seem mysterious and complicated. The supermarket tabloids are always reporting some new threat to your health. There is indeed a long list of possible threats to health, but trying to keep track of them all overlooks two important facts. First, these threats often aren't adequately proven. Second, even if they do prove to be true, they aren't that important. For instance, grilled foods may pose cancer-causing risks, but only if you eat such meals more than 30 times a year. We suggest moderating the amount of grilled foods you eat, but not necessarily discontinuing grilled foods. Many people find a benefit in controlling caffeine intake, particularly in the evening, but this is a minor problem compared with drinking alcohol.

Here we've tried to emphasize only the important and the proven. As we said before, only a few areas require your attention.

Is It Really as Simple as Postponing Aging?

Current thinking about health preservation has the primary goal of postponing or delaying aging. There's no better way to postpone aging than early prevention—by vigorous exercise, not smoking, and maintaining ideal body mass—and doctors today are becoming more interested in preventive medicine. Studies have shown that if prevention is begun before ages 30 to 40 and continued throughout life, aging is postponed by 10 to 16 years on average. Fewer lifetime risks to health means slower accumulation of damage, which means more gradual loss of function. To be sure, some infirmities are not known to be caused by prior health risks, including chronic neurological diseases such as Parkinson's and a small number of cancers. Doctors sometimes think of these, which we do not know how to prevent, as "bad luck" diseases, and they remind us that we can't prevent or cure everything all of the time.

In the following sections, we elaborate on the concept of postponing aging, present some compelling new data, and report some transformative results. This is a new era in understanding aging and how to slow it down and understanding health and how to prolong it.

We recognize that the discussions that follow can be challenging, particularly when they displace old dogmas. You may want to browse through these discussions, look at the figures, and come back later for a deeper reading.

If you have a new health problem, look it up in Part II of this book now.

Defining "Morbidity" and "Mortality"

Some key terms that will help you understand the new perspectives are:

Morbidity, an unfamiliar term to many people, encompasses all that is meant by "aging." Morbidity is everything about diminished health that is not death. It includes sickness, frailty, weakness, disease, infirmity, injury, disability, blindness, deafness, aging, and depression. Morbidity increases with age. Morbidity is all of the infirmities that precede death. If you can understand the term "morbidity," you can understand how and why we age, and how we can postpone aging. The five figures in this section will help.

Mortality, on the other hand, represents an irreversible single terminal event—death. Mortality is a simple way to describe the duration of an individual human life.

Compressing or Expanding Morbidity?

By 1980, people, on average, were living longer and, therefore, also became increasingly health impaired and frail in their later years. This was termed the "failure of success." It seemed that the more progress was made by medical advances in keeping people alive, the sicker the people became.

In 1980, the authors of this book and our colleagues hypothesized that if we could postpone illness and the effects of aging more than we were already postponing death, we could compress the illness portion of life between a later onset and a more slowly increasing age at death. Lifetime morbidity—the portion of a person's life that was spent ill or infirm—could be decreased, not increased. The failures of success could be fewer and rarer. This scenario, the "compression of morbidity," could result in better health.

However, there were some problems with this hypothesis.

In 1980, no one had developed a way to quantify morbidity. Without such a simple measurement, the compression of morbidity hypothesis could not be tested.

The conventional wisdom in 1980 was that mortality was the most important health outcome and that life expectancy was the most useful measurement. Morbidity was too hard to study, took too long to measure, and was too confusing to score. However, several research groups in the 1980s, including one that included the authors, developed patient "self-report" questionnaires that defined morbidity based on the subject's ability to carry out Activities of Daily Living (ADLs).

ADLs include getting up, walking, eating, hygiene, reach, grip, dressing and grooming, running errands, and other general activities. The scoring range includes "normally"(0), "with some difficulty"(1), "with much difficulty"(2), "unable to do"(3). Scoring an eight-item questionnaire thus might generate a score ranging from zero to 24. A typical 20-year-old has Health Assessment Questionnaire Disability Index (HAQ-DI) units of only a little above zero; the 40-year-old, about 0.1; a 60-year-old, about 0.5; and an 80-year-old, about 1.0 HAQ-DI units. A score of 3.0 represents total disablement. Repeating the assessments at yearly intervals provides a picture of individual human aging.

The HAQ-DI morbidity metric, developed by the authors and our Stanford colleagues, has been used for tens of thousands of subjects in hundreds of studies in scores of languages since 1980. The HAQ and similar instruments gave us a metric for morbidity for the first time and have enabled the quantitative study of human aging, which, for us, is simple but momentous. You would doubtless prefer to have your own lifetime morbidity to be most like the one shown by the bottom line in Figure 1, with infirmity beginning later in life and lasting for a shorter time.

This figure depicts a life diagram of morbidity from birth to death. The next four figures summarize results from our two 30-year longitudinal studies of morbidity and mortality. The metric for mortality is age at death in years. The metric for morbidity is expressed in Health Assessment Questionnaire Disability Index (HAQ-DI) units (0 = No difficulty – 3.0 = Disabled).

The three lines in Figure 1 illustrate different life scenarios of morbidity, from birth, at the left, to death, at the right. The top line and attached shaded area represent "Present Morbidity" projected from about 1980. Birth is at age zero on the left; then the baseline runs through young adulthood in a prolonged period of minimal morbidity. The person is functionally intact and unimpaired. At perhaps age 56 in the figure, morbidity becomes readily observable and continues to increase over the rest of life, with death at an average age of 78 years and including perhaps 22 years of progressive morbidity.

The "Life Extension" scenario on the second line shows morbidity at the same age, 56 years, but a typical life has been extended to 82 years by, for example, using new drugs to using seat belts while driving on safer roads in sturdier cars, with morbidity continuing to increase over a projected duration of 26 years. More morbidity accumulates over these additional years of extended life, and total lifetime morbidity increases. This has been termed the "expansion of morbidity."

In the third scenario, the onset of morbidity has been postponed to age 65 by, for example, reduction in the health risks of smoking and obesity. Death, however, has only been postponed by one year, to age 79. Morbidity has been compressed from both directions, from a postponed age at onset and from a more slowly increasing age at death. Morbidity, or impaired life, is reduced from 22 to 14 years. Eight additional years of good health!

Important data have come from a number of longitudinal studies, including the Runners Study, whose results are shown in Figure 2.

This study, and the study in Figure 3, were sponsored and monitored by the National Institutes of Health, approved by the Stan-

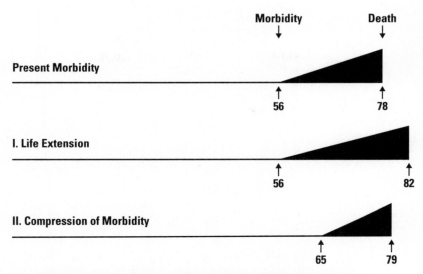

Figure 1. Human Aging: Alternative Scenarios for Lifetime Morbidity

ford University Human Subjects committee, were carried out over 30 continuous years by over 25 epidemiologists and support staff at Stanford University, and published in major peer-reviewed medical journals, with results extended every several years. Progress was reported at major conferences and in the lay press yearly.

This study documents postponement of aging by over 16 years in senior long-distance runners, a greater postponement than found in previous studies of any intervention. The controls and the established mechanisms by which exercise postpones morbidity and mortality establish the link between the exercise and these results.

In this lipid-lowering study at Stanford University, 961 long-term, long-distance runners and control individuals—from parallel groups of subjects of the same ages and genders, from similar sources not selected for robust exercise activity—the runners exercised more than 10 times the minutes each week as those in the control group and had done so for over 12 years.

The Runners Study began in 1984 with recruitment of 538 runners over age 50 and 423 age-matched (averaging 58 years) control subjects. The runners were recruited from a runners club in the Palo Alto, California, area, generally ran over 2,000 miles yearly, and had been running an average of 12 years before they were invited to join the study.

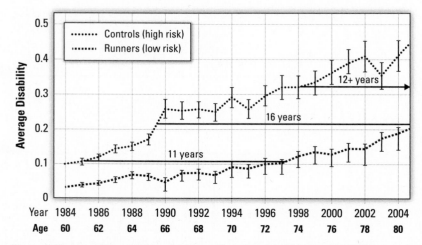

Figure 2. Runners (low risk) versus Controls (average risk). Morbidity (Disability) Scores: Runners (n = 538) and Controls (n = 423); 1984–2005, ongoing. Disability (HAQ-DI) was postponed by over 16 years in the runners group. Conclusion: Persons with lifelong, vigorous exercise practices are likely to be rewarded by a longer, stronger life. Vertical "error bars" define the means of values at each year of age.

The people in the control group were drawn randomly from the same communities, were age-matched to the runners, and many (about 25%) also ran recreationally, although less intensively; the control group averaged only 10% of the yearly mileage of the runners.

This study intentionally allowed the runners, who had a greater than average interest in health maintenance, to self-select into the runners group. Those in the control group were healthy, educated, and age and gender-matched. They were not obese or smokers; nor were the runners. The study identified and corrected for selection biases.

How did these remarkable results come about? Lifelong, regular, vigorous aerobic exercise is an extremely effective intervention. Relatively few persons exercise this vigorously for this long.

Another study, at The University of Pennsylvania (UPenn), was designed to confirm the Runners Study, but with older subjects, additional variables of smoking and obesity, and more subjects.

In the UPenn study, we studied people who were about 10 years older than those in the Runners Study so that we could better examine health changes over the age of 80. An HAQ-DI of 0.3 units (moderate disability) was postponed by 10 years in low-risk subjects compared with high risk.

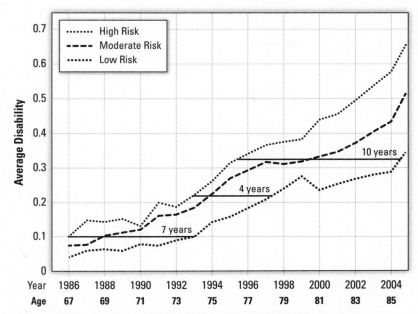

Figure 3. The University of Pennsylvania Study: 1986–2005 (ongoing). Exercise, Smoking Cessation, and Weight Control: Disability Delayed by 10 Years

The study was funded by the National Institutes of Health, monitored by the Stanford University Human Subjects Committee, and results published periodically in major peer-reviewed medical journals and presented at national conferences.

We enrolled 2,237 UPenn alumni in 1986. About 90% were male, representative of student populations at elite universities before World War II, when they were in college. We recruited the subjects with the help of the UPenn Alumni Association, which also helped us follow them over a long time and stimulated the subjects to participate in the long-term study.

The three study groups were based on the number of risk factors (zero, one, two, or three) at the beginning of the study: smoking, obesity, and lack of exercise. We used the same study team and questionnaire end points as in the Runners Study.

Results confirmed those of the Runners Study. The HAQ-DI score was postponed by 10 years in low-risk subjects compared with high risk. The UPenn subjects were typical of their classmates.

What happened greatly exceeded pre-study projections. Decreasing health risk factors reduced by a great amount the lifetime consequences from health risks, including some bad outcomes, such as premature heart attacks and strokes, emphysema, diabetes, and other chronic conditions.

Extremely good outcomes were achieved in the studies: aging was postponed by 16 years in the Runners Study and by 10 years in the UPenn students with good health habits as compared to their classmates.

We studied the death rates of participants in the Runners Study to confirm that the runners died each year at a lower rate than those in the control group. Mortality was assessed in the runners and control groups from 1984 to 2009, and the surviving subjects continue to be tracked. The primary follow-up is the National Death Index (NDI), a database of all deaths in the United States.

After 25 years of follow-up, 48% of the controls and only 28% of the runners had died. After 10 years of follow-up, those in the control group had four times the rate of death of the runners.

Deaths among the runners were postponed by 7 years as compared with the controls, while morbidity was postponed by 16 years. Morbidity was compressed by 7 years.

In the UPenn study, results of mortality outcomes showed a life extension of three to four years in the low-risk group compared with the high-risk group; this difference began early in the study and was maintained thereafter over two decades. The life extension is highly significant. In these study groups, 80% died by the last data point (2013), so mortality data are nearly complete. The control groups had fewer health risks and higher socioeconomic status than U.S. population averages. (We have included a short list of studies and papers that have documented these results in the Additional Reading appendix at the end of the book.)

What the Emerging Metrics Tell Us

Questionnaires that have helped to revolutionize the assessment of human aging have measured a similar metric: difficulty in activities of daily living (ADL).

These measurements of quality of life (morbidity) complement our measurement of the quantity of life (mortality). They provide a functional definition of the elusive term "morbidity." They define and advocate patient-reported outcomes without the filter of the investigator. They standardize morbidity outcomes across many diseases and pathologies. These studies are game changers, and the impact of the morbidity metric has been profound.

The conventional wisdom that mortality rates are the best measure of national health and that the doctor always knows best has

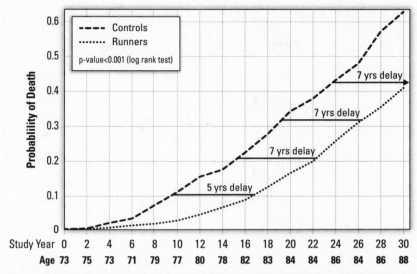

Figure 4. Regular, Vigorous, Long-Term Exercise: Mortality in the Runners Study (1984–2016, ongoing). Mortality in controls (higher risk) and Runners Club (lower risk) was assessed from 1984 to 2016. Death as confirmed by the National Death Index (NDI) was postponed by 7 years in runners compared with controls.

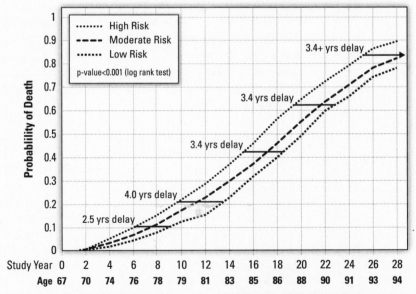

Figure 5. Reduction in Inactivity, Smoking, and Obesity: Mortality in the University of Pennsylvania Study. Death is postponed by 3 to 4 years in low-risk compared with high-risk alumni.

been challenged by this increasing use of patient-reported functional outcomes. Outcome assessment metrics improve research rigor in clinical trials, longitudinal studies, and population health. They permit assessment when there are multiple causes of decline in function, as in the study of human aging.

We can't eliminate aging, but we can delay it. We have science-based proof. We know how, and while it takes discipline and diligent effort, it isn't all that hard. As an added benefit, we can save money by being healthier, as individuals and as a society.

What We've Learned about Aging and Morbidity

In the 1970s, the conventional wisdom was that an expansion of morbidity was occurring as people lived longer into the ages of greater infirmity. People had longer lives but worsening health: the failure of success.

Morbidity, as defined by quantitative data on ADL, is detectable after the age of 20 to 30 years and slowly progresses over the rest of life. Physical function can improve somewhat in those who increase training activities at any age and from any level of function. Improvements are more modest when the subject is older or has more disability.

Aging early in life results from microbiological and molecular processes that are largely unobservable, and the progress of aging at this early stage is imperceptible. The rate of aging is affected by injuries, training interruptions, forced inactivity, depression, diseases, and other life events. Other contributors to functional decline include accumulation of disease-related infirmity and the slowing of defense mechanisms of the body, such as cardiac output and nerve function.

The greatest compression of morbidity may also be a consequence of suicide, murder, or airplane crashes at an early age. None of these represent an ideal lifespan.

Social changes have greatly affected both morbidity and mortality. Changes in habits over time tend to partially cancel each other out. In the 1980s and 1990s, the United States reduced cigarette use more than any other country, which decreased both morbidity and mortality. On the other hand, after 2000, people in the United States dramatically increased their average body mass index (BMI), increasing morbidity and mortality. Over the past three decades, people began jogging by the millions, increasing physical activity, but spent twice as much time looking at TV, computers, tablets, phones, and so on, decreasing physical activity.

Compression of morbidity is readily, even dramatically, achievable for most persons, but not for all illnesses. There are illnesses without known risk factors, cancers without known causes, and Gompertz Law remains unchanged: the force of mortality is very strong and nearly all human beings will die before their 116th birthday, although hundreds will live past 115.

We began our longitudinal studies of aging in 1984 and 1986, currently ongoing after 33 and 31 years, to test the compression of morbidity hypothesis. The studies allow us to directly compare morbidity and mortality in the same groups of study participants. We found that postponement of disability in those with fewer health risks is far greater than postponement of mortality, documenting that compression of morbidity does occur for those who decrease their health risks from smoking, obesity, and inactivity. The postponement of morbidity documented in these studies is substantially greater than previously thought.

We might now infer some principles of successful postponement of aging. An intervention cannot be successful without targeting major health risks. The intervention needs to be preventive, initiated well before the time of expected consequences. The greatest effectiveness is likely to come from physical exercise, begun early, practiced hard, and continued for a lifetime. Other major health risks whose elimination postpones aging include cigarette smoking and elevated BMI.

Additional interventions where postponement of aging seems possible include use of seat belts, airbags, safer roads, medication to treat high blood pressure (hypertension) and to lower harmful cholesterol, and low-dose aspirin. All these have been established to have large effects on both mortality and morbidity. At this time, however, none has been proven to delay morbidity longer than mortality and, hence, to compress morbidity.

The conventional wisdom of human aging has been fueled by unrealistic expectations, suspension of disbelief, and sometimes superficial science. We have moved beyond miracle elixirs and fountains of youth, skin creams, and plastic surgery. But current medical approaches to increasing the life span too often leave discussion of the results of aging—decreased size, strength, and vitality; diabetes; liver disease; cataracts; or decreased libido—in the fine print.

Our perspective is that a healthy life requires an early start to prevention. The accumulated damage and progressive decline in our bodies over time makes full reversal of established aging processes unlikely. A more conservative and more plausible strategy

Table 4: Your Master Plan for Preserving Your Health	Exercise	Diet and Nutrition	Not Smoking	Alcohol Moderation	Weight Control
Potentially Fatal Disease					
Heart Attack and Stroke	X	X	X		X
Lung Cancer			X		
Breast Cancer		X			X
Colon Cancer	X				
Mouth Cancer			X		
Liver Cancer			X	X	
Esophageal Cancer			X	X	
Cervical Cancer					
Emphysema			X		
Cirrhosis		X		X	
Diabetes	X	X			X
Trauma				X	
Nonfatal Disease					
Osteoarthritis	X				X
Hernias	X		X		X
Hemorrhoids	X				X
Varicose Veins	X		X		X
Thrombophlebitis	X		X		X
Gallbladder Disease		X			X
Stomach Ulcers		X	X	X	
Dental Problems		X	X		
Osteoporosis	X	X			
Falls and Fractures	X	X		X	

Avoiding Injury	Screening Tests	Estimated Risk Reduction	Notes
		70%	Diet: low in saturated fat and salt, high in fiber; vitamin E and aspirin as advised; treat high blood pressure.
		90%	Smoking causes nearly all cases.
	X	50%	Screening: self-examination, annual doctor's exam, mammography.
	X	50%	Aspirin or similar drugs as advised. Screening: colonoscopy, fecal blood tests.
		90%	Smoking (pipes and cigars) causes nearly all cases.
		50%	Alcohol causes many cases.
		50%	Smoking causes many cases.
	X	90%	Screening: Pap smears.
		90%	Smoking causes nearly all cases.
		90%	Alcohol, together with poor nutrition, causes nearly all cases.
		50%	Much diabetes occurring late in life can be prevented entirely.
X		75%	Failure to wear seat belts and drunk driving are the largest factors.
		50%	You can prevent the disability, not necessarily the arthritis.
		50%	Poor muscle tone, a big belly, and coughing are a bad combination.
		50%	Sitting around while overweight causes much of the problem; hygiene is also important.
		50%	Inactivity lets the fluid drop to the lowest point; using leg muscles helps blood flow in legs.
		50%	The factors for this condition can also cause blood clots in the legs.
		40%	Dietary fat and obesity are the causes in many cases.
		70%	Aspirin and some other pain-relieving drugs can cause stomach problems.
	X	80%	Diet: low in sugar. Screening: dental checkups. Brush and floss.
		50%	Diet: high in calcium. Exercise: weight-bearing. Estrogen and other drugs may help, if recommended by physician.
X		50%	Keep your body and bones strong; make your environment friendly.

calls for the postponement of aging rather than its reversal. Hence, useful interventions might best be employed before serious damage occurs and continued for life, with the goal of decreasing the rate of physical and mental decline.

Aging is a longitudinal problem, and postponing its damage requires the use of the kind of longitudinal data we have been discussing. Short-term data cannot illuminate long-term problems.

Doctors and researchers have made progress in understanding aging, but much work remains if we are ever to understand the full impact of bad behavioral health habits or the full benefits of the changes we advocate. Our perception is that we will need to peel back the causal onion for quite some time before we find what is in the center.

The Power of Prevention: How It Works

You can now put together a simple master plan for illness prevention. First, prevent the fatal illnesses mentioned at the beginning of this chapter. Second, prevent the nonfatal illnesses.

For a summary of the ways in which you can substantially reduce risks for 24 serious and very common conditions, see Table 4 on pages 44–45. You may be surprised to learn how many different health problems you can prevent. If you do everything right to reduce your risk for individual conditions, you can reduce your risk for all diseases combined by about 70%. That's the power of prevention!

The Habit of Health

An old joke maintains that everything pleasurable is illegal, immoral, or fattening. This is exactly the wrong attitude. Health is pleasurable; ill health is not. Good health habits have their own immediate reward. If changing your behavior for health is making you feel less well, you're doing something wrong. Exercise makes you feel better. Good diets make you feel better. Avoiding nicotine makes you feel better. Having a reasonable body weight makes activities easier and more pleasurable.

CHAPTER 2

Home Medicine Chest

You can prepare for most minor illnesses by keeping a few remedies and supplies in your home. To save money, buy only the items you will need often, and buy the inexpensive brands. Table 5 on page 48 lists the products we recommend that you keep on hand. You can do almost all the home care described in this book with these items.

This chapter discusses dosages and side effects of some common medicines. Keep in mind the following points about drugs:

▲ Always read the manufacturer's information for every product because that information can change. Talk to your doctor or pharmacist if you have questions.

▲ Medications eventually go bad, so you should replace them at least every three years. Label nonprescription medicines with the date of purchase so that you can remember when you got them. Many have an expiration date on them; it is usually safe to go by that. Check your medicine cabinet regularly; you may find items that have expired or that you don't need.

▲ Keep all drugs out of the reach of children. No bottle is totally childproof.

▲ All drugs can cause side effects, even when you use them properly. Many common medicines have unavoidable side effects, such as drowsiness.

▲ Don't assume that a drug is safe just because it doesn't require a prescription. Misusing over-the-counter drugs can be dangerous.

▲ The drugs in this chapter may relieve symptoms, but they aren't cures. If you can get along without drugs, you're usually better off.

▲ For most medicines, different brands are available. Look for the best price. A brand-name drug is not necessarily better than a less costly generic or store-brand drug.

Hundreds of over-the-counter medicines are available at your supermarket or drugstore. For most medicines, several nearly identical products exist as competing brands, which has posed a problem for us. If we discuss drugs and treatments by chemical name, the terms can be long and confusing; if we use brand names, we may

Table 5: Home Pharmacy

Medication or Tool	Use
Essential	
Blood Pressure Cuff (p. 50)	To monitor blood pressure
Bandages and Adhesive Tape (p. 50)	To close and protect minor wounds
Antiseptic Cleansers (p. 52) (3% hydrogen peroxide, iodine)	To cleanse minor wounds
Thermometer (p. 53)	To measure body temperature
Pain and Fever Medications (p. 54) (acetaminophen, aspirin, ibuprofen, naproxen, or ketoprofen)	To relieve pain, to lower fever
Prescription Narcotic Pain Relievers (p. 57)	To relieve serious pain, for a while
Antacids (nonabsorbable) (p. 59)	To relieve upset stomach
Skin Soothers (baking soda) (p. 61)	To treat skin irritation and soak wounds
Recommended for families with small children	
Syrup of Ipecac (p. 61)	To induce vomiting in cases of poisoning from drugs or plants
Liquid Acetaminophen (p. 55)	To relieve pain and fever in young children
Optional	
Antihistamines and Decongestants (p. 62)	To treat allergy symptoms
Nose Drops and Sprays (p. 63)	To treat a runny nose
Cold Tablets (p. 64)	To treat cold symptoms
Cough Syrups (p. 66)	To treat coughing
Laxatives (p. 67)	To treat constipation
Diarrhea Remedies (p. 68)	To treat diarrhea
Sodium Fluoride (p. 68)	To prevent dental problems
"Artificial Tears" Eye Drops (p. 69)	To treat irritated eyes
Zinc Oxide (p. 70)	To treat hemorrhoids
Antifungal Preparations (p. 71)	To treat skin fungus
Hydrocortisone Cream (p. 71)	To treat rashes
Sunscreen Agents (p. 72)	To prevent sunburn
Wart Removers (p. 72)	To remove some warts
Elastic Bandages (p. 73)	To treat sprains and strains
Vitamin Preparations (p. 74)	To supplement "average" diets

appear to favor a particular product, when there are equally satisfactory alternatives. Hence, we give you some clues to reading the list of ingredients on the package so that you can figure out what the drug is likely to do. We don't list all available drugs, but we do mention some representative alternatives. The brand names listed in this chapter are vigorously marketed and should be available almost everywhere. They aren't necessarily superior to alternatives containing similar formulas we haven't listed.

Blood Pressure Cuff

These cuffs are for people who are concerned about developing high blood pressure or are taking medication for high blood pressure. They may save some visits to your doctor to have your pressure checked. You can use these tests for reassurance as well as to guide treatment. If your blood pressure if over 140/90 (some would say 120/80) on several occasions, you should check it out with your doctor. Follow the doctor's advice for treatment, lifestyle changes, and follow-up appointments. See page 294.

We suggest that you invest in one of the newer wrist blood pressure cuffs that are battery-powered, durable, and automatic; they are very easy and quick to use. Snap it on your wrist, pull the Velcro tight, and push the button. After the beep, read the blood pressure and write it down if you are making a chart.

When you visit the doctor, check your results with the doctor's assistant's results to confirm that they are about the same.

These cuffs usually cost about $40–$60 and should last for many years. You'll probably recoup your money on the first doctor visit you can avoid.

Bandages and Adhesive Tape

Purpose
To close and protect minor wounds.

Bandages really don't "make it better." Sometimes it's better to leave a minor wound open to the air than to cover it. Still, a home medical shelf wouldn't be complete without a package of assorted adhesive bandages. To fashion larger bandages, you also need adhesive tape and gauze. Bandages are useful for covering tender blisters, keeping dirt out of wounds, and keeping the edges of a cut together. They have some cosmetic value in keeping the wound out of sight.

Use
For smaller cuts and sores, use a bandage from the package. Leaving the bandage on for a day or so is usually long enough; change the bandage daily or if it gets wet if you wish to keep the wound covered longer. For cuts, apply the bandage perpendicular to the cut, and draw the skin toward the cut from both sides to relax skin tension before applying the bandage. The bandage should then keep the edges together during healing. For larger injuries, make a bandage from a roll of sterile gauze or from sterile 2"x2" (5x5 cm) or 4"x4" (10x10 cm) gauze pads, and firmly tape it in place with adhesive tape. Change the bandage daily. If you see white fat protruding from the cut, see your doctor.

Side Effects
If the wound isn't clean when you cover it with a bandage, you may hide a developing infection from early discovery. Clean the wound with antiseptics and keep it clean. Change the bandage if it becomes wet. Some people are allergic to adhesive tape and should use nonallergenic paper tape. If adhesive tape is left on for a week or so, it will irritate almost anyone's skin, so give the skin a rest.

Some people leave a bandage on too long because they're afraid of the pain as they remove it—particularly if hair is

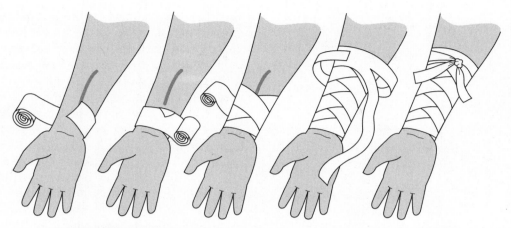

Wraparound bandage. This type of bandage makes a neat, long-lasting wrap for a large wound. It is easier to tape the end of the bandage, but if you have no tape, you can tie the bandage as shown.

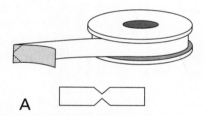

A

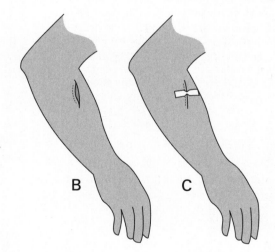

Butterfly bandage. This type of bandage allows a short, shallow wound to heal quickly.

(A) Fold a length of adhesive tape in two and snip off the folded corners.

(B) Make sure the wound is clean and that one edge is not lying over the other.

(C) Tape the wound together so that its edges meet and the narrow part of the bandage lies over the cut.
Use this only in the first six hours after injury; otherwise bacteria may grow in the wound.

See also Broken Ribs (page 100) to learn how to identify and splint a cracked rib.

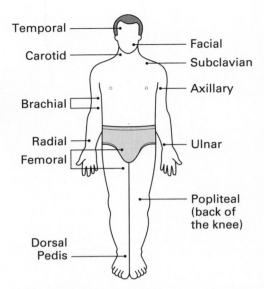

Temporal — Facial
Carotid — Subclavian
— Axillary
Brachial —
Radial — Ulnar
Femoral —
— Popliteal (back of the knee)
Dorsal Pedis —

Pressure points. If a bandage doesn't stop a person's wound from bleeding, slow the flow of blood to that part of the body by squeezing on a pressure point. Choose the nearest pressure point between the wound and the person's heart. The most commonly used pressure points are **inside the upper arm** and **inside the thigh**.

stuck to the tape. For painless removal, apply nail polish remover to the back of the adhesive tape (not the pad that covers the wound) and let it soak for five minutes. This will dissolve the adhesive and release both the skin and hair.

Antiseptic Cleansers

Purpose
To cleanse minor wounds.

A dirty wound often becomes infected. If dirt or foreign bodies are trapped beneath the skin, they can fester and delay healing. Only a few germs are introduced at the time of a wound,

but they may multiply to a great many over several days. An antiseptic removes the dirt and kills the germs. A solution of 3% hydrogen peroxide, which foams and cleans as you work it into the wound, is a good cleansing agent, and iodine is a reasonably good agent with which to kill germs. A strong baking soda solution will draw fluid and swelling out of a wound and will act to soak and clean it at the same time. Plain soap and water will help and are handy and inexpensive.

Most of the time, the solutions' cleansing action is more important than germ killing because many preparations (Listerine, Zephiran, Bactine, etc.) really aren't very good at killing germs. Antibiotic creams (such as Bacitracin and Neosporin) are expensive, usually unnecessary, and of questionable effectiveness. First-aid sprays are a waste of money.

Give careful attention to the initial cleaning of a wound and scrub out any embedded dirt particles. Do this even though it hurts and bleeds. For small, clean cuts, use soap and water followed by iodine, and then soap and water again. Betadine is a nonstinging iodine preparation. For larger wounds, use hydrogen peroxide with vigorous scrubbing.

Dosage
Most hydrogen peroxide is sold at 3% strength. Don't use a hydrogen peroxide solution stronger than 3%, such as that used for bleaching hair. Pour the solution on the wound and scrub with a rough cloth. Wash it off and repeat. Continue until you can see no dirt beneath the level of the skin. If you can't get the wound clean, go to a doctor.

Paint or wipe iodine onto the wound and the surrounding area. Wash it off within a few minutes, leaving a trace of the iodine color on the skin.

To soak a wound in a baking soda solution, use one tablespoon (15 ml) in one cup (250 ml) of warm water. If a finger or toe is injured, you can soak it in the cup. For other wounds, soak a washcloth with the solution and place over the wound as a compress. Generally, a wound should be soaked for five to ten minutes at a time, twice a day. If the skin is puckered and "waterlogged" after the soak, it has been soaked too long. You can place cellophane or plastic wrap over the cloth compress to retain heat and moisture longer.

Side Effects

Hydrogen peroxide is safe on the skin but can bleach hair and clothing, so try not to spill it.

Iodine can burn the skin if left on full strength, so be careful. Iodine is also poisonous if swallowed; keep it away from children. Some people are allergic to iodine; discontinue use if you get a rash.

Baking soda is completely safe as long as it's used on the skin, not swallowed.

Thermometer

Purpose

To measure body temperature.

Fever is an important clue in diagnosing illness, and a very high body temperature may lead to problems. The best places to measure body temperature are the rectum and the mouth. Rectal temperatures are about 0.5°F (0.25°C) higher than oral (mouth) temperatures and usually reflect the body's condition more accurately. Oral temperatures can be affected by hot or cold foods, routine breathing, and smoking.

Digital thermometers are now the standard. Contact thermometers—strips of plastic held against the forehead—aren't as accurate. Digital thermometers have the advantage of quicker readings than mercury thermometers, which is useful for younger children. They're more expensive than mercury thermometers, but safer. It is better to replace your old glass thermometers with digital devices if you have not already done so. We have seen perforated eardrums from the incorrect use of ear thermometers and don't recommend them.

Thermometers are designed in different ways to make taking oral and rectal temperatures easier. Generally, oral thermometers have a longer bulb at the business end, providing a greater surface area for a faster reading. Rectal thermometers may have a shorter, rounder bulb to facilitate entry into the rectum.

Rectal thermometers are best for young children because it's hard for children to hold an oral thermometer under the tongue. Lubricants, such as Vaseline, can make inserting rectal thermometers easier. Place the child on his or her stomach and hold one hand on the buttocks to prevent movement. Insert the thermometer an inch or so (2–3 cm) inside the rectum. Underarm thermometers are reliable for young infants. The disposable plastic skin patches that have been marketed as thermometers are not consistently reliable.

Side Effects

The mercury in older thermometers is poisonous, so take care not to bite down while having your oral temperature taken. Better, dispose of them—carefully—and replace them with a digital model.

Pain and Fever Medications

Purpose

To relieve pain and to lower fever. Sometimes, to help relieve itching.

Five major over-the-counter drugs do these tasks: acetaminophen, aspirin, ibuprofen, naproxen, and ketoprofen. Acetaminophen probably is the safest; the other four can cause severe or even fatal bleeding of the stomach, although only rarely if just a few tablets are taken. On the other hand, acetaminophen doesn't reduce inflammation; aspirin, ibuprofen, naproxen, and ketoprofen do, if taken in substantial dosage. Aspirin should not be used to treat fever in children and teenagers because of the risk of Reye's syndrome, a rare but serious problem of the liver and brain. Ibuprofen and naproxen are better than the others for relief of menstrual cramps.

In high doses, ketoprofen appears to be more toxic than the four main drugs, so use it sparingly as a last choice. Do not exceed the recommended dose.

Some over-the-counter pain medication makers conceal the key drug in the pain relief medication somewhere in the fine print under "active ingredients," and refer obliquely to the amount of analgesic, or pain reliever, present in each tablet. It's often surprisingly hard to find out what is in the drug just from the ingredients listed on the box. There are really only five drugs, but many manufacturers. Each company wants its product to seem unique in a crowded marketplace,

so companies develop many minor variations on a similar theme and try to develop distinctive advertising.

For example, Excedrin is half aspirin and half acetaminophen. Excedrin Extra Strength adds caffeine to the mix; this improves pain relief but may make you jittery. Some pain relievers include other ingredients. For example, an antacid may be added (as in Bufferin) in an attempt to cut down on stomach distress. Other than these variations, there's little medical reason to prefer one product over another in most cases. If you like a particular formulation, use it. If you want to save money, read the labels carefully and look for the best buys.

On some over-the-counter pain medication bottles, you may see the initials U.S.P., which stand for "United States Pharmacopeia." Although not an absolute guarantee that the drug is the best, it does mean that the drug has met certain standards in composition and physical characteristics. The same is true of the designation N.F., which stands for "National Formulary."

Finally, remember that acetaminophen, ibuprofen, naproxen, and ketoprofen are available by doctor's prescription at up to twice the strength of the nonprescription formulas. If you have the stronger type of one drug in your medicine cabinet, don't confuse it with the weaker over-the-counter formula. And don't combine them unless your doctor agrees.

Acetaminophen

Acetaminophen is available in several brand-name preparations (Tylenol, Datril, Liquiprin, Tempra, etc.). In the UK, it's known as Paracetamol. It's slightly less predictable than aspirin, somewhat less powerful, and doesn't have the anti-inflammatory action that makes aspirin valuable in treatment of arthritis and some other diseases. On the other hand, it doesn't cause ringing in the ears or upset stomach, common side effects with aspirin. Nor can it cause Reye's syndrome, a rare but serious potential side effect of aspirin when taken by children with chicken pox or the flu.

Dosage
Acetaminophen is used in doses identical to those of aspirin. For adults, two 325 mg tablets every three to four hours is standard. In children, 65 mg per year of age every four hours is satisfactory. There is no additional benefit from taking higher amounts. Like aspirin, acetaminophen comes combined with other ingredients in products that offer little advantage over acetaminophen.

Side Effects
People seldom experience side effects from acetaminophen. If you suspect a side effect, call your doctor. A variety of rare toxic effects have been reported, but none are definitely related to the use of this drug. A major overdose can cause liver failure, and this can be fatal. Keep the bottle where children can't reach it. If you abuse alcohol, severe liver toxicity can occur at as little as 4,000 to 6,000 mg a day. Never exceed 4,000 mg per day under any circumstances.

Liquid Ibuprofen and Liquid Acetaminophen for Small Children
Aspirin is almost never recommended for small children because of the possibility of Reye's syndrome. Most pediatricians now recommend that parents use liquid ibuprofen rather than liquid acetaminophen because it is less toxic in case of accidental overdose.

Dosage
Liquid ibuprofen and liquid acetaminophen come in varying strengths, so read the label on your bottle for the correct dosage. Although the bottle will say that one dose will last for about four hours, our experience has been that it is closer to three hours. From noon to midnight, awaken the child if necessary. After midnight, the fever will usually decrease by itself and become less of a problem, so missing a dose is less important. But check the child's temperature at least once during the night to make sure. Remember, you must keep repeating the dose as long as there is fever, but check with your doctor after ten days.

Nonsteroidal Anti-inflammatory Drugs (NSAIDs)
Aspirin
Aspirin is an ordinary and extraordinary drug. It's good for everyday problems, but it can be life-saving in your middle or later years. More expensive aspirin preparations may use coated tablets for easier swallowing or faster dissolving, but this usually doesn't make them more effective than cheaper brands.

If an aspirin bottle contains a vinegary odor when opened, the pills have begun to deteriorate and should be discarded. Aspirin usually has a shelf life of at least three years, although shorter periods may sometimes occur.

Dosage
In adults, the standard dose for pain relief is two tablets taken every three to

four hours as required. The maximum effect occurs in about two hours. Each standard tablet is 5 grains, or 325 mg. If you use a nonstandard concoction, you'll have to do the arithmetic to calculate equivalent doses. The terms "extra strength," "arthritis pain formula," and the like merely indicate a greater amount of aspirin per tablet. This is medically trivial. You can take more tablets of the cheaper aspirin and still save money. When you read that a product "contains more of the ingredient that doctors recommend most," you may be sure that the product contains a little bit more aspirin per tablet, perhaps 400 to 500 mg instead of 325.

Here are some hints for good aspirin usage. Aspirin treats symptoms; it doesn't cure problems. Thus, for symptoms such as headache or muscle pain or menstrual cramps, don't take it unless you hurt. On the other hand, for control of fever, you'll be more comfortable if you repeat the dose every four hours during the day because this prevents fever from going up and down. The afternoon and evening are the worst times for fever, so try not to miss a dose during these hours.

If you need aspirin for relief from some symptom over a prolonged period, check the symptom with your doctor. Relief from pain or fever is not improved if you increase the dose, and you're more likely to irritate your stomach, so take only the standard dose (650 mg every four hours), even if you still have some discomfort.

To control inflammation, as in serious arthritis, the dose of aspirin must be high, often up to 16 tablets daily, and must continue over a prolonged period.

A doctor should monitor such treatment; problems sometimes occur.

Avoid giving aspirin to children or teenagers with a fever because of the possibility they may later develop Reye's syndrome, a potentially fatal disease of the liver and brain. We strongly recommend acetaminophen instead.

Aspirin prevents complications of high blood pressure in pregnant women and prevents heart attacks and thrombotic strokes. These are major and unique benefits. The dose for this use is very low: 81 mg (one low-dose adult aspirin) every day or every other day. Review the discussion on page 23, and check with your doctor. Most men over 50 and women over 65 should be on it.

Side Effects

In addition to Reye's syndrome in children, aspirin can cause an upset stomach or ringing in the ears in adults and children. If your ears ring, reduce the dose.

Serious gastrointestinal hemorrhage or a perforated (ruptured) stomach can occur; aspirin more than doubles your risk of a bleeding ulcer. If your stomach is upset, try taking aspirin a half hour after meals, when the food in the stomach will act as a buffer. Coated aspirin (such as Ecotrin) can help protect the stomach. However, a small number of people don't digest coated aspirin and so receive no benefit. Buffers are sometimes added to aspirin to protect the stomach and may help a little. If you take a lot of aspirin, you may want to ask your doctor about new prescription drugs that may be safer, though more expensive.

Asthma, nasal polyps, deafness, serious bleeding from the digestive tract, ulcers, and other major problems have been associated with aspirin.

Ibuprofen

Ibuprofen (Advil, Motrin, Nuprin, etc.) is about as toxic to the stomach as aspirin, and more so than acetaminophen. It doesn't cause ringing in the ears like aspirin or cause severe liver disease as acetaminophen may in rare cases. It appears to be almost impossible to commit suicide by overdose with ibuprofen. But concern has been raised about kidney problems (mild and reversible), and ibuprofen is sometimes more expensive than the alternatives. It's the best over-the-counter preparation for menstrual cramps.

Dosage

Ibuprofen comes in 200 mg tablets, and the maximum recommended dose is 1,200 mg (six tablets) per day. This is about one half the recommended dose for the prescription equivalent, but this dose is effective for minor problems and shouldn't be exceeded without a doctor's advice. Avoid giving to children.

Side Effects

Gastrointestinal upset is the most frequent problem and is reason to stop or to call the doctor. Serious gastrointestinal hemorrhage or a perforated stomach can result. The rare patient with aspirin allergy may also be allergic to ibuprofen. Read the label carefully.

Naproxen and Ketoprofen

Naproxen (Naprosyn and Anaprox by prescription; Aleve over-the-counter) and ketoprofen (Orudis) are also available without prescription. Naproxen has a longer "half-life" than other pain relievers, so you need to take it only twice a day. It is effective against pain, fever, and inflammation. Ketoprofen is similar and does not offer any new benefits; it may be more toxic.

Dosage

Naproxen and Aleve comes in 200 mg tablets. Read the label carefully. Because naproxen is slightly more toxic to the stomach than ibuprofen, don't take more than three tablets in 24 hours or more than two if you're over 65 years old. Ketoprofen comes in 12.5 mg tablets. Do not take more than six tablets in 24 hours.

Side Effects

Stop taking the drug and call your doctor if you experience gastrointestinal upset. Avoid giving to children. Do not use if you have an allergy to aspirin.

Prescription Narcotic Pain Relievers

Purpose

To relieve serious pain, for a while

This has been a stealth epidemic of misguided treatment approaches, gullible addicts and abusers, greedy suppliers, and many deaths that did not have to occur. Some who abuse the drugs are "street" users while others are prescription users who sometimes obtain illegal or forged prescriptions.

The epidemic crept into medical practice over the past two decades to an undesirable level and is now recognized nationally. Recent estimates cite tens of thousands of deaths per year in the United States alone. Over 4 million Americans have used these drugs "recreationally." There are many such drugs, including codeine, Vicodin, Tylenol with Codeine "3" or "4", Percodan, Percocet, and Fentanyl, which have been around for a long time. They are prescribed for toothaches, sprained limbs, back pain post-op, migraine headaches, other headaches, dental procedures, and other minor pain syndromes.

Ironically, their growing use apparently came from a new medical specialty—pain-based medicine, which took the position that the doctor's first obligation, for all patients, is to relieve pain. The new mantra: every doctor visit should involve a discussion of pain, a medical note on pain, and far too often, a narcotic pain reliever.

From one perspective, this is an important subject that had been neglected; from another, it is profoundly harmful and has led to an epidemic of mass overmedication and neglect of simpler and less toxic remedies, and has distracted from finding treatments targeted at the cause rather than a cover-up of a problem.

These drugs impair your body's greatest defense mechanism: pain. Pain keeps you away from the burner on a hot stove, tells you what not to do with that injured body part, and reminds you if you forget. These medicines impair thought processes and cause constipation, inactivity, muscle atrophy, loss of strength, depression, and decreased muscle mass, among many other problems. The resulting general mental slow-down affects the elderly in particular, causing a decline in social interactions and depressed cognition. The Surgeon General and the Food and Drug Administration have repeatedly warned of profound ill effects to public health. The U.S. Senate has heard testimony on the 44 senior deaths daily in the United States attributable to prescription opioids. Others would cite even higher numbers, including physical neglect, hypostatic pneumonias, suicide, as well as the illegal resale of these drugs. The epidemic is a major public health problem and has continued to grow over the last two decades. Importantly, there are safer and far less toxic approaches to chronic pain syndromes.

Nor are opioids really helpful in relieving minor pain syndromes or arthritis. They don't fight inflammation and don't speed healing. The pain relief is about that of non-opioid acetaminophen for most people. They cause habituation, which means a possible need to increase dosage over time. The standard advice is to use them in as low a dose as possible for as short a time as possible. Still, a lot of people are on the slippery slope to addiction.

To be sure, some pain does require strong medications, sometimes for a long time, and these must be conveniently accessible to those who truly need them. Kidney stones, heart attacks, labor and delivery, bone cancer, and major trauma come to mind. Not strained limbs.

In our family of several generations, as well as in our practices, we have encountered many such problems. In our family, we find that a bandage frequently stops pain, that a sling or a splint can help the sprain or strain, and that cold packs work pretty well for acute trauma.

The nonsteroidal anti-inflammatory drugs (NSAIDs), particularly with stomach protection measures such as antacids and other drugs, are much better than opioids for inflammatory arthritis. There is much to be said for massage, cold packs, and music.

Pain is not the "fifth vital sign" after pulse, blood pressure, respiratory rate, and temperature. Indeed, it is not a vital sign at all. In this book, we suggest some ways to manage rib fractures and other injuries without pain medications. As reported above, prescription opiate-based pain relievers are a direct cause of tens of thousands of deaths a year in the United States. This tragic number is on the order of magnitude of suicides, homicides, motorcycle accidents and other major threats to life.

These deaths are truly unnecessary. They come from intentional or unintentional overdoses, respiratory depression, tolerance to ever higher doses, drugs in combinations, addictions, combination with alcohol, and so on. We regret that some of the blame for this tragic epidemic comes from the medical profession. Do not seek out prescription pain relievers. If they don't seem right for you, seek another opinion and, if necessary, a third.

If you have leftover pain medicines after a medical problem has passed, get rid of them. If you can't find a secure place to discard, check with your doctor's office; most have places to discard medications and needles safely. You can also find instructions on the proper way to dispose of medications and a list of locations that take back expired and unneeded medications at fda.gov.

Antacids

Purpose
To relieve or prevent upset stomach, heartburn, and GERD (gastroesophageal reflux disease).

Nonabsorbable Antacids
Maalox, Di-Gel, Gelusil, and Mylanta are examples of nonabsorbable antacids. They're an important part of the home pharmacy. They help neutralize stomach acid and thus decrease heartburn, ulcer pain, gas pains, and stomach upset. Because they aren't absorbed by the body, they usually don't upset the acid-base balance of the body and are quite safe.

Almost all these antacids are available in both liquid and tablet form. For most purposes, the liquid form is superior. It coats more of the surface area of the gullet and stomach than the tablets do. Indeed, if not well chewed, tablets may be almost worthless. Still, during work or play, a bottle can be cumbersome, and a few tablets in a shirt pocket or handbag may be convenient for midday doses.

Absorbable Antacids
Baking soda, Alka-Seltzer, Rolaids, and Tums contain absorbable antacids. The main ingredient in these products is sodium bicarbonate (Alka-Seltzer, baking soda), dihydroxyaluminum sodium carbonate (Rolaids), or calcium carbonate (Tums). These medicines are more powerful acid neutralizers than nonabsorbable antacids, and they come in convenient tablet form. Calcium carbonate is also an excellent source of supplemental calcium and can help prevent osteoporosis.

Reading the Labels

Nonabsorbable antacids contain magnesium or aluminum or both. As a general rule, magnesium causes diarrhea and aluminum causes constipation. Different brands are slightly different mixtures of the salts of these two metals, designed to avoid both diarrhea and constipation. A few brands also contain calcium, which can be mildly constipating.

Different products differ in taste. While potency may vary, most people will ultimately select the particular antacid that has a taste they can tolerate and that doesn't upset their bowels. Keep trying different brands until you're satisfied.

Dosage

The standard adult dose is two tablespoons (30 ml) or two well-chewed tablets. Use one-half the adult dose for children ages six to twelve, and one-fourth the adult dose for children ages three to six. The frequency of the dose depends on the severity of the problem. For stomach upset or heartburn, one or two doses will often suffice. For gastritis, several doses a day for several days may be needed. For ulcers, medication may be needed for six weeks or more, taken as frequently as every hour or so. A doctor should supervise this type of program.

If you wish to use baking soda as an antacid, use one teaspoon (5 ml) in a glass of water every four hours as needed—but only occasionally. Baking soda is absorbable and can upset the body's acid-base balance.

Side Effects

In general, the only problem is the effect on bowel movements. Maalox tends to loosen stools slightly; Mylanta is about average. Adjust the dose and change brands as needed. Check with your doctor before using these compounds if you have kidney disease, heart disease, or high blood pressure. Some brands contain significant quantities of salt and should be avoided by people on a low-salt diet. Di-Gel has the lowest salt content of the popular brands.

Be careful if you take baking soda by mouth. First, there's a lot of sodium in it. It can cause problems if you have heart trouble or high blood pressure or are on a low-salt diet. Second, if you take baking soda regularly for many months, there's some evidence that it may result in calcium deposits in the kidneys and thus cause kidney damage.

Talk with your doctor before using antacids to treat side effects of other medications, such as aspirin, naproxen, ibuprofen, or ketoprofen, as they may mask a serious problem, such as ulcers.

Stomach Acid Blockers

Cimetidine (Tagamet), famotidine (Pepcid AC), ranitidine (Zantac), and nizatidine (Axid AR) are prescription drugs widely used for stomach ulcers and have been approved for over-the-counter use in lower doses to treat heartburn. Rather than neutralize stomach acid like antacids, they act to block the body's production of the acid. Most people won't need these medicines, but you can consider them if antacids aren't effective. If you take other medications, check with your doctor before taking Tagamet; it can increase the potency of a number of other medications, including some taken for blood thinning (warfarin), asthma (theophylline), and seizures. Pepcid AC may be slightly better in this regard. Don't exceed the recommended dose.

Your doctor may recommend stronger medications, called proton pump inhibitors, if necessary. These drugs—for instance, Prilosec, Protonix, and Nexium—reduce the stomach acid levels more than the older drugs mentioned above, but most people do not need them. These drugs are generally well tolerated; Prilosec is now available without a prescription.

Skin Soothers

Baking Soda

Baking soda (sodium bicarbonate, $NaHCO3$) is a very useful household chemical. It has three principal medical uses:

▲ As a weak solution, it acts to soothe the skin and reduce itching; thus, it's helpful in conditions ranging from sunburn to poison oak to chicken pox. This is the use we discuss on this page.

▲ As a strong solution, it will draw fluid and swelling out of a wound and will act to soak and clean the wound at the same time. (See Antiseptic Cleansers, page 52.)

▲ If taken by mouth, it serves as an antacid and may help alleviate heartburn or stomach upset. Because the sodium in baking soda is absorbed by the body, however, we strongly recommend using another antacid instead.

Dosage

To soothe the skin, use from two tablespoons to a half cup (30–120 ml) in a bath of warm water. Blot the skin gently after the bath and allow the solution to dry on the skin. Repeat this procedure as often as necessary.

Side Effects

There are none as long as the baking soda is applied only to the skin.

Skin Creams and Moisturizing Lotions

There's little to be said about the various artificial materials—for example, Lubriderm, Vaseline, Alpha Keri—that people apply to their skin in an attempt to temporarily improve its appearance or retard its aging. The various claims of such products are not science-based, and long-term benefits have not been demonstrated.

Sometimes dry skin can actually cause symptoms, thus becoming a medical problem. Remember that bathing or exposure to detergents may contribute to the drying of skin. Decreasing the frequency of baths or showers, wearing gloves when working with cleansing agents, and other similar measures may be as important as using any lotion or cream.

Moisturizing creams and lotions may make your skin feel better to you; this is the "soothing" action. Use such creams as the product labels state. They have essentially no side effects, except that a rare person will be allergic to the lanolin in some of these products.

Syrup of Ipecac

Purpose

To induce vomiting if someone has been poisoned by a plant or a drug. Vomiting will empty the stomach of any poison that has not already been absorbed. Syrup of ipecac is especially useful if you have small children.

Our colleague, Dr. Robert Pantell, author of *Taking Care of Your Child*, notes that although syrup of ipecac is not recommended for routine use by many organizations, it has been approved by the FDA to continue as an over-the-counter preparation for emergency use to cause vomiting in poisoning. Before use, call the poison control center, your physician, or the emergency department.

Don't use ipecac or anything else to induce vomiting if the poison swallowed is a petroleum-based compound (for example, gasoline, cleaning/polishing products) or a strong acid or alkali. Call the Poison Control Center immediately. See Poisoning (page 86) for more advice on poisoning.

Because of the possibility of aspiration (inhaling foreign matter into the lungs)—particularly in children—the use of ipecac has decreased in recent years, replaced mostly by "pumping out" the stomach through a nasogastric tube. Unfortunately, quite a lot of time can pass before you get to the emergency room or doctor's office, during which the possible poison is being absorbed into the body. Ipecac is faster. A finger in the back of the throat is even faster, but both have a slight risk of aspiration. (If going to the emergency room, you might have someone call ahead so the ER is ready for you and to ask what the ER's standard procedure is.)

It's far better to keep toxic chemicals out of a child's reach than to have to use ipecac. When you buy ipecac, use the purchase as a reminder to check the house for toxic materials that a child might reach; move them to a safer place. If your child does swallow something, the sooner the stomach is emptied, the milder the problem will be, with the exceptions listed previously. There's no time to buy ipecac after your child has swallowed poison; therefore, you should have it on hand just in case you ever need it.

Dosage
One tablespoon (15 ml) of ipecac may suffice for a small child; two to four teaspoons (10–20 ml) are necessary for older children and adults. Follow the dose with as much warm water as can be given, until vomiting occurs. Repeat the dose in 15 minutes if you haven't had any results.

Side Effects
Ipecac is an uncomfortable medication, but it's not hazardous unless vomiting causes material to be thrown down the windpipe into the lungs. This can cause pneumonia, so do not induce vomiting in a victim who is unconscious or nearly unconscious. *Do not cause vomiting of volatile materials, such as petroleum compounds or drain cleaner, that can be inhaled into the lungs and cause damage.* We believe that this can be an important medicine, and even life-saving in some cases. Not all doctors agree with us, however, so talk with your own doctor or the emergency room about its risks and benefits.

Antihistamines and Decongestants for Allergies

Purpose
To treat allergy symptoms; these agents can also reduce itching.

Chlor-Trimeton, Sinarest, Actifed, Allegra, Claritin, Benadryl, Sudafed, and

Dimetapp are among the many over-the-counter drugs designed for treatment of minor allergic symptoms. They're similar to the cold compounds described on page 64, but they less frequently contain pain and fever agents like aspirin, acetaminophen, naproxen, ibuprofen, or ketoprofen. Usually these drug compounds contain an antihistamine and a decongestant agent, and sometimes acetaminophen. These ingredients can be identified from the label.

If you tolerate one of these drugs well and get relief, you may continue to take it for several weeks (for example, through hay fever season) without seeing a doctor. However, decongestants taken as nose drops or nasal spray should be used more sparingly and only for short periods, as detailed in Nose Drops and Sprays (right).

Reading the Labels

The decongestant is usually pseudoephedrine or phenylpropanolamine. If the compound name is not familiar, the suffix "-ephrine" or "-edrine" usually identifies a decongestant. The antihistamine is often chlorpheniramine, diphenhydramine, or brompheniramine. If not, the antihistamine is sometimes identifiable on the label by the suffix "-amine."

Dosage

Take according to product directions. Reduce the dose if you note side effects, or try another compound.

Side Effects

These are usually minor and disappear after the drug is stopped or dosage is decreased. Agitation and insomnia usually indicate too much of the decongestant. Drowsiness usually indicates too much antihistamine. Avoiding the substances to which you are allergic is far superior to taking drugs. Drugs, to a certain degree, inevitably impair your functioning. However, the newer "nondrowsy" antihistamines, such as Allegra or Claritin, are less prone to cause drowsiness and represent a treatment advance. Consider these especially if you are driving or using heavy equipment.

Nose Drops and Sprays

Purpose

To treat a runny nose.

A runny nose is often the worst symptom of a cold or allergy. Because this complaint is so common, remedies are big business, and there are many advertised as decreasing your nasal drip: Afrin, Neo-Synephrine, Vicks, Sinarest, and other drops or sprays.

The active ingredient in these compounds is a decongestant drug, often ephedrine or phenylephrine. These preparations are "topical," meaning that you apply them directly to the inflamed tissue. You can then feel the membranes shrinking down and "drawing," and you will note a decrease in the amount of secretion. However, some problems are associated with using these compounds.

The major drawback is that the relief is temporary. Usually the symptoms return in a couple of hours, so you repeat the dose. This is fine for a while. But the drugs work by causing the muscles in the walls of the blood vessels to shrink, decreasing blood flow. After many applications, these small muscles become fatigued and fail to respond. Finally, they're so fatigued that they relax entirely, and the situation becomes worse than it was in the beginning. This is medically termed "rebound vasodilation" and can occur if you use these drugs steadily for three days or more. Many patients interpret these increased symptoms as a need for more medication, but taking more only makes the problem worse. Therefore, *use nose drops or sprays for only three days at a time.* After several days' rest, you may use them again for three more days.

Dosage

These drugs are almost always used in the wrong way. If you don't bathe the swollen membranes on the side surface of the inner nose, you won't get the desired effect. If you can taste the drug, you've applied it to the wrong area. Apply small amounts to one nostril while lying down on that side for a few minutes so that the medicine will bathe the membranes. Then apply the agent to the other nostril while lying on that side (see drawing right). Treat four times a day if needed, but don't continue for more than three days without interrupting the therapy.

Side Effects

Rebound vasodilation from prolonged use is the most common problem. If you apply these agents incorrectly and swallow a large amount of the drug, you may experience a rapid heart rate and an uneasy, agitated feeling. The drying effect of the drug can result in nosebleeds.

Try to avoid the substances to which you're allergic rather than treating the consequences of exposure. Often, simple measures like changing a furnace filter,

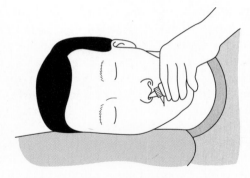

Applying nose drops or spray. Apply small amounts to one nostril while lying down on that side for a few minutes. If you can taste the drug, you've applied it to the wrong area.

using a vaporizer, or using an air conditioner to filter the air will improve allergic symptoms.

Cold Tablets

Purpose

To relieve some symptoms of colds and flu.

Actifed, Chlor-Trimeton, Drixoral, Contac, Dimetapp, and dozens of other products are widely advertised as being effective against the common cold. Surprisingly, many give satisfactory symptomatic relief. We don't think that these compounds add much to standard treatment with acetaminophen and fluids, but some people believe otherwise. We don't discourage their use for short periods.

These compounds usually have three basic ingredients. The most important is a fever and pain reducer: acetaminophen, aspirin, or ibuprofen. In addition, these contain a decongestant drug to shrink the swollen membranes and the small blood vessels, and an antihistamine to block any allergy and to dry mucus.

Reading the Labels

The decongestant is often pseudoephedrine or phenylpropanolamine. If not, the suffix "-ephrine" or "-edrine" will usually identify this component of the compound. The antihistamine is often chlorpheniramine (Chlor-Trimeton, etc.) or diphenhydramine. If not, the antihistamine is usually (but not always) identifiable on the label by the suffix "-amine."

Occasionally a "belladonna alkaloid" is added to these compounds to enhance other actions and reduce stomach spasms. In the small doses used, there's little effect from such a drug. It is listed as "scopolamine," "belladonna," or something similar. Other ingredients that may be listed contribute little. Don't use products with caffeine if you have heart trouble or difficulty sleeping.

These products take the much promoted "combination-of-ingredients" approach. As a rule, single drugs are preferable to combinations of drugs; they allow you to be more selective in treatment of symptoms, and consequently you take fewer drugs. The ingredients in combination products are available separately, and these individual products should be considered as alternatives. For example, the major ingredient in combination products is usually aspirin or acetaminophen. Pseudoephedrine is an excellent decongestant and is available without prescription in 30 mg and 60 mg tablets. Chlorpheniramine, a strong antihistamine, is available with-

out a prescription in the standard 4 mg size. When possible, consider applying medicine directly to the affected area, such as nose drops or sprays for a runny nose.

Finally, note that the commonly prescribed cold medicines (Sudafed, Actifed, Dimetapp) are really just more concentrated and expensive formulations of the same types of drugs that are available over the counter (often even under the same names). Is it worth a trip to the doctor just for that?

Dosage

Try the recommended dosage. If you feel no effect, you may increase the dosage by one-half. Don't exceed twice the recommended dosage. Remember that you're trying to find a compromise between desired effects and side effects. Increasing the dosage gives some chance of increased beneficial effects, but it guarantees a greater probability of side effects.

Side Effects

Drugs that put one person to sleep will keep another awake. The most frequent side effects of cold tablets are either drowsiness or agitation. The drowsiness is usually caused by the antihistamine component, and the insomnia or agitation results from the decongestant component. You can try another compound that has less or none of the offending chemical, or you can reduce the dose. There are no frequent serious side effects; the most dangerous is drowsiness if you intend to drive or operate machinery.

In rare cases, the "belladonna" component will cause dry mouth, blurred vision, or inability to urinate. You may experience aspirin's usual side effects—upset stomach, ringing in the ears, or, rarely, bleeding from the stomach.

Cough Syrups

Purpose
Cough medication is a confusing area, with many products from which to choose. To simplify, consider two major categories:

▲ Expectorants are usually preferable because they liquefy the secretions the body produces while fighting illness and allow the body's defenses to get rid of the bad material by coughing it up more easily.

▲ Cough suppressants should be avoided if the cough is bringing up any material or if there's a lot of mucus. In the late stages of a cough, when it's dry and hacking, compounds containing a cough suppressant may be useful.

We prefer cough compounds that don't contain an antihistamine, which dries mucus and can harm as much as help.

Reading the Labels
Guaifenesin (Robitussin, Benylin expectorant, Vicks, etc.), potassium iodide, and several other frequently used chemicals cause an expectorant action.

Cough-suppressant action comes principally from narcotics, such as codeine. Over-the-counter cough suppressants legally may not contain codeine. They often contain dextromethorphan hydrobromide (DM), which is not a narcotic but is a close chemical relative.

Many commercial mixtures contain a little of everything and may have some cold compound ingredients as well.

We'll discuss guaifenesin (Robitussin, Benylin expectorant, Vicks, etc.) and dextromethorphan (Vicks Formula 44, Robitussin-DM, etc.) specifically; follow the label instructions for other agents.

Guaifenesin
Guaifenesin draws more liquid into the mucus that triggers a cough. Thus, the cough medicine liquefies these mucus secretions so that they may be coughed free. The resulting cough is easier and less irritating. For a dry, hacking cough remaining after a cold, the lubrication alone often soothes the inflamed area. Guaifenesin doesn't suppress the cough reflex but encourages the natural defense mechanisms of the body. There's controversy over its effectiveness, but it appears to be safe. It isn't as powerful as the codeine-containing preparations, but for routine use, we prefer it to prescription drugs. Pepper and garlic, not usually thought of as medicines, have a similar effect.

Reading the Labels
Guaifenesin is also available in combination with decongestants and cough suppressants; the decongestants may carry a "-PE" suffix for "phenylephrine" and the cough suppressants a "-DM" for "dextromethorphan."

Dosage
Follow the directions on the label. Call your doctor if you have a sick and coughing child less than one year old.

Side Effects
No significant problems have been reported. If you use preparations containing other drugs, you may feel side effects from the other components of the combination.

Dextromethorphan (DM)
Robitussin-DM, Triaminic-DM, Vicks Formula 44, and others contain dextromethorphan, a drug that "calms the cough center." The drug makes the areas of the brain that control coughs less sensitive to the stimuli that trigger coughs. No matter how much you use, it will seldom decrease a cough by more than 50%. Thus, you usually can't totally suppress a cough. This is actually good for you because the cough is a protective reflex. Dextromethorphan is best used with dry, hacking coughs that are preventing sleep or work.

Dosage
See the directions on the label. Adults may require up to twice the recommended dosage to obtain any effect, but don't exceed this amount. A higher dose may produce problems, not further benefit.

Side Effects
Drowsiness is the only side effect that has been frequently reported.

Laxatives

Purpose
To treat constipation.

We prefer a natural diet, with natural vegetable fiber residue, to the use of any laxative. But if you must use a laxative, the most attractive alternative is psyllium as a bulk laxative to hold water in the bowel and soften the stool.

Metamucil, FiberCon, and similar preparations contain substances refined from the psyllium seed. They can help both diarrhea and constipation. Psyllium draws water into the stool, forms a gel or thick solution, and thus provides bulk. It isn't absorbed by the digestive tract; it only passes through. Thus, it's a natural product and essentially has no side effects. However, it doesn't always work. Glycerin suppositories work also to draw water into the stool and often have a very gentle action.

Dosage
One teaspoon (5 ml), stirred in a glass of water and taken twice daily, is a typical dose. A second glass of water or juice should also be taken. Psyllium is also available in more expensive, individual-dose packets for use when you don't have a measuring spoon. The effervescent versions mix a bit more rapidly and taste better to some people.

Side Effects
If you take a bulk laxative without sufficient water, the gel that is formed could conceivably lodge in your esophagus (the tube that leads from the mouth to the stomach). Sufficient liquid will prevent this problem.

There are other laxatives, less frequently needed, that are less natural. These include fecal softeners such as Colace, Dialose, and Doxidan; bowel stimulants such as Correctol, Dulcolax by mouth or rectal suppository, Imodium, Ex-Lax, coffee, and milk of magnesia; and that old family standby, mineral oil. Do not use mineral oil if you have trouble swallowing. All are safe if used in moderation, but can lead to "laxative habit" in which they become necessary for good bowel movements.

Diarrhea Remedies

Purpose
To treat diarrhea.

For occasional loose stools, no medication is required. A clear liquid diet (for example, water or ginger ale) is the first remedy for any diarrhea: it rests the bowel and replaces lost fluid. When diarrhea persists, products with loperamide or bismuth are often helpful.

If these don't control the diarrhea, stronger agents containing substances such as paregoric may be prescribed. Long-term or severe diarrhea may require the help of a doctor and antibiotic treatments.

To prevent or treat "traveler's diarrhea."

It's better to use antibiotics, such as tetracycline, doxycycline, or others, than to take the older "stopper-uppers" such as Lomotil. Consult your doctor before your trip to get a prescription. Sometimes you can just do this by phone. Some doctors suggest that you begin the antibiotic at the beginning of the trip. We think it is better to take the medicine with you and to begin treatment if you develop any loose stools at all.

Imodium

Imodium A-D generally has replaced other nonprescription medicines for slowing down the bowel and decreasing the number of stools. It should not be used by children. Donnagel and Parepectolin also find wide use.

Dosage
Follow the directions on the label.

Side Effects
If used to excess, these drugs can possibly cause constipation. Rare side effects include dry mouth, dizziness, drowsiness, and vomiting.

Bismuth Subsalicylate (Pepto-Bismol, Kaopectate)

Dosage
Follow the label directions. For children under age three, call the doctor for dosage.

Side Effects
Bismuth may cause a temporary, harmless darkening of the tongue and/or stool.

Sodium Fluoride

Purpose
To protect teeth from decay.

Take care of your teeth; they help you chew. There's good evidence that preventive measures can save teeth. Brush your teeth with a toothpaste that contains fluoride, as recommended by your dentist. Many doctors feel that daily flossing is the most important way to prevent adult tooth decay. Adult tooth loss is usually due to plaque buildup, gum disease, and bone loss. Water jets (such as Waterpik) remove food products from between the teeth, but they're less effective than proper flossing.

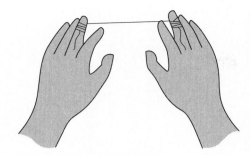

Dental flossing. Wrap floss around your two middle fingers. Use your index fingers to guide the floss into the spaces between your teeth. This way you don't need to wrap the floss tightly. Rub the floss up and down against the teeth's surfaces. If you prefer, tie the floss into a 12-inch loop and you may find it much easier to use.

Sodium Fluoride Supplements

If your water supply is fluoridated, your fluoride intake is adequate and you don't need to supplement your diet. The ground water in many areas is naturally fluoridated. Find out if your water is fluoridated; your local health department usually has the answer. If it isn't fluoridated, you should supplement your children's diet with fluoride. All authorities agree that fluoride is needed through age 10, and probably longer. Adults probably don't require dietary fluoride, although having a dentist paint teeth with sodium fluoride paste is thought to be helpful, as is use of a fluoride toothpaste. Fluoride is effective in preventing tooth decay in persons of all ages. Please support your local health department in fluoridation of water. The occasional person or organization that opposes fluoridation is not aware of the strong science base.

Dosage

Fortunately, it's relatively easy to supplement with fluoride when the water supply isn't treated. Buy a large bottle of soluble fluoride tablets. Most tablets are 2.2 mg and contain 2 mg of fluoride; the rest is a soluble sugar.

If the water supply has low fluoride content, children under the age of 3 need approximately 0.25 mg per day, ages 3 to 6 need 0.5 mg, and ages 6 to 10 need 1 mg. If the water is partially fluoridated, check doses with your dentist. The tablets can be chewed or swallowed. They may also be taken in milk; they don't alter its taste. In states where fluoride is available only by prescription, request a prescription from your doctor or dentist on a routine visit.

Side Effects

Too much fluoride will mottle the teeth (make gray spots) and won't give them additional strength, so don't exceed the recommended dosage. At the recommended dosage, there are no known side effects; fluoride is a natural mineral present in many natural water supplies.

"Artificial Tears" Eye Drops

Purpose

To treat irritated eyes.

The tear mechanism normally cleans, soothes, and lubricates the eye. Occasionally, the environment can overwhelm this mechanism, or not enough tears flow. In these cases, the eye becomes "tired," feels dry or gritty, and may itch. A number of compounds that may aid this problem are available.

There are two general classes of eye preparations. One class contains compounds intended to soothe the eye

(Murine, Prefrin, etc.). Added to these compounds may be decongestants that shrink blood vessels and thus "get the red out" (Visine, Murine Plus, Visine LR). Their capacity to soothe is debatable. The use of decongestants to get rid of a bloodshot appearance is totally cosmetic. Such preparations possibly interfere with the normal healing process, so we don't recommend them.

The other class of preparations makes no claims of special soothing effects and contains no decongestants. Their purpose is to lubricate the eye, to be "artificial tears." These chemical solutions are similar to those of the body, so that no irritation occurs. Ophthalmologists prefer such preparations for minor eye irritation. Murine lubricating eye drops is one example.

Dosage

Use as frequently as needed in the quantity required. You can't use too much, although usually a few drops give just as much relief as a bottleful. If your eyes are constantly dry, check with your doctor because it may indicate an underlying problem. Usually the symptom of dry eyes lasts only a few hours and is readily relieved. Too much sun, wind, or dust usually causes the minor irritation.

Side Effects

No serious side effects have been reported. Visine and other drugs containing decongestants tend to sting a bit.

None of these drugs treats eye infections or injuries or removes foreign bodies from the eye. In Part II, Common Problems, we give instructions for more severe eye complaints (pages 150–159).

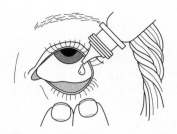

Inserting eye drops. Gently pull down the lower lid. Drip the solution into the sac formed by the lid, not on the eyeball itself. Blink a few times.

Zinc Oxide

Purpose

To treat hemorrhoids.

Zinc oxide powders and creams soothe the irritated area while the body heals the inflamed vein. They also help toughen the skin over the hemorrhoids so that it's less easily irritated. Many people get relief with Preparation H, Anusol, or others, but these offer little advantage.

Reading the Labels

We don't advocate the use of creams that contain ingredients identified by the suffix "-caine" because repeated use of these local anesthetics can cause further irritation.

Dosage

Apply as needed, following label directions. Don't trap bacteria beneath the creams; apply them after a bath when you have carefully cleaned and dried the area. Remember to clean the area thoroughly with soap and water each day.

Side Effects

Essentially none.

Antifungal Preparations

Purpose

To treat fungus infecting the skin, mouth, throat, and vagina.

Fungal infections of the skin usually aren't serious, so treatment isn't urgent. In general, the fungus needs moist, undisturbed areas to grow and will often disappear with regular cleansing, drying, and application of powder to keep the area dry. Clean and dry the area twice daily.

If you need a medication, there are effective nontoxic agents available. For athlete's foot, try one of the zinc undecylenate creams or powders, such as Desenex. In difficult cases, tolnaftate (Tinactin, etc.) and clotrimazole (Lotrimin, etc.) are useful for almost all skin fungus problems, but they are more expensive.

Miconazole (e.g., Monistat 7) is effective and safe for yeast infections (candida monilia) of the mouth, throat, and vagina. If you experience no relief after a week, see the doctor.

Dosage

For athlete's foot, use as directed on the label. For other skin problems, selenium sulfide is effective. It's available by prescription in a 2.5% solution but also over the counter in a 1% solution as Selsun Blue shampoo. Use the shampoo as a cream and let it dry on the skin; repeat several times a day to compensate for the solution's weaker strength.

Side Effects

There are very few. Selenium sulfide can burn the skin if used to excess, so decrease application if you notice any irritation. Selenium may discolor hair and will stain clothes. Be very careful when applying any of these products around the eyes. Don't take them by mouth.

Hydrocortisone Cream

Purpose

To temporarily relieve skin itching and rashes such as poison ivy and poison oak.

Brand names of over-the-counter hydrocortisone cream include Caldecort, Cortizone-10, and Benadryl Itch Stopping Cream. These are strong, local anti-inflammatory preparations. Used for a short period, these creams are safe and almost totally nontoxic. They'll clear up many minor rashes, but they "suppress" a condition rather than "cure" it.

Dosage

Rub a very small amount into the rash. If you can see any cream remaining on the skin, you've used too much. Repeat as frequently as needed, which often is every two to four hours.

Side Effects

Over the long term, these creams can cause skin atrophy (thinning of the skin), so limit their use to a two-week period. After this time, check with your doctor. Theoretically, these creams can make an infection worse, so be careful about using them if it is possible the rash might be infected. Don't use these creams around the eyes, and don't take them by mouth.

Sunscreen Agents

Purpose

To prevent sunburn.

Dermatologists continually remind us that sun is bad for the skin. Exposure to the sun accelerates skin aging and increases the chance of skin cancer. Advertisements, on the other hand, keep extolling the virtues of a suntan. As Americans, we spend much of our youth trying to achieve a pleasing skin tone and disregard the later consequences.

Sunscreen agents can prevent burning but allow you to be in the sun. If your skin is unusually sensitive to the sun's effects, it's best to block the rays; this is achieved with a strong sunscreen agent, like PreSun, or any PABA-containing agent with a high sunscreen number. The rating numbers on the label are a good guide to the blocking power of the different agents. The higher the number, the better the blocking power. Suntan lotions that aren't sunscreen agents block relatively little solar radiation.

The length of time an agent stays on the skin is important. Even the strongest cream or lotion won't help after it has washed off, so look for the nonwater-soluble products if you plan to be in and out of the water.

Remember that beach umbrellas, loose clothing, broad-brimmed hats, and sitting in the shade are sunscreens!

Dosage

Apply evenly to exposed areas of skin as directed on the label.

Side Effects

Very rare skin irritation and allergy have been reported.

Wart Removers

Purpose

To remove some warts.

Warts are a curious little problem. The capricious way in which they form and disappear has led to countless myths and home therapies. They can be surgically removed, burned off, or frozen off, but they'll also go away by themselves or after treatment by hypnosis. Warts are caused by a virus and are a reaction to a minor local viral infection. If you get a wart, you're likely to get more. When one disappears, the others often go away also. The exception is plantar warts, on the sole of the foot, which won't go away by themselves and sometimes not even with home treatment. The doctor may be needed.

Over-the-counter chemicals, such as Compound W and Wart-Off, are moderately effective for treatment of warts. They contain a mild skin irritant. With repeated application, they slowly burn off the top layers of the wart and eventually the virus is destroyed.

Dosage

Apply repeatedly, as directed on the product label. Persistence is necessary.

Side Effects

These products are effective because they are caustic to the skin. Be careful to apply them only to the wart, and be very careful around your eyes or mouth.

Elastic Bandages

Purpose

To treat sprains and similar injuries.

Any family periodically needs elastic (Ace, etc.) bandages. You'll probably need both a narrow width and a broad width. If problems recur, the one-piece devices designed specifically for knees and ankles are sometimes more convenient. All these bandages primarily provide gentle support, but they also act to reduce swelling. The support given is minimal, and it's possible to reinjure the body part despite the bandage. Thus, an elastic bandage isn't a substitute for a splint, a cast, or a proper adhesive-type dressing. Perhaps the most important function of these bandages is to remind yourself that you have a problem so that you're less likely to reinjure yourself.

Application

When wrapping the bandage, start at the far end of the area to be bandaged and work toward the trunk of the body, making each loop a little looser than the one before. Thus, a knee bandage should be tighter below the knee than above, and an ankle bandage should be tighter on the foot than on the lower leg. Many people think that because a bandage is elastic, it must be stretched. That's wrong. The stretchability is to allow the person to move. Simply wrap the bandage as you would a roll of gauze.

Continue using the bandage as support well past the time of active discomfort to allow complete healing and to help prevent reinjury; this usually takes about six weeks. During the latter part of

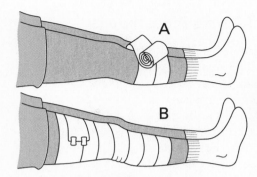

Wrapping an elastic bandage.

(A) Start wrapping the bandage on the far side of the joint (in this case, the knee). Don't stretch the bandage as you wrap.

(B) Wrap past the joint, firmly at first, then more loosely the farther up you go. Use the clips that come with most elastic bandages to fasten the loose end.

this period, you can stop using the bandage except during activities that will likely stress the injured part. Remember that reinjury is still possible while these bandages are being used.

The newer "bandages" for the knee and ankle slip on and provide better support but are a little more expensive. For even better protection, knee braces with metal hinges on the sides provide more support.

Side Effects

The simple elastic bandage or knee brace can cause trouble when it is too tight. Problems arise when circulation in the limb beyond the bandage is impaired. The bandage should be firm but not tight. The limb shouldn't swell, hurt, or be cooler beyond the bandage. The skin shouldn't have any blue or purple color.

Vitamin Preparations

The use of vitamin supplements has always been controversial. In the past, there was theoretical reason to believe that supplements might have benefits; there were also good reasons to believe that these benefits might only be theoretical. Classic diseases of vitamin deficiency (scurvy, beriberi, pellagra, etc.) are rare and occur only in people whose diets are inadequate in virtually every respect, or who have diseases or take medications that interfere with natural vitamins. Most past research on vitamin intake studied diet only and didn't directly address the issue of supplements to the diet. This research suggested that a well-balanced diet should provide adequate amounts of vitamins and minerals.

On the other hand, it's now known that there are specific situations in which vitamin supplements are appropriate. There are good studies indicating that supplements may be useful in individuals with "average" diets outside the special circumstances mentioned above. Here's a summary of current information on vitamin supplements.

▲ Vitamin A: Multiple studies of prevention of a variety of conditions have been inconclusive.
▲ Vitamin C: A Canadian study indicated that people over age 55 who took vitamin C supplements (at least 300 mg daily for five years) have a 70% lower risk for eye cataracts, but most other studies of a variety of conditions have been disappointing or have shown only minor benefit.

▲ Vitamin D: Most pediatricians recommend vitamin D supplements for infants who are breast-feeding.
▲ Vitamin E: Some studies suggest that vitamin E supplements (400 International Units [IU]) may reduce the risk of heart disease by preventing the oxidation of LDL cholesterol. Some other studies, however, have been negative. The Canadian study that looked at vitamin C supplements and cataracts also investigated vitamin E supplementation (400 IU daily) and found a lower risk of cataracts.
▲ Folic acid: In combination with vitamin B_6 and B_{12}, folic acid may reduce the chances of a heart attack by reducing blood levels of homocysteine. Because of this, increasing numbers of doctors encourage use of folic acid and multivitamins. Several studies have demonstrated that the use of a folic acid supplement (1 mg per day) before and during early pregnancy greatly reduces the risk of severe defects of the nervous system in the baby. Since 1998, folic acid has been required in breads and cereals, and spinal cord birth defects have greatly reduced in frequency.
▲ Multivitamins and minerals: One study suggested that the use of a multivitamin and mineral preparation by healthy adults over 65 reduced the number of illness days by more than half. This supplement contained vitamin A, beta-carotene, thiamine, riboflavin, niacin, vitamin B_6, folic acid, vitamin B_{12}, vitamin C, vitamin D, vitamin E, iron, zinc, copper, selenium, iodine, calcium, and magnesium. The amount of each

vitamin or mineral was similar to the current recommended daily allowances except for beta-carotene and vitamin E, which were above the usual recommended allowances.

The use of vitamin supplements for purposes other than those indicated above is entirely optional. They're unlikely to cause problems when taken in reasonable dosages, but consider the cautions listed below. If you do buy vitamins, the cheaper "house" brands usually are of similar quality to those that are heavily advertised.

Dosage

Multivitamin preparations usually contain the current recommended daily allowance of each vitamin. Other dosages are indicated above.

Side Effects

Vitamin A, vitamin D, and vitamin B_6 (pyridoxine) can cause severe problems when taken in excessively large doses. Large doses of vitamin C have been reported to be associated with kidney problems in rare instances. Other vitamins have not been studied as extensively, but serious side effects appear to be very rare.

PART II

Common Problems

CHAPTER 3

Emergencies

Emergencies require prompt action, not panic. What action you should take depends on the facilities available and the nature of the problem.

If there are massive injuries or if the victim is unconscious, you must get help immediately. Go to the emergency room if it is close. Have someone call ahead if you can.

If you can't reach the emergency room quickly, you can usually obtain help by calling 911. Calling for help is especially important if you think that someone has swallowed poison. Poison control centers and emergency rooms can often tell you over the phone how to counteract the poison, thus beginning treatment as early as possible. Please do not use the "911" number for problems that are not emergencies; keep the lines clear for real emergencies.

The most important thing is to *be prepared*. Work out a procedure for medical emergencies. Develop and test it before an actual emergency arises. Have the telephone numbers written down in the front of this book or stored in your cellphone. Know the best way to reach the emergency room by car. If you plan emergency action ahead of time, you'll decrease the likelihood of panic and increase the probability of receiving the proper care quickly.

Call an Ambulance?

An ambulance isn't always the fastest way to reach a medical facility. It must travel to both your location and back and often isn't twice as fast as a private car. If the victim can readily move or be moved and a private car is available, use the car and have someone call ahead.

On the other hand, the ambulance brings with it a trained crew that knows how to lift a victim to minimize the chance of further injury. Intravenous fluids and oxygen are usually available; splints and bandages are provided; and in some instances, lifesaving resuscitation may be employed on the way to the hospital. Thus, care by ambulance attendants may most benefit a person who:

▲ Is gravely ill
▲ May have a back or neck injury
▲ May be having a heart attack
▲ Is short of breath

In our experience, ambulances are too often used as expensive taxis. An ambulance may be needed more urgently at another location, so use good judgment in deciding to call for one. Your community's EMT (emergency medical technician) program can be a great resource; use it wisely.

Emergency Signs

The decision charts for the common problems covered in Part II of this book assume that no emergency signs are present. *Emergency signs overrule the charts and dictate that you must seek medical help immediately.* Be familiar with the following emergency signs.

Major Injury

Common sense tells us that a person with a broken leg or large chest wound deserves immediate attention. Emergency facilities exist to take care of major injuries. They must be used promptly.

Possible Neck or Spinal Injury

Do not move the patient before skilled help arrives unless absolutely required. Injury can be made worse if the patient is moved before being adequately splinted.

No Pulse or Breath

Someone whose heart or lungs aren't working needs help right away. Call 911. If you know CPR (cardiopulmonary resuscitation), start it after you call for help or ask someone else to call. If the person is choking, see Choking (page 82).

Unconsciousness

The person who is unconscious needs emergency care immediately.

Bleeding That Can't Be Stopped

Most wounds will stop bleeding if pressure is applied. This is the most important part of first aid for such wounds. A wound that continues to bleed despite the application of pressure requires attention in order to prevent unnec-

Seizures

An extremely high fever can cause a seizure or convulsion. Such seizures are relatively common in normal, healthy children, especially those between six months and four years of age. Although a seizure may appear dramatic, there is little danger to the child. Usually a fever-related (febrile) seizure lasts a few minutes and causes no lasting effects. (Sometimes there is brief weakness or even paralysis in an arm or leg.) Less than half of all children who have one such seizure ever have another. Repeated seizures, or a seizure that lasts more than 30 minutes, may suggest more serious medical conditions.

If a child with a fever has seizures, do the following:

▲ Protect his or her head from hitting the floor or hard objects. Place the child on a bed.
▲ Keep the child's airway open (see drawing on page 80), and do rescue breathing as needed.
▲ Do not force an object or your fingers into a person's mouth. This is likely to result in injury. It's not possible for the child to "swallow the tongue," and serious tongue bites are rare.
▲ Start to lower the child's fever with sponging. Never give a person having seizures anything by mouth.
▲ **Get immediate medical attention.** Call 911.

essary loss of blood. The average adult can tolerate the loss of several cups of blood with little ill effect, but children

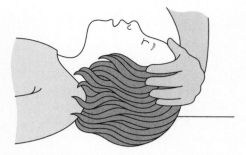

Open airway. If a child is having a febrile (fever-related) seizure, pull the head back slightly. Do not force anything into the mouth.

can tolerate only smaller amounts, relative to their body size.

Stupor or Drowsiness

A decreased level of mental activity short of unconsciousness is termed "stupor." A practical way of determining if the severity of stupor or drowsiness needs urgent treatment is to note the victim's ability to answer questions. If the victim is not sufficiently awake to answer questions concerning what has happened, then urgent action is necessary. Children are more difficult to judge, but the child who cannot be aroused needs immediate attention.

Emergency First Aid

We haven't tried to teach complex first-aid procedures such as CPR (cardiopulmonary resuscitation) in this book. To use such procedures correctly, you need hands-on instruction and practice. Community organizations such as the American Red Cross and the American Heart Association offer training.

Disorientation

Disorientation is described in terms of time, place, and person—that is, according to whether the person can answer these questions correctly:

▲ What is the date?
▲ Where are we?
▲ Who are you?

A person who doesn't know his or her identity is in more trouble than a person who doesn't know where he or she is, and that person is in more trouble than a person who can't give the correct date.

Disorientation may be part of a variety of illnesses and is especially common when the person has a high fever. The person who previously has been alert and then becomes disoriented and confused deserves immediate medical attention.

Shortness of Breath

We discuss shortness of breath more extensively in its own section (page 262). As a general rule, emergency attention is needed if the person is short of breath even though resting. However, in young adults, the most frequent cause of shortness of breath at rest is the hyperventilation syndrome, which is not a serious concern (page 298). Nevertheless, if you can't confidently determine that shortness of breath is due to the hyperventilation syndrome, then the reasonable course of action is to seek immediate aid.

Cold Sweats

As an isolated symptom, sweating isn't likely to be serious. It's the normal response to elevated temperature. It's also the natural response to stress, either psychological or physical. Most people have experienced sweaty palms when "put on the spot" or stressed psychologically. Also, sweating may occur with breaking a fever, and this kind of sweating is usually not serious.

In contrast, a "cold sweat" in a person complaining of chest pain, abdominal pain, or lightheadedness indicates a need for immediate attention; this may be a serious illness.

Severe Pain

Surprisingly, severe pain by itself rarely determines if a problem is serious and urgent. Most often, pain is associated with other symptoms that indicate the urgency of the condition. The most obvious example is pain associated with major injury—like a broken leg—which itself clearly requires urgent care.

The severity of pain is subjective and depends on the individual; often the magnitude of the pain is altered by emotional and psychological factors. Nevertheless, severe pain demands urgent medical attention, if for no other reason than to relieve the pain.

Much of the art and science of medicine is directed at the relief of pain, and the use of emergency procedures to secure this relief is justified even if the cause of the pain eventually proves to be minor. However, the person who frequently complains of severe pain from minor causes is in much the same situation as the boy who cried "wolf": calls for help will inevitably be taken less and less seriously by the doctor. This situation is a dangerous one, for the person may have difficulty obtaining help when it is most needed.

Heat Stroke

Exposure to a warm and humid environment, especially while not drinking enough fluids, can cause "heat exhaustion." Symptoms include weakness, headache, dizziness, thirst, nausea, and vomiting. The person's temperature may be elevated, but not above 101°F (38°C). The skin is sweaty because the body is trying to cool off. Move the person into a cool place and have him or her drink lots of water.

"Heat stroke," also called sunstroke, is an **emergency**. It arises when the body is no longer able to cool off. A person with heat stroke has dry skin. Body temperature rises quickly when sweating stops, often topping 105°F (40.5°C). A person suffering heat stroke no longer complains of heat or thirst and may be confused or delirious, lose consciousness, or have seizures.

The person with heat stroke needs immediate medical care. You must rapidly cool the person's body by ice baths, ice packs, wet sheets, or any other means possible. Brain damage and other injuries may result if the victim's temperature doesn't go down. Treatment in the emergency room can be very effective.

Choking

Your dinner companion can't breathe, can't talk, and is turning blue. He's gasping for air and puts his hand to his throat. These signs tell you he's choking. Do you know what to do?

Choking on a foreign object, usually food, is all too common. The most frequent setting for choking in adults is the evening meal, often in a restaurant or at a party. This situation increases the risk of choking in several ways: First, the victim is likely to have been drinking alcoholic beverages, and this may slow the reflexes that normally keep food from going down the wrong way. Second, the victim is likely to be distracted from the business of eating by conversation or entertainment. Finally, this is the time that solid meats such as steak are most commonly eaten, and these meats are usually the culprits in adult choking.

Children stick a much wider variety of objects into their mouths, are likely to do so at any time of the day or night, and are much less likely to complicate the situation with alcohol. Nevertheless, a child is still most likely to choke on food. The most likely foods are hot dogs, grapes, peanuts, and hard candy.

Home Treatment

Choking is an emergency, but emergency medical services—doctors, EMTs, ambulances, emergency rooms, hospitals—play virtually no role in its treatment. In almost every case, the victim's fate will be decided by the time such help can respond. Either someone knowledgeable steps forward and relieves the

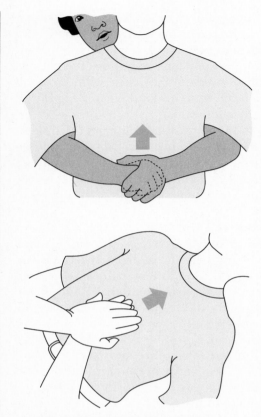

Abdominal-thrust (Heimlich) maneuver for adults. The figures show proper hand positions. *Top:* standing position. *Bottom:* prone position.

choking, or there's a very good chance the person won't survive.

You can be that knowledgeable someone. The most effective way to relieve choking is with the abdominal-thrust, or Heimlich, maneuver. Pushing on the lungs from below rapidly raises the air pressure inside the lungs and behind the foreign object that is causing the choking. This results in the forceful expulsion of the object from the throat back into the mouth. Done properly, an abdominal-thrust maneuver does not

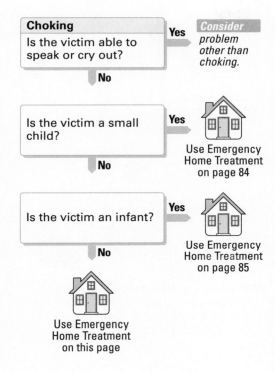

Choking
Is the victim able to speak or cry out?
Yes → *Consider* problem other than choking.
↓ **No**

Is the victim a small child?
Yes → Use Emergency Home Treatment on page 84
↓ **No**

Is the victim an infant?
Yes → Use Emergency Home Treatment on page 85
↓ **No**

Use Emergency Home Treatment on this page

pose great risk of doing harm. Still, it's not the kind of thing you want to do to someone who won't benefit from it. The most important sign that a person should be treated with the abdominal-thrust maneuver is the inability to talk. If the person in difficulty can speak, forget about the abdominal-thrust maneuver.

For Adults

1. Stand behind the choking victim and place your arms around him or her. Make a fist and place it against the victim's abdomen, thumb side in, between the navel and the breastbone.

2. Hold your fist with your other hand, and push upward and inward, four times quickly.

If the victim is pregnant or obese, place your arms around his or her chest and your hands over the middle of the breastbone. Give four quick chest thrusts.

If the victim is lying down, roll the victim over onto his or her back. Place your hands on the abdomen and push in the same direction on the body that you would if the victim were standing (inward and toward the upper body).

If the victim is much taller or heavier than you, make the victim lie on the floor and use the lying-down method described above.

3. If the victim doesn't start to breathe, open the mouth by moving the jaw and tongue, and look for the swallowed object. If you can see the object, sweep it out with your little finger. If you try to remove an object you can't see, you may only push it in more tightly.

4. If the victim doesn't begin to breathe after the object has been removed from the air passage, use mouth-to-mouth resuscitation.

5. Call for help, and repeat these steps until the object is dislodged and the victim is breathing normally.

For Small Children

1. Kneel next to the child, who should be lying on his or her back.

2. Position the heel of one hand on the child's abdomen between the navel and the breastbone. Deliver 6 to 10 thrusts inward and toward the upper body.

3. If this doesn't work, open the mouth by moving the jaw and tongue and look for the swallowed object. *If you can see the object,* sweep it out of the throat using your little finger. If you try to remove an object you can't see, you may only push it in more tightly.

4. If the child doesn't begin to breathe after the object has been removed, use mouth-to-mouth resuscitation.

5. Call for assistance, and repeat these steps until the object is dislodged and the child is breathing normally or until help arrives.

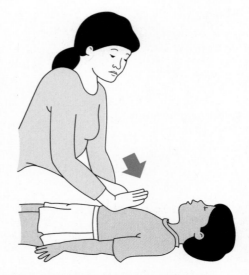

Abdominal thrust for choking children. Place the bottom of your hand between the child's navel and breastbone. Deliver six to ten quick thrusts. If this doesn't work, go to step 3.

For Infants

1. Hold the infant along your forearm, facedown, so that the head is lower than the feet.

2. Deliver four rapid blows to the back, between the shoulder blades, with the heel of your hand.

3. If this doesn't work, turn the baby over and, using two fingers, give four quick upward thrusts to the chest.

4. If you're still not successful, open the infant's mouth by moving the jaw and tongue and look for the swallowed object in the throat. *If you can see the object,* try to sweep it out gently with your little finger. If you try to remove an object you can't see, you may do more harm by pushing it in more tightly or triggering the child's gag reflex.

5. If the baby doesn't begin to breathe after the object has been removed, use mouth-to-nose-and-mouth resuscitation.

6. Call for assistance, and repeat these steps until the object is dislodged and the baby is breathing normally.

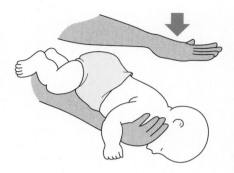

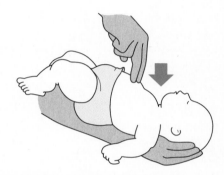

Abdominal thrust for choking infants. If four rapid blows to the infant's back don't work, deliver four quick thrusts to the infant's chest as shown above.

Poisoning

Although poisons may be inhaled or absorbed through the skin, for the most part they are swallowed. The term "ingestion" refers to swallowing.

Most poisoning can be prevented. Children almost always swallow poison accidentally. Don't allow children to reach potentially harmful substances like these:

▲ Medications*
▲ Insecticides
▲ Caustic cleansers
▲ Organic solvents
▲ Fuels
▲ Furniture polishes
▲ Antifreezes
▲ Drain cleaners

* Induce vomiting

The last item is the most damaging: drain cleaners like Drano are strong alkali solutions that can destroy any tissue they touch.

Keep all drugs in child-resistant bottles. Because there are no totally childproof bottles, keep drugs out of small children's reach. Aspirin overdoses have been responsible for more childhood deaths than any other medication.

Identifying the Problem

Treatment must be prompt to be effective, but identifying the poison is as important as speed. *Don't panic.* Try to identify the swallowed substance without taking up too much time. If you can't or if the victim is unconscious, go to the emergency room right away. If you can identify the poison, call the doctor or Poison Control Center immediately and get advice on what to do. Always bring the container with you to the hospital. Life-support measures come first in the case of an unconscious victim, but doctors must identify the ingested substance before they can begin the proper treatment.

Many significant medication overdoses are due to suicide attempts. Any suicide attempt is an indication that the person needs help, even if he or she has physically recovered from the overdose itself and is in no immediate danger.

Home Treatment

All cases of poisoning require professional help. Someone should call for help immediately. If the victim is conscious and alert and the ingredients swallowed are known, there are two types of treatment: those in which vomiting should be induced, and those in which it should not. Inducing vomiting is only truly safe if the ingested substance is a drug or a plant.

Do not induce vomiting if the victim has swallowed any of the following:

▲ **Acids:** battery acid, sulfuric acid, hydrochloric acid, bleach, hair straightener, etc.
▲ **Alkalis:** Drano, drain cleaners, oven cleaners, etc.
▲ **Petroleum products:** gasoline, furniture polish, kerosene, lighter fluid, etc.

These substances can destroy the esophagus or damage the lungs as they are vomited. Neutralize them with milk while contacting the physician. If you don't have milk, use water or milk of magnesia.

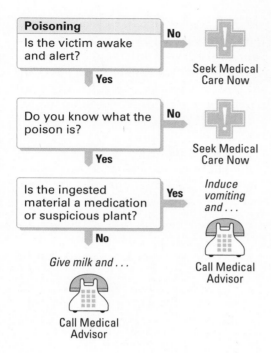

Poisoning
Is the victim awake and alert?

No → Seek Medical Care Now

Yes ↓

Do you know what the poison is?

No → Seek Medical Care Now

Yes ↓

Is the ingested material a medication or suspicious plant?

Yes → *Induce vomiting and . . .* Call Medical Advisor

No ↓

Give milk and . . . Call Medical Advisor

Food Poisoning

Food poisoning is often blamed for stomach or bowel problems that don't have any obvious explanation ("Must have been something I ate"). Actually, the most common type of food poisoning is that due to streptococcal or staphylococcal bacteria; this type is usually mild. Serious illness can result from food poisoning due to other bacteria such as clostridial (botulism), cryptosporidium, and certain E. coli; fortunately these occur rarely. Treat symptoms as described in the appropriate sections: Diarrhea (page 268) and Nausea and Vomiting (page 266). The main symptom of botulism is paralysis, starting with the muscles of the eyes, mouth, and throat, and then involving the entire body—that's obviously an emergency!

Vomiting is a safe way to remove medications or plants from the stomach. It's more effective and safer than a stomach pump and doesn't require the doctor. Vomiting can sometimes be achieved immediately by touching the back of the throat with a finger; this is usually the fastest, and thus the best, way.

A somewhat old-fashioned way to induce vomiting is to give two to four teaspoons (10–20 ml) of syrup (not extract) of ipecac (page 61), followed by as much liquid as the victim can drink. Vomiting usually follows within 20 minutes. Mustard mixed with warm water also works. If there is no vomiting within 25 minutes, repeat. Collect what comes up for the doctor to examine.

Before, during, and after first aid for poisoning, contact the Poison Control Center.

If an accidental poisoning has occurred, make sure that it doesn't happen again. Put poisons where children cannot reach them. Dispose of old medications properly. You can find instructions and "take back" locations at fda.gov.

What to Expect at the Doctor's Office

Significant poisoning is best managed at the emergency room. Treatment of the conscious victim depends on the particular poison and whether the person has vomited most of it back out. If indicated, the stomach will be emptied by vomiting or by a stomach pump. Victims who are unconscious or have swallowed a strong acid or alkali will require admission to the hospital.

CHAPTER 4

Common Injuries

Cuts

Most cuts (lacerations) affect only the skin and the fatty tissue beneath it and heal without permanent damage. However, injury to internal structures such as muscles, tendons, blood vessels, ligaments, or nerves can bring permanent damage. Your doctor can decrease this chance. These are the signs that normally call for a cut to be examined by a doctor:

▲ Bleeding that you can't control with pressure—this is an emergency (page 79)
▲ Numbness or weakness in the limb beyond the wound
▲ Inability to move fingers or toes

Signs of infection—such as pus oozing from the wound, fever, or extensive redness and swelling—won't appear for at least 24 hours. Bacteria need time to grow and multiply. If these signs appear, you must consult a doctor.

Stitches

The only purpose of stitching (suturing) a wound is to pull the edges together to hasten healing and minimize scarring. Stitches injure tissue to some extent, so they aren't recommended if the wound can be held closed without them. Stitching should be done within eight hours of the injury. Otherwise, the edges of the wound are less likely to heal together and germs are more likely to be trapped under the skin. Stitching is often required in young children who are apt to pull off bandages, or in areas that are subject to a great deal of motion, such as the fingers or joints.

Difficult Cuts

Unless the cut is very small or shallow, call your doctor about cuts in these areas:

▲ On the chest, abdomen, or back unless the cut is clearly minor
▲ On the face—facial wounds can be disfiguring
▲ On the palm—hand wounds can be difficult to treat if they become infected

Home Treatment

Cleanse the wound. Soap and water will do, but be vigorous. You may also use 3% hydrogen peroxide (page 52) or a commercial antiseptic such as Merthiolate. Make sure no dirt, glass, or other foreign material remains in the wound.

The edges of a clean, minor cut can usually be held together by "butterfly" bandages or, preferably, by Steri-Strips—strips of sterile paper tape (page 50). Apply either of these bandages so that the edges of the wound join without "rolling under."

Pain medication (page 54) can of course help reduce discomfort but is often not needed.

See the doctor if the edges of the wound can't be kept together, if signs of infection appear (pus, fever, extensive redness and swelling), or if the cut isn't healing well within two weeks.

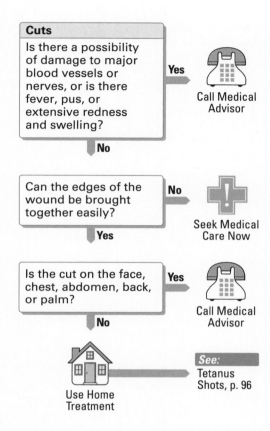

Cuts

Is there a possibility of damage to major blood vessels or nerves, or is there fever, pus, or extensive redness and swelling?

Yes → Call Medical Advisor

No ↓

Can the edges of the wound be brought together easily?

No → Seek Medical Care Now

Yes ↓

Is the cut on the face, chest, abdomen, back, or palm?

Yes → Call Medical Advisor

No ↓

Use Home Treatment

See: Tetanus Shots, p. 96

What to Expect at the Doctor's Office

The wound will be thoroughly cleansed and explored to be sure that no foreign particles are left and that blood vessels, nerves, and tendons are undamaged. Since the doctor may use an anesthetic to numb the area, report any possible allergy to local anesthetics (Xylocaine, for example). The doctor will give a tetanus shot (page 96) and antibiotics if needed.

Lacerations that may require a surgical specialist include those with injury to tendons or major vessels, especially those in the hand, and those on the face.

Stitches

Your doctor will tell you when stitches are to be removed. You can often perform this simple procedure at home with a clean pair of small, sharp scissors or a fingernail clipper.

1. Clean the skin and the stitches. Sometimes a scab must be removed by soaking.
2. Gently lift the stitch away from the skin by grasping a loose end of the knot with tweezers.
3. Cut the stitch as close to the skin as possible, so that a minimum amount of the stitch that was outside the skin will be pulled through. This reduces the chance of infection.
4. Lift the tweezers to pull the stitch out.

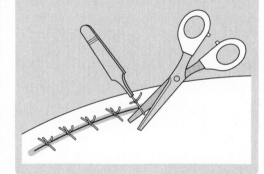

Puncture Wounds

Nails, pins, tacks, and other sharp objects can cause puncture wounds of the skin. Since puncture wounds rarely need stitches, the important questions are:

▲ Are the underlying tissues injured?
▲ Is anything (dirt or object) left in the wound?
▲ Does the victim need a tetanus shot?

Most minor puncture wounds involve the extremities—arms, hands, legs, and especially feet. A deep puncture elsewhere on the body could cause internal injury that is not obvious, so call the doctor for advice. A puncture wound on the hand can be serious if it gets infected. Call the doctor for a wound on the hand unless it is very minor.

A nail, ice pick, or other large object is more likely to cause underlying injury than a narrow item like a needle. The rare signs of serious injury are:

▲ Blood pumping vigorously from the wound—possible injured artery
▲ Numbness or tingling in the limb beyond the wound—possible injured nerves
▲ Difficulty moving the limb beyond the wound—possible injured tendon

These symptoms require **emergency** care.

Puncture wounds can become infected, especially if foreign material remains inside—a splinter, needle, or piece of glass. See the doctor if you have any question about whether the wound is free of foreign material. Signs of infection include:

▲ Fever
▲ Extensive redness
▲ The formation of thick, yellowish pus
▲ Swelling of the area around the wound

These are signs to see a doctor and usually take 24 hours or more to develop.

Home Treatment

Don't apply pressure to the wound unless it bleeds heavily or pumps in a way suggesting an artery has been injured. Let the wound bleed as much as possible to remove foreign material.

Clean the wound with soap and water or 3% hydrogen peroxide (page 52). Soak the wound in warm water or a baking soda solution several times a day for four or five days (page 53). This helps keep the skin puncture open so that germs or foreign debris can drain from it.

Seek medical care if you see signs of infection or if the wound hasn't healed after two weeks.

Make sure you are immunized against tetanus (page 96).

What to Expect at the Doctor's Office

The doctor will examine the wound to assess the extent of the puncture, injury to underlying tissues, and possible infection. He or she may have X-rays taken or explore the wound surgically. Be prepared to tell the doctor about possible allergies to local anesthetics, such as Xylocaine. Most doctors recommend home treatment. Antibiotics are rarely prescribed.

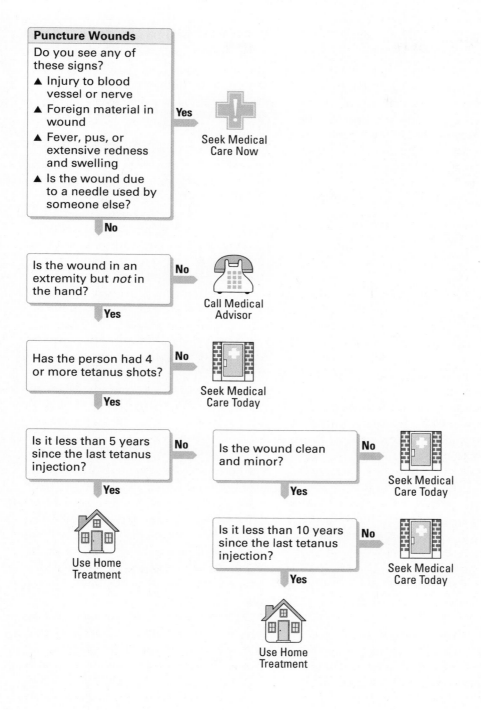

Puncture Wounds

Do you see any of these signs?
- ▲ Injury to blood vessel or nerve
- ▲ Foreign material in wound
- ▲ Fever, pus, or extensive redness and swelling
- ▲ Is the wound due to a needle used by someone else?

Yes → Seek Medical Care Now

No ↓

Is the wound in an extremity but *not* in the hand?

No → Call Medical Advisor

Yes ↓

Has the person had 4 or more tetanus shots?

No → Seek Medical Care Today

Yes ↓

Is it less than 5 years since the last tetanus injection?

No → Is the wound clean and minor?

Yes ↓

Use Home Treatment

Is the wound clean and minor?

No → Seek Medical Care Today

Yes ↓

Is it less than 10 years since the last tetanus injection?

No → Seek Medical Care Today

Yes ↓

Use Home Treatment

Animal Bites

Rabies is a very serious viral infection carried in the saliva of animals. It can be transmitted to humans through a bite or scratch. Although 3,000 to 4,000 animals with rabies are found in the United States each year, only one or two people get the disease.

A rabid animal may behave in strange ways:

▲ Not running from humans as you would expect
▲ Attacking without provocation
▲ Drooling or foaming at the mouth
▲ Walking around in the daytime if it is normally nocturnal

Avoid animals that act out of the ordinary.

The main carriers of rabies are skunks, foxes, bats, and raccoons. Rabies is less common in cattle, dogs, and cats. The disease is extremely rare in squirrels, chipmunks, rats, and mice. Cats and dogs pose the greatest risk of rabies to people because of their frequent contact with humans and the large number of bites reported each year. For the sake of your pets, your neighbors, and yourself, immunize your cats and dogs against rabies.

If you have been bitten by a wild animal, or by a dog or cat whose immunization history you don't know, call your doctor to decide whether you need antirabies treatment.

If you have been bitten by a pet dog or cat, and the animal's owner has its shots up-to-date and will observe the animal for sickness, you don't need to go to the doctor.

Home Treatment

Treat animal bites as you would other wounds. Turn to Cuts (page 88), Scrapes and Abrasions (page 94), Puncture Wounds (page 90), or Tetanus Shots (page 96) for the appropriate treatment.

If a wild animal causes the bite, call animal control officials. Trying to trap a wild animal may expose you or others to additional risk.

A pet whose shots are up-to-date is unlikely to have rabies. Still, you should arrange to have the animal observed for the next 15 days to make sure it does not develop the disease. You can usually rely on pet owners to watch the animal. If the owner is uncooperative, call animal control officials. If the animal develops rabies during the observation period, bite victims must be treated immediately.

Many localities require that you report animal bites promptly to the health department.

What to Expect at the Doctor's Office

The doctor must balance the remote possibility of rabies exposure with the risks of treatment. An unprovoked attack by a wild animal, or a bite from an animal that appears to be rabid, may require the rabies vaccine and antirabies serum. A bite caused by an animal that escaped may require treatment to be safe.

Doctors give rabies vaccine in five injections—one immediately and four over the next 28 days. The vaccine may cause local skin reactions, fever, headache, and nausea. Severe reactions are rare. The antirabies serum used today

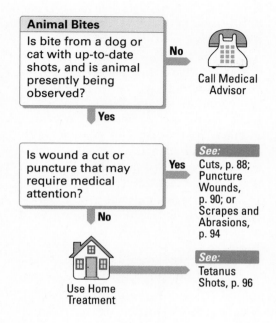

Animal Bites

Is bite from a dog or cat with up-to-date shots, and is animal presently being observed?

No → Call Medical Advisor

Yes ↓

Is wound a cut or puncture that may require medical attention?

Yes → *See:* Cuts, p. 88; Puncture Wounds, p. 90; or Scrapes and Abrasions, p. 94

No ↓

Use Home Treatment → *See:* Tetanus Shots, p. 96

is of human origin and causes few side effects.

The doctor may give you a tetanus shot, although tetanus from an animal bite is rare. Usually you don't need antibiotics.

Scrapes and Abrasions

Scrapes and abrasions are shallow wounds. Several layers of the skin may be torn or even totally scraped off, but the wound doesn't go far beneath the skin. Abrasions are usually caused by falls onto the hands, elbows, or knees, but skateboard and bicycle riders can get abrasions on just about any part of the body. Because abrasions expose millions of nerve endings, all of which send pain impulses to the brain, they're usually much more painful than cuts.

Home Treatment

Remove all dirt and foreign matter. Washing the wound with soap and warm water is the most important step in treatment. You can also use 3% hydrogen peroxide to cleanse the wound (page 52). Most scrapes will scab rather quickly; this is nature's way of "dressing" the wound.

Adhesive bandages may be used as necessary for a wound that continues to ooze blood; they must be removed if they get wet (page 50). Antibacterial ointments (Neosporin, Bacitracin, etc.) are optional; their main advantage is in keeping bandages from sticking to the wound.

Loose skin flaps, if they aren't dirty, may be left to help form a natural dressing. If the skin flap is dirty, cut it off carefully with nail scissors. (If it hurts, stop! You're cutting the wrong tissue.)

Watch the wound for signs of infection—pus, fever, or severe redness or swelling—but don't be worried by redness around the edges; this is an indication of normal healing. Infection won't be obvious in the first 24 hours; fever may indicate a serious infection.

Pain can be treated for the first few minutes with an ice pack in a plastic bag enclosed in a towel applied over the wound as needed. Do not put ice directly on the area since that can cause frostbite. The worst pain subsides fairly quickly, and acetaminophen or other over-the-counter pain medication can then be used if needed (page 54).

See the doctor if signs of infection appear or if the scrape or abrasion isn't healed within two weeks.

What to Expect at the Doctor's Office

The doctor will make sure that the wound is free of dirt and foreign matter. Soap and water and 3% hydrogen peroxide (page 52) will often be used. Sometimes a local anesthetic (Xylocaine, for example) is required to reduce the pain of the cleansing process. Tell the doctor of possible allergies to anesthetics.

An antibacterial ointment such as Neosporin or Bacitracin is sometimes applied after cleansing. Betadine is a painless iodine preparation that is also occasionally used (page 52). Tetanus shots aren't required for simple scrapes, but if the patient is overdue for a shot, it is a good chance to get caught up (page 96) and avoid a future doctor visit to get the shot.

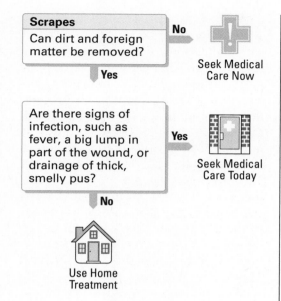

Scrapes

Can dirt and foreign matter be removed?

No → Seek Medical Care Now

Yes ↓

Are there signs of infection, such as fever, a big lump in part of the wound, or drainage of thick, smelly pus?

Yes → Seek Medical Care Today

No ↓

Use Home Treatment

Tetanus Shots

People may come to the doctor's office or emergency room to get a tetanus shot even though it isn't needed. This section's decision chart illustrates the essentials of the current U.S. Public Health Service recommendations. It can save you and your family several visits to the doctor. See the advice on immunization (pages 30 and 32) and Cuts (page 88).

The question of whether or not a wound is "clean" and "minor" may be troublesome. Wounds caused by sharp, clean objects such as knives or razor blades have less chance of becoming infected than those in which dirt or foreign bodies have penetrated and lodged beneath the skin. Abrasions and minor burns won't result in tetanus. The tetanus germ can't grow in the presence of air, so the skin must be cut or punctured for the germ to reach an airless location.

Immunization

If you've never received a basic series of three tetanus shots, you should see your doctor. Sometimes a different kind of tetanus shot is required if you haven't been adequately immunized. This shot is called "tetanus immune globulin" and is used when immunization isn't complete and there is a significant risk of tetanus. It is more expensive, more painful, and more likely to cause an allergic reaction than the tetanus booster. So keep a record of your family's immunizations in the back of this book and know the dates.

During the first tetanus shots (usually a series of three injections given in early childhood), the person develops a resistance to tetanus over a three-week period. This immunity then slowly declines over many months. After each booster, immunity develops more rapidly and lasts longer. If you have had an initial series of five tetanus injections, immunity will usually last at least 10 years after every booster injection. Nevertheless, if a wound has contaminated material beneath the skin and isn't exposed to the air, and if you haven't had a tetanus shot within the past five years, a booster shot is advised to keep the level of immunity as high as possible.

Tetanus immunization is very important because the tetanus germ is quite common and the disease (lockjaw) is so severe. Be absolutely sure that each of your children has had the basic series of three injections and appropriate boosters. Because the immunity lasts so long, adults usually get away with a long period between boosters, but immunization of children should be "by the book."

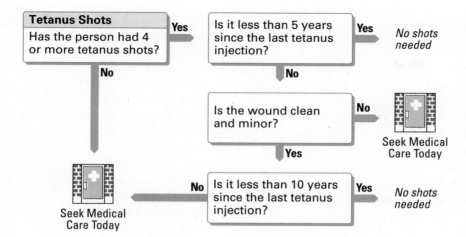

Tetanus Shots

Has the person had 4 or more tetanus shots?

— **Yes** → Is it less than 5 years since the last tetanus injection?
  — **Yes** → *No shots needed*
  — **No** → Is the wound clean and minor?
    — **No** → Seek Medical Care Today
    — **Yes** → Is it less than 10 years since the last tetanus injection?
      — **Yes** → *No shots needed*
      — **No** → Seek Medical Care Today

— **No** → Seek Medical Care Today

Broken Bone?

You may find it hard to tell a broken bone from an injury to soft tissues, such as ligaments and tendons. Like a sprain or a strain, fractures can be painful. In most cases, the bone fragments remain aligned after the fracture, so you can't tell by sight whether a bone is broken; usually, neither can a doctor.

Besides obvious deformity of a limb (which requires medical attention), here are some signs of a serious fracture:

▲ If the fracture injures nearby nerves or blood vessels, a limb can be cold, pale, or numb—signs to call the doctor.

▲ Paleness, sweating, dizziness, and thirst are signs of shock. The person with these **emergency signs** needs immediate medical attention (page 79).

▲ Sprains and other soft-tissue injuries usually allow some use of a limb, but fractures are often more disabling. While sprains and strains improve over a day or two, a broken bone may remain painful and unable to bear weight.

▲ Although soft-tissue injuries cause bruises under the skin, major bruising is more likely with a fracture.

Fortunately, few fractures are emergencies. In most fractures the bone pieces are in place and don't require setting. No harm is done if you wait a day or two before the doctor puts a cast on a broken arm or leg. After all, the cast doesn't cause healing; it just keeps the bones in place as they heal.

For broken ribs you can't do much more than tape and rest the affected ribs. Use only two or three short strips of 1"–2" adhesive tape, taping them in line with the affected rib, with a little tension on the skin to hold the rib together. Change the tape every two days and inspect the skin for blisters or sores underneath. If you find either, give the tape a rest. (See Broken Ribs, page 100.)

If you have shortness of breath after a chest injury, you may have hurt a lung. See the doctor right away.

For a possible skull fracture, see Head Injuries (page 108).

Home Treatment

An ice pack on the injured area will help reduce pain and swelling. Wrap it in a towel to avoid frostbite. Rest and protect the limb for at least 48 hours.

Splinting an injured limb is a good way to rest the bone, especially if you are taking the person for medical care. Here are some guidelines for splinting:

▲ Immobilize the joints above and below the painful area. For example, to splint an injury of the lower arm, you must stop the elbow and wrist from moving.

▲ You can use any stiff material as a splint—a piece of wood, folded magazine, umbrella, or rolled-up newspaper.

▲ Don't wrap the limb so tightly that you cut off circulation.

After 48 hours of rest, carefully test the limb. See if you can use it and whether it is painful when moved. See the doctor for any injury that is still painful.

Take acetaminophen, aspirin, ibuprofen, or naproxen as little as possible for as short a time as possible for pain.

Broken Bone?

Do you see any of these signs?

▲ Limb is cold, blue, or numb
▲ Pelvis or thigh might be broken
▲ Victim is sweaty, pale, dizzy, or thirsty
▲ Limb is crooked

Yes →

Seek Medical Care Now

No ↓

Do you see any of these signs?

▲ Limb that can't bear weight or be used
▲ A lot of bleeding and bruising in the injured area
▲ Fracture near a joint in a child

Yes →

Seek Medical Care Today

No ↓

Use Home Treatment

What to Expect at the Doctor's Office

A technician or assistant usually takes an X-ray of the injured area before you see the doctor. A crooked limb must be set, or straightened, which may require general anesthesia. The doctor may put pins in the bone during surgery to hold pieces together as they heal.

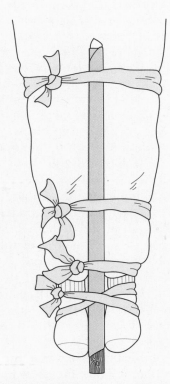

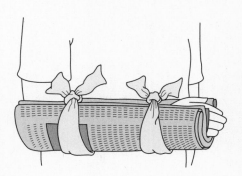

Splints. If a person may have a broken limb, it's important to keep that limb from shifting as you apply home treatment or go to the hospital.

Left: Forearm splint made of rolled newspapers and strips of cloth.

Above: Splint for one leg anchored by the other leg and by a board wrapped with a towel.

Broken Ribs

Broken ribs are surprisingly common injuries that can usually be taken care of at home. Some of our family members have had them after falls on ice in Antarctica, off horses in Botswana, playing touch football, and in our bathroom at home. Sometimes, particularly in children or teens, the injury may be just a bruise or a "greenstick" fracture in which the break doesn't go completely through the rib (similar to the way an immature, or green, tree branch splits when bent). We've used the process described here to good effect many times.

The goals of home treatment are to check for danger signs such as shortness of breath or coughing up blood, which can suggest injury to the underlying lung or air leaking from the lung to the pleural space around the lung. If there is possible injury to more than three ribs or to other parts of the body, have it checked out at the doctor's office or emergency room. Usually you will not encounter these complications.

If these problems are not present, use home treatment and strap the rib with one-inch adhesive tape. If this does not relieve discomfort within an hour, seek medical care the same day. The biggest problem with strapping a rib is that it can immobilize the chest wall too much, limiting deep breathing, which can result in pneumonia. You only want to strap the broken rib or ribs; you do this by applying the adhesive tape strips directly in line with the rib that may be fractured. If the suspected fractures are on both sides of the chest, or if pain is still severe after 24 hours despite home therapy, it is time to get medical care.

Home Treatment

The steps in home treatment are simple and sensible. Get a black magic marker. Push on the chest all over with a finger or thumb, looking for sore spots. If you find one or more of these tender areas, mark them with an "x" Next, locate the rib above and below the mark and put more marks on the skin over the rib, about 4 inches or more in each direction. Draw a line on the skin over the rib to connect the marks. If the tenderness you had found is not over a rib, it is not likely to be a broken rib.

If the tender place is on a rib, walk your fingers out from the tender place four inches in each direction, following the line you have just drawn. Make marks along the suspect rib toward the breastbone and toward the spine, about 8–10 inches apart. Push firmly on these

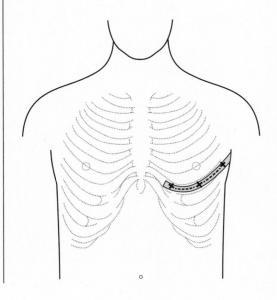

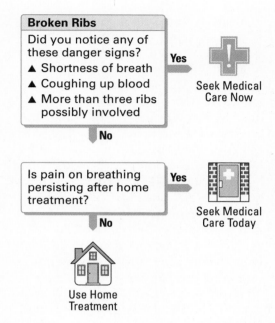

Broken Ribs

Did you notice any of these danger signs?
- ▲ Shortness of breath
- ▲ Coughing up blood
- ▲ More than three ribs possibly involved

Yes → Seek Medical Care Now

No ↓

Is pain on breathing persisting after home treatment?

Yes → Seek Medical Care Today

No ↓

Use Home Treatment

two spots but not on the original tender spot, causing the rib to bow a little. If the bowing causes pain at the original tender spot, the rib is almost certainly broken.

Now put one-inch adhesive tape, about 8–10 inches long, along the rib over the marks. Put gentle pressure on the tape so that it pulls together the skin over the probable break just a little but not enough to irritate the skin. Now do the same thing with two more strips of tape, lapping them a half-inch over the original strip on each side. Ask the patient to take a deep breath and ask if the pain is gone or much better. If it is, you have confirmed a broken rib and strapped it, all without needing an X-ray, and without immobilizing the chest, in less than five minutes.

After two days—or sooner if there is pain under the tape—remove the tape, inspect the skin, and replace the tape, more gently, if there is redness or blistering under the tape. Usually the patient won't need the tape for more than a week or so, but full healing of a broken rib takes 4–6 weeks. The patient usually shouldn't need pain medicines. If pain continues for more than a week, returns, or the patient develops any of the danger signs on the chart, he or she may need a medical visit and perhaps an X-ray.

Ankle Injuries

Ligaments are tissues that connect the bones of a joint to provide stability during the joint's action. When the ankle is twisted severely, either the ligaments or the bone must give way. If the ligaments give way, they may be stretched (strained), partially torn (sprained), or completely torn (torn ligaments). If the ligaments don't give way, one of the bones around the ankle will break (fracture).

Strains, sprains, and even some minor fractures of the ankle will heal well with home treatment. Some torn ligaments do well without a great deal of medical care; operations to repair them are rare. For practical purposes, the immediate attention of the doctor is necessary only when the injury has been severe enough to cause obvious fracture to the bones around the ankle or to cause a completely torn ligament. This is indicated by a deformed joint with abnormal motion.

Swelling

The typical ankle sprain swells either around the bony bump at the outside of the ankle or about two inches (5 cm)

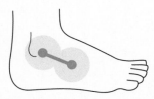

Ankle swelling. The highlighted area shows the ligament that gets stressed when you "turn your ankle."

in front of and below it. The amount of swelling doesn't differentiate among sprains, tears, and fractures. The common chip fractures around the ankle often cause less swelling than a sprain. Sprains and torn ligaments usually swell quickly because there is bleeding into the tissue around the ankle. The skin will turn blue-black in the area as the blood is broken down by the body.

A swollen ankle that isn't deformed doesn't need prolonged rest, casting, or X-rays. Home treatment should be started promptly. Detection of any damage to the ligaments may be difficult immediately after the injury if much swelling is present. Because it is easier to do an adequate examination of the foot after the swelling has gone down and because no damage is done by resting a mild fracture or torn ligament, there is no need to rush to the doctor.

Pain

Pain tells you what to do and not to do. If it hurts, don't do it. If pain prevents any standing on the ankle after 24 hours, see a doctor. If little progress is being made so that pain makes weight-bearing difficult after 72 hours, see the doctor.

Home Treatment

RICE is the key word:

▲ Rest
▲ Ice
▲ Compression
▲ Elevation

Rest the ankle and keep it elevated. Apply ice in a towel to the injured area and leave it there for at least 30 minutes. If there is any evidence of swelling after the first 30 minutes, then apply ice in a

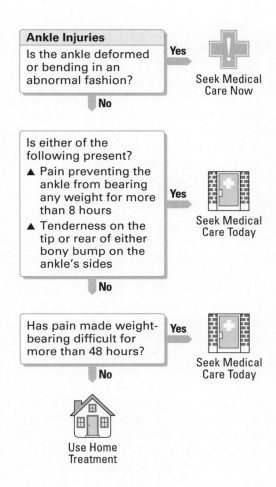

Ankle Injuries

Is the ankle deformed or bending in an abnormal fashion?

Yes → Seek Medical Care Now

No

Is either of the following present?
▲ Pain preventing the ankle from bearing any weight for more than 8 hours
▲ Tenderness on the tip or rear of either bony bump on the ankle's sides

Yes → Seek Medical Care Today

No

Has pain made weight-bearing difficult for more than 48 hours?

Yes → Seek Medical Care Today

No

Use Home Treatment

towel for 30 minutes on and 15 minutes off through the next few hours. If the ankle stops being painful while elevated, you may cautiously try to put weight on that leg. If the ankle is still painful when bearing weight, you should avoid putting weight on that leg for the first 24 hours. Heat may be applied, but only after 24 hours.

An elastic bandage can help but may not prevent reinjury if you resume full activity (page 73). Don't stretch the bandage so that it's very tight and interferes with blood circulation. You generally shouldn't try taping on children; if it's done incorrectly, it may cut off circulation to the foot.

The ankle should feel relatively normal in about 10 days. Be warned, however, that full healing won't take place for four to six weeks. If strenuous activity, such as organized athletics, is to be pursued during this time, the ankle should be taped by someone experienced in this technique.

Over-the-counter pain medication (page 54) can of course help to reduce discomfort.

What to Expect at the Doctor's Office

The doctor will examine the motions of the ankle to see if they are abnormal and may have an X-ray taken. If there is no fracture or only a minor chip fracture, it is likely that a continuation of home treatment will be recommended. For other fractures, a cast will be necessary or, rarely, an operation to put the bones back together. An operation may be required to repair a torn ligament.

Knee Injuries

The ligaments of the knee may be stretched (strained), partially torn (sprained), or completely torn (torn ligaments). Unlike ankle ligament injuries, torn ligaments in the knee need to be repaired surgically as soon as possible after the injury occurs. If surgery is delayed, the operation is more difficult and less likely to be successful. For this reason, the approach to knee injuries is more cautious than for ankle injuries. If there is any possibility of a torn ligament, go to the doctor.

Fractures in the area of the knee are less common than around the ankle, and they always need to be cared for by a doctor.

Knee injuries usually occur during sports, when the knee is more likely to experience twisting and side contact. (Deep knee bends stretch ligaments and may contribute to injuries; they should be avoided.) Serious knee injuries occur when the leg is planted on the ground and a blow is received to the knee from the side. If the foot can't give way, the knee will. There is no way to totally avoid this possibility in athletics. The use of shorter spikes and cleats helps, but knee braces and supports give little protection.

Abnormal Motion

When ligaments are completely torn, the lower leg can be wiggled from side to side or front to back when the leg is straight. Compare the injured knee to the opposite knee to get some idea of what amount of side-to-side motion is normal. If the knee slides front to back (called "the drawer sign"), this is even more serious, since it suggests a tear of the ligament in the front of the knee (ACL). If you think your knee motion may be abnormally loose, see a doctor.

If the cartilage within the knee has been torn, normal motion may be blocked, preventing it from being straightened. Although a torn cartilage doesn't need immediate surgery, it deserves medical attention.

Pain and Swelling

The amount of pain and swelling doesn't indicate the severity of the injury. The ability to bear weight, to move the knee through the normal range of motion, and to keep the knee stable when wiggled is more important.

Typically, strains and sprains hurt immediately and continue to hurt for hours and even days after the injury. Swelling tends to come on rather slowly over a period of hours but may reach rather large proportions. When a ligament is completely torn, there is intense pain immediately, which subsides until the knee may hurt little or not at all for a while. Usually there is significant bleeding into the tissues around the joint when a ligament is torn; swelling tends to come on quickly and be obvious, even impressive, to the eye.

The best policy when there is a potential injury to the ligament is to avoid any major activity until it is clear that this is a minor strain or sprain. Home treatment is intended only for minor strains and sprains.

Home Treatment

RIP is the key word: rest, ice, and protection. Rest the knee and elevate it. Apply an ice pack, enclosed in a towel, for at

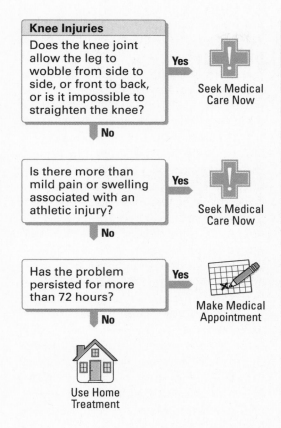

Knee Injuries

Does the knee joint allow the leg to wobble from side to side, or front to back, or is it impossible to straighten the knee?

Yes → Seek Medical Care Now

No ↓

Is there more than mild pain or swelling associated with an athletic injury?

Yes → Seek Medical Care Now

No ↓

Has the problem persisted for more than 72 hours?

Yes → Make Medical Appointment

No ↓

Use Home Treatment

least 30 minutes to minimize swelling. If there is more than slight swelling or pain despite the fact that the knee was immediately rested and cold was applied, see the doctor. If this isn't the case, apply the ice treatment on the knee for 30 minutes and then off for 15 minutes for the next several hours. Limited weight-bearing may be attempted during this time with a close watch for increased swelling and pain.

Heat can be applied after 24 hours. By then, the knee should look and feel relatively normal; after 72 hours, this should clearly be the case. If not, see the doctor. Remember, however, that a strain or sprain isn't completely healed for four to six weeks and requires protection during this healing period. Elastic bandages won't prevent reinjury but will ease symptoms a bit and remind the injured person to be careful with the knee (page 73).

Over-the-counter pain medication (page 54) can, of course, help to reduce discomfort.

What to Expect at the Doctor's Office

The knee will be examined for abnormal motion. A massively swollen knee may have blood removed from the joint with a needle. Torn ligaments need surgical repair. X-rays may be taken but usually aren't helpful. For injuries that appear minor, home treatment will be advised. Over-the-counter pain medications are sometimes, but not often, required (page 54).

Arm Injuries

The ligaments of the wrist, shoulder, and elbow joints may be stretched (strained) or partially torn (sprained), but complete tears are rare. Fractures may occur at the wrist, are less frequent around the elbow, and are uncommon around the shoulder. Injuries often occur during a fall, when the weight of the body is caught on the outstretched arm.

Wrists
The wrist is the most frequently injured joint in the arm. Strains and sprains are common, and the small bones in the wrist may be fractured. Fractures of these small bones may be difficult to see on an X-ray. The most frequent fracture of the wrist involves the ends of the long bones of the forearm and is easily recognized because it causes an unnatural bend near the wrist. Physicians refer to this as the "silver fork deformity."

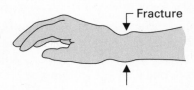
Fracture

Elbows
"Tennis elbow" is the most frequent elbow injury; if you think this is the problem, consult Elbow Pain (page 234). Other injuries are much less frequent and usually result from falls, automobile accidents, or contact sports. A common problem in children under five years of age is partial dislocation due to adults pulling on the arm.

Shoulders
The collarbone (clavicle) is a frequently fractured bone; fortunately, it has remarkable healing powers. There is usually a pronounced swelling over the collarbone at the site of the fracture. An inability to raise the arm on the affected side is common; the shoulders may also appear uneven. Bandaging the arm to the chest or use of a figure-of-eight bandage is the only treatment required. The figure-of-eight bandage usually comes from the drugstore complete with instructions. The figure-of-eight bandage lets you use the arm better.

Shoulder separation, often seen in athletes, is perhaps the most common injury of the shoulder. It is a stretching or tearing of the ligament that attaches the collarbone to one of the bones that forms the shoulder joint. It causes a slight deformity and extreme tenderness at the end of the collarbone on the top of the shoulder. Sprains and strains of other ligaments occur, but complete tearing is unusual, as are fractures. Dislocations of the shoulder are rare but are best treated early.

Severe fractures and dislocations are best treated early. These usually cause deformity, severe pain, and limited movement. Other fractures won't be harmed by delayed treatment if the injured limb is rested and protected. Complete tears of ligaments are rare; strains and sprains will heal with home treatment.

Home Treatment
RICE is the key word: rest, ice, compression, and elevation. Rest the arm and apply ice wrapped in a towel for at least 30 minutes. If the pain is gone and there is no swelling at the end of this time,

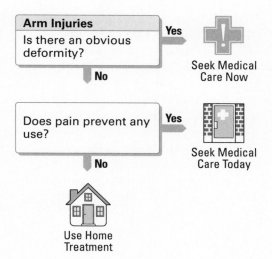

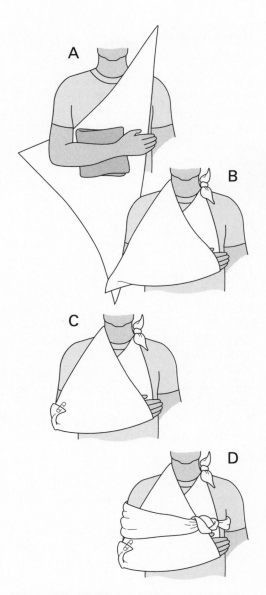

you can stop the ice treatment. A sling for shoulder and elbow injuries and a partial splint for wrist injuries will elevate, protect, and rest the injury while allowing the patient to move around. Continue ice treatment for 30 minutes on and 15 minutes off through the first eight hours.

Heat can be applied after 24 hours. The injured joint should be usable with little pain within 24 hours and should be almost normal by 72 hours. If not, see the doctor. Complete healing takes from four to six weeks, and activities with a likelihood of reinjury should be avoided during this time. Over-the-counter pain medication (page 54) can help.

What to Expect at the Doctor's Office

An examination and sometimes X-rays will be performed. A cast or sling may be applied. Pain medication is sometimes given, but acetaminophen or other over-the-counter medication (page 54) is usually adequate. Certain fractures, especially those around the elbow, may require surgery.

Tying an arm sling. (A) Use a triangular piece of cloth (or a folded square sheet). A small folded towel adds support.

(B) Tie as shown.

(C) A safety pin will hold it securely.

(D) To add even greater security, tie another strip of cloth around the chest and arm as shown.

Head Injuries

The skull is a strong container that protects and carefully cushions the valuable contents inside. Head injuries are potentially serious, but few lead to long-term problems. Doctors divide head injuries into two basic types:

▲ Injury to the bone, skin, and other tissues of the skull
▲ Injuries to the brain, blood vessels, and other tissues within the skull

Treat cuts, abrasions, and other wounds of the head as you would other trauma to the skin (pages 88 and 94). See the doctor if you suspect a fracture of a skull bone, or if you see blood or clear fluid in the ears or nose following head injury.

A head injury that causes concussion or loss of consciousness requires **emergency** care. See the doctor as well if there may be bleeding or severe bruising within the head, suggested by these signs:

▲ Loss of alertness: increasing lethargy, unresponsiveness, abnormally deep sleep, coma
▲ Unequal pupil size after head injury (though about one in four people has slightly unequal pupils all the time)
▲ Severe vomiting or "projectile vomiting," which may be ejected several feet

In severe head injury, two or more signs are often present at once. Vomiting is usually forceful, repeated, and progressively worse.

In rare cases, slow bleeding inside the head forms a blood clot that causes chronic headache, persistent vomiting, or personality changes months after the injury.

Careful observation is the most important part of diagnosing head injury. You can usually do this at home as well as, if not better than, a hospital staff member. A family member is more likely to pay closer attention to the person with a head injury and know what is normal for him or her.

Home Treatment

Stop the bleeding of skin wounds by applying pressure directly on the wound, preferably with a sterile dressing. Ice applied to a bruised area may reduce swelling, but "goose eggs" often form anyway.

The initial observation period is crucial. Symptoms of bleeding inside the head usually appear within 24 to 72 hours after injury. Check the person every 2 hours during the first 24 hours, every 4 hours for the second 24 hours, and every 8 hours for the third day.

Because many injuries occur during the evening, the injured person will usually be asleep several hours after the accident. You can look in on the sleeping person periodically to check his or her pulse, pupils, and arousability. If the person has a minor head bump and no sign of brain injury, nighttime checking is usually not necessary.

What to Expect at the Doctor's Office

The doctor will ask about the nature of the accident and assess the patient's appearance and vital signs. He or she will do a physical exam and check for

Head Injuries

Have you seen any of the following?

▲ Unconsciousness
▲ Victim cannot remember injury
▲ Seizure
▲ Visual problems
▲ Bleeding from or around eyes, ears, or mouth
▲ Changes in behavior (irritability, lethargy, sleep)
▲ Fluid draining from nose
▲ Persistent vomiting
▲ Irregular breathing or heartbeat
▲ Child under 2 years of age, or possibly being abused
▲ Victim under influence of alcohol or drugs

Yes → Seek Medical Care Now

No ↓

Is there a cut? — **Yes** → *See:* Cuts, p. 88

No ↓

Use Home Treatment

other injuries. If internal bleeding is possible, the patient may be kept in the hospital for observation. The doctor will avoid giving drugs, such as sedatives or strong pain medication, that may hide signs.

Bleeding within the skull is hard to diagnose. Skull X-rays are seldom helpful. CT scans and MRIs can be helpful but are expensive and may miss early accumulations of blood. With severe injuries, the victim may require X-rays of the neck to check for possible injury to the cervical spine.

Burns

Burns are injuries caused most commonly by heat. They can also result from chemicals, electricity, or radiation.

Heat burns are ranked according to the depth of skin injury:

▲ **First-degree burns** are superficial, resulting in red and tender skin. They are painful but rarely serious. The common sunburn is a first-degree burn. Even when first-degree burns affect a large area of skin, they seldom result in long-term problems. Usually you don't need to see a doctor.

▲ **Second-degree burns** are deeper, producing blisters of the skin. Scalding with hot water or a very severe sunburn are common types of second-degree burns. They are painful and may be serious if a large area of skin is affected. However, second-degree burns rarely result in infection or scarring. See a doctor for second-degree burns covering an area larger than the hand or affecting the face or hands. Otherwise, treat the burn at home.

▲ **Third-degree burns** destroy all skin layers and extend into deeper tissues. They do not hurt because nerve endings have been destroyed (but they may be surrounded by a painful second-degree burn). A third-degree burn usually involves obviously charred skin. Such burns can lead to fluid loss, infection, and scarring. All third-degree burns need medical attention.

One of the most common burns is sunburn. Sunburn is preventable, by avoiding tanning salons or prolonged exposure to the sun, and by using a sunscreen (page 72).

Sunburn is most painful 6 to 48 hours after sun exposure. Injured skin may peel 3 to 10 days after the burn. In rare cases, people with sunburn have visual problems. If this happens, call your doctor. Otherwise, you don't need to see the doctor for a sunburn unless there is very severe pain or blistering.

Home Treatment

For heat burns, immediately apply cold water or ice wrapped in a towel to the affected area. This stops the burning, limits the injury, and eases pain. Cool running water is fine. Apply cold until pain is relieved, or for about an hour. But do not apply cold so long that the burned area becomes numb; frostbite can occur. Reapply cold if needed.

For sunburn, cool compresses or cool oatmeal baths (Aveeno, etc.) may be helpful. Ordinary baking soda (one-half cup in a tub of water) is just as useful.

Anesthetic creams and sprays can relieve pain, but they may also slow healing, and they can cause irritation or allergic reactions in some people. Antibiotic creams such as Neosporin or Bacitracin probably do no harm to a burn, but they won't help a lot either. Don't apply butter, cream, or ointments such as Vaseline.

Use an over-the-counter pain reliever (page 54).

Don't break blisters. If blisters break by themselves, leave the overlying skin

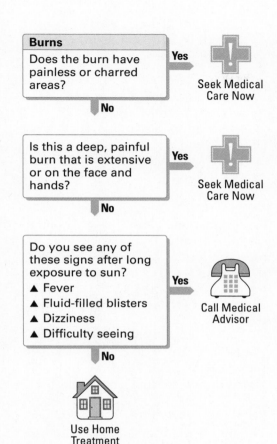

Burns

Does the burn have painless or charred areas?

Yes → Seek Medical Care Now

No ↓

Is this a deep, painful burn that is extensive or on the face and hands?

Yes → Seek Medical Care Now

No ↓

Do you see any of these signs after long exposure to sun?
▲ Fever
▲ Fluid-filled blisters
▲ Dizziness
▲ Difficulty seeing

Yes → Call Medical Advisor

No ↓

Use Home Treatment

in place. Keep the area clean, and protect yourself against the cause of blisters next time.

A burn that is painful for more than 48 hours requires medical attention.

What to Expect at the Doctor's Office

The doctor will assess the size and severity of the burn and determine whether the victim needs antibiotics, hospitalization, or skin grafts. Pain relievers may be prescribed.

The doctor may apply a dressing and/or an antibacterial ointment. Change the dressing regularly according to directions. Check the burn often for signs of infection.

Severe burns may require hospitalization. Third-degree burns may require skin grafts.

Infected Wounds

If a wound becomes infected, bacteria can grow in the bloodstream—a serious condition that doctors call "septicemia." This is why it's so important to clean a wound thoroughly and keep it clean.

Normally, after skin is hurt, the body begins to heal by forming a scab. These are the signs of *normal* healing:

▲ The wound may seep serum, which is yellowish and clear. (People often mistake serum for pus, which is thick, smelly, and never appears on the first day or so.)
▲ The edges of the wound will be pink or red.
▲ The wound may feel warm or itch.

The normal healing time depends on the type of wound. A minor wound requires about this amount of time:

▲ On the face—3 to 5 days
▲ On the chest and arms—5 to 9 days
▲ On the legs—7 to 12 days

Larger wounds, or those that gape, requiring new skin or tissue to grow across an open space, need more time to heal. Children heal faster than adults. If a wound fails to heal within the expected time, call the doctor.

In contrast, an infected wound may fester within the skin, causing pain and swelling. Infection usually takes two to three days to develop. If you have an infection, it's a good idea for a doctor to examine the wound unless it is clearly minor. Sometimes a festering wound will break open and pus will drain out. This is good, often allowing the wound to heal well.

Overall, you should see the doctor for any of the following:

▲ An increase in pain, redness, or swelling around the wound a day or more after the injury
▲ Drainage of pus (not serum) from the wound
▲ Fever (see page 284) and a general sick feeling

Home Treatment

Keep the wound clean. Leave it open to the air if possible. You may bandage the wound if it is oozing blood or serum or is unsightly or likely to get dirty. Since children pick at scabs, a bandage may be a good idea for them. Change the bandage daily.

Each day, gently soak and clean the wound in warm water. This will help remove debris and keep the scab soft. Watch the wound for signs of infection.

What to Expect at the Doctor's Office

The doctor will examine the wound for infection, and an assistant will take your temperature. The doctor may take sample blood or fluid from the wound for laboratory tests. The doctor may prescribe antibiotics.

If the wound is festering, the doctor may drain it with a needle or scalpel. This is not very painful and actually relieves discomfort.

For severe infections you may need to stay in the hospital.

Infected Wounds

Are any of the
following present?

▲ Fever above 99.9°F
(37.7°C) and a
general ill feeling

▲ An increase in pain,
redness, or swelling
a day or more after
the injury

▲ Thick, smelly pus
draining from the
wound

Yes →

Seek Medical
Care Today

No

Use Home
Treatment

Is It Blood Poisoning?

There is a folk saying that red streaks
running up the arm or leg from a
wound indicate blood poisoning and
that the patient will die when the
streaks reach the heart. In fact, such
streaks are only an inflammation of
the lymph channels carrying away the
debris from the wound. They will stop
when they reach local lymph nodes
in the armpit or groin and do not, by
themselves, indicate blood poisoning.

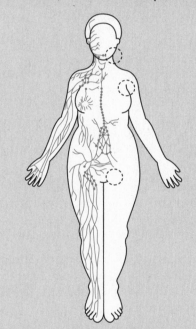

Lymph system. The left side of this figure
shows the lymph channels through the body.
The circles on the right side show the lymph
node locations; swelling or pain in these
areas can be an important symptom.

Insect Bites or Stings

Most insect bites are trivial, but some bites or stings may cause reactions. Local reactions consist of pain, swelling, and redness at the site of the bite or sting. They are uncomfortable but don't pose a serious hazard.

In contrast, systemic reactions (those that involve the whole body) may occasionally be serious and may require emergency treatment. There are three types of systemic reactions. All are rare.

▲ An **asthma attack** is the most common, causing difficulty in breathing and perhaps audible wheezing.
▲ **Hives** or extensive skin rashes following insect bites are less serious but indicate that a more severe reaction might occur if the patient is bitten or stung again.
▲ **Fainting** or loss of consciousness rarely occurs and suggests that the collapse is due to an allergic reaction. This is an **emergency** (page 88).

If the person has had any of these reactions in the past, he or she should be taken immediately to a medical facility if stung or bitten.

If the local reaction to a bite or sting is severe or a deep sore is developing, a doctor should be consulted by telephone. Children often have more severe local reactions than adults.

Spider Bites

Bites from poisonous spiders are rare. The female black widow spider accounts for many of them. This spider is glossy black with a body approximately one-half inch (1 cm) in diameter, a leg span of about two inches (5 cm), and a characteristic red hourglass mark on the abdomen. The black widow spider is found in woodpiles, sheds, basements, or outdoor privies. The bite is often painless, and the first sign may be cramping abdominal pain. The abdomen becomes hard and boardlike as the waves of pain become severe. Breathing is difficult and accompanied by grunting. There may be nausea, vomiting, headache, sweating, twitching, shaking, and tingling sensations in the hands. The bite itself may not be prominent and may be overshadowed by the systemic reaction.

Brown recluse spiders, which are slightly smaller than black widows and have a white violin pattern on their backs, cause painful bites and serious local reactions but aren't as dangerous as black widows. Hobo spiders are similar in size and consequences to the brown recluse but are found mainly in the Northwest.

This book has separate sections on the bites of Ticks (page 200) and Chiggers (page 202).

Home Treatment

Apply something cold, such as ice or cold packs, promptly. Delay in cold applications results in a more severe local reaction. Acetaminophen or other over-the-counter pain relievers may be used (page 54). Antihistamines, such as chlorpheniramine (Chlor-Trimeton) or diphenhydramine (Benadryl), can be helpful in relieving the itch somewhat (page 62). If the reaction is severe or if the pain doesn't diminish in 48 hours, consult the doctor by telephone.

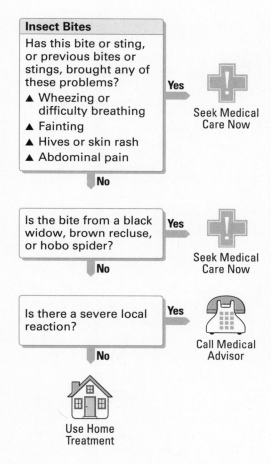

Insect Bites

Has this bite or sting, or previous bites or stings, brought any of these problems?
- ▲ Wheezing or difficulty breathing
- ▲ Fainting
- ▲ Hives or skin rash
- ▲ Abdominal pain

Yes → Seek Medical Care Now

No ↓

Is the bite from a black widow, brown recluse, or hobo spider?

Yes → Seek Medical Care Now

No ↓

Is there a severe local reaction?

Yes → Call Medical Advisor

No ↓

Use Home Treatment

What to Expect at the Doctor's Office

The doctor will ask what sort of insect or spider has inflicted the wound and will look for signs of systemic reaction. If a systemic reaction is present, adrenalin by injection is usually necessary. Rarely, measures to support breathing or blood pressure will be needed; these measures require an emergency room or hospital.

If the problem is a local reaction, the doctor will examine the wound for signs of dead tissue or infection. Occasionally, the wound will need to be drained surgically. In other cases, pain relievers or antihistamines may make the patient more comfortable. Adrenalin injections are occasionally used for very severe local reactions.

If a systemic reaction has occurred, the doctor may give shots to try to desensitize the patient's body to the insect's poison. People with serious allergies to insect bites can buy emergency kits (such as EpiPen) to cut off systemic reactions.

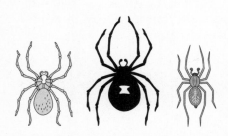

Poisonous spiders. *Left:* Brown recluse, shown from above. *Center:* Black widow, shown from below. *Right:* Hobo, shown from above. All appear at approximate actual size.

Snake Bites

North America's poisonous snakes come in two groups: coral snakes and pit vipers, which include rattlesnakes, copperheads, and cottonmouths. At least one species of poisonous snake is found in each of the contiguous United States except Maine, Delaware, and Michigan.

Of the 45,000 snake bites reported each year in the United States, only 20% are made by poisonous snakes. Those snakes don't inject venom with every bite. All told, fewer than 20 people actually die from snake bites each year. The major damage caused by poisonous snake bites is loss of function in an arm or leg.

Home Treatment
Experts agree that the most important steps for snake bites are:

1. Correct identification of the snake
2. A quick trip to the hospital

Pit Viper Bites
Most experts believe that trying to suck the venom out of the wound makes sense if you can do it within three minutes after the bite. Use a suction cup, if possible, but in emergencies, you can use your mouth, quickly spitting out the venom and blood. Experts don't agree on the benefit of making cuts over the bite in an attempt to remove venom. Don't apply cold to the bite. Don't lie flat; keep the bite lower than the heart. It is helpful for the patient not to use the arm or leg with the bite and to rest, but these actions aren't as important as getting to medical care as soon as possible.

Doctors don't agree on the use of tourniquets for pit viper bites. Tourniquets that are too tight and left in place too long may actually cause worse damage and even lead to amputation. If you use a tourniquet, follow these guidelines:

▲ Tourniquets are useful only on an arm or leg, not on the trunk or the face.
▲ Place the tourniquet 4 to 6 inches (10–15 cm) above the bite.
▲ Make the tourniquet snug, but not tight enough to cut off blood flow, and loosen it for at least 2 minutes every 15 minutes.

Coral Snake Bites
Neither a tourniquet nor suction is useful. It's probably good to wash the area around the wound right away. But the most important task is to find medical help as quickly as possible.

What to Expect at the Doctor's Office
Hospitals are equipped with antivenin kits to counteract snake venoms. The doctor will want to know what sort of snake made the bite and if the patient has ever had a bad reaction to antivenin. Further treatment will depend on the condition of the patient. As stated above, most snake bites, even from poisonous snakes, are not fatal.

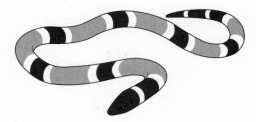

Snake Bites

Did the bite come from a coral snake?

Yes → Seek Medical Care Now

No ↓

Did the bite come from a pit viper?

Yes → *If the bite occurred less than 3 minutes before, suck out the poison, and . . .*

Seek Medical Care Now

No ↓

Have you identified the type of snake?

Yes → *See:* Puncture Wounds, p. 90

No ↓

Seek Medical Care Now

Coral snakes. Coral snakes, which are poisonous, can be identified by ring pattern—red rings between yellow rings. Some nonpoisonous snakes have rings of the same colors as coral snakes—red, yellow, and black—but in a different arrangement.

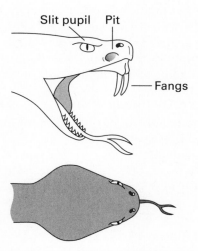

Slit pupil   Pit

Fangs

Pit vipers. *Top:* The pit viper's "pits" are small depressions located between the eye and nostril on either side of the snake's head.

Bottom: Venom glands on either side of the head (inside the mouth) create the distinctive triangular head shape the pit viper has when viewed from above.

Fishhooks

The problem with fishhooks is, of course, the barb. Meant to keep the fish hooked, it has the same effect when people are caught. Nevertheless, a fishhook usually can be removed without a doctor's help, unless it is in someone's eye. *Never try to remove hooks that have actually penetrated the eyeball;* this is a job for the doctor.

The patient's confidence and cooperation are needed in order to avoid a visit to the doctor. A pair of electrician's pliers with a wire-cutting blade should be part of your fishing equipment. The advantage of the doctor's office is the availability of a local anesthetic.

Home Treatment

Occasionally, the hook will have moved all the way around so that it lies just beneath the surface of the skin. If this is the case, often the best technique is simply to push the hook on through the skin, cut it off just behind the barb with wire cutters, and remove it by pulling it back through the way it entered (shown in the drawing below). This may be somewhat painful but most children are able to tolerate it.

On other occasions, the hook will be embedded only slightly and can be re- moved by simply grasping the shank of the hook (pliers help), pushing slightly forward and away from the barb, and then pulling it out.

If the barb isn't near the surface or if you don't have pliers or wire cutters, use the method illustrated below. The hook is usually removed quickly and almost painlessly.

1. Put a loop of fish line through the bend of the fishhook so that, at the appropriate time, a quick jerk can be applied and the hook can be pulled out directly in line with the shaft of the hook.

2. Holding on to the shaft, push the hook slightly in and away from the barb so as to disengage the barb.

3. Holding this pressure constant to keep the barb disengaged, give a quick jerk on the fish line and the hook will pop out.

If you aren't successful, push the hook all the way through and out so that the barb can be cut off with wire cutters.

Be sure that the person's tetanus shots are up-to-date (page 96). Treat the

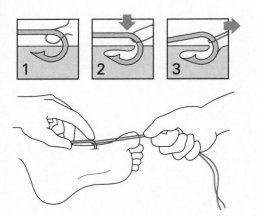

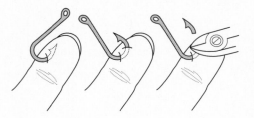

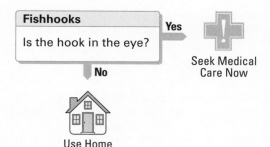

Fishhooks

Is the hook in the eye?

Yes → **Seek Medical Care Now**

No ↓

Use Home Treatment

wound as in the Home Treatment section for Puncture Wounds (page 90). If all else fails, a visit to the doctor should solve the problem.

What to Expect at the Doctor's Office

The doctor will use one of the three methods described to remove the hook.

If necessary, the area around the hook can be numbed with a local anesthetic before the hook is removed. Often, however, injecting a local anesthetic is more painful than just removing the hook without the anesthetic.

If the hook is in the eye, it's likely that the doctor will recommend the help of an eye specialist (ophthalmologist), and it may be necessary to remove the hook in the operating room.

Removing a Splinter

A splinter under the skin can often be pulled out with tweezers. If some material remains, you can usually dislodge it by picking away at the overlying skin with a clean needle. Sterilize the needle first by dipping it in rubbing alcohol or holding it in a match flame. Another option is to soak the area of skin twice a day in a cup of very warm, but not hot, water mixed with one tablespoon (15 ml) of baking soda (page 52); the splinter will probably come out by itself in a day or two. Don't let a splinter wound become infected.

Smashed Fingers

Smashing fingers in car doors or desk drawers, or with hammers or baseballs, is all too common. If the injury involves only the end segment of the finger (the terminal phalanx) and doesn't involve a significant cut, the help of a doctor is seldom needed. Blood under the fingernail (subungual hematoma) is a painful problem that you can treat.

Joint Fractures

Fractures of the bone in the end segment of the finger aren't treated unless they involve the joint. Many doctors feel that it is unwise to splint the finger even if there is a fracture of the joint. Although the splint will decrease pain, it may also increase the stiffness of the joint after healing. However, if the fracture isn't splinted, the pain may persist longer, and you may end up with a stiff joint anyway. Discuss the advantages and disadvantages of splinting with your doctor.

Dislocated Nails

Fingernails are often dislocated in these injuries. It isn't necessary to have the entire fingernail removed. The nail that is detached should be clipped off to avoid catching it on other objects. Nails will take from four to six weeks to grow back.

Home Treatment

If the injury doesn't involve other parts of the finger and if the finger can be moved easily, apply an ice pack for swelling and use acetaminophen, aspirin, ibuprofen, or naproxen for pain (page 54).

Blood under a Nail

Pain caused by a large amount of blood under the fingernail can often be relieved simply.

This home (or emergency room) remedy sounds terrible but is very simple and can sometimes save the nail.

1. Bend open an ordinary paper clip and hold it with a pair of pliers.

2. Heat one end of the paper clip with the flame from a butane lighter or gas stove, steadying the hand holding the pliers with the opposite hand.

3. When the tip is very hot, touch it to the nail; it will melt its way through the fingernail, leaving a clean, small, painless hole. There is no need to press down hard. Take your time, lifting the paper clip to see if you are through the nail; usually the blood will spurt a little when you are through. Reheat the paper clip if necessary.

The blood trapped beneath the nail can now escape through the small hole, and the pain will be relieved as the pressure is released. If the hole closes and the blood reaccumulates, the procedure can be repeated using the same hole once again.

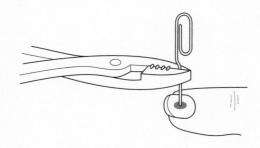

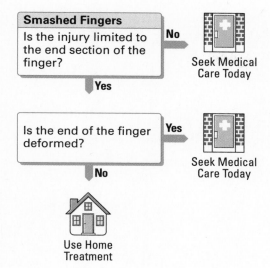

Smashed Fingers

Is the injury limited to the end section of the finger?

No → Seek Medical Care Today

Yes

Is the end of the finger deformed?

Yes → Seek Medical Care Today

No

Use Home Treatment

What to Expect at the Doctor's Office

The doctor will examine the finger. An X-ray is likely if it appears that more than the end segment is involved. If there is a fracture involving the last joint of the finger, you should expect a discussion of the advantages and disadvantages of splinting the finger. Often the injured finger is splinted by bandaging it together with an adjacent finger. If the finger is splinted, exercise it periodically to keep it mobile. Severe finger injuries may occasionally require surgery.

Ingrown Nails

Ingrown nails can be treated at home. Cut the nail straight across so that its corner can grow outside the skin. Let the nail grow free by firmly pushing the skin back from the corner with a Q-tip twice a day. Keep the area clean. For hangnails, keep them clean. Don't chew on them.

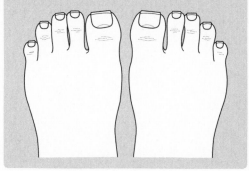

CHAPTER 5

Ear, Nose, Throat, Eye, and Mouth Problems

Is It Viral, Bacterial, or Allergic?

The first part of this chapter discusses upper respiratory problems, including colds and flu, sore throats, ear pain or stuffiness, runny nose, cough, hoarseness, swollen glands, and nosebleeds. A central question is important to each of these complaints: Is it caused by a virus or bacteria, or is it an allergic reaction?

In general, the doctor has more effective treatment than is available at home only for bacterial infections. Viral infections and allergies don't improve with treatment by penicillin or other antibiotics. To request a "penicillin shot" for a cold or allergy is to ask for a drug reaction, risk a more serious "superinfection," and waste time and money. Unnecessary use of antibiotics is a major cause of the growing problem of antibiotic-resistant bacteria.

Among common problems well treated at home are:

▲ The common cold, often termed by doctors a "viral URI" (upper respiratory infection)
▲ The flu, when uncomplicated
▲ Hay fever
▲ Mononucleosis—infectious mononucleosis or "mono"

Medical treatment is commonly required for:

▲ Strep throat

▲ Ear infection
▲ Viral gastroenteritis (sometimes)

How can you tell these conditions apart? Table 6 and the decision charts for the symptoms discussed in this chapter will usually suffice. Here are some brief descriptions that may also help.

Viral Syndromes

Viruses usually involve several portions of the body and cause many different symptoms. Three basic patterns (or syndromes) are common in viral illnesses; however, overlap among these three syndromes is not unusual. Your illness may have features of each.

Viral URI. This is the "common cold." It includes some combination of the following: sore throat, runny nose, stuffy or congested ears, hoarseness, swollen glands, and fever. One symptom usually precedes the others, and another symptom (usually hoarseness or cough) may remain after the others have disappeared.

The Flu. Fever may be quite high. Headache can be excruciating. Muscle aches and pain (especially in the lower back and eye muscles) are equally troublesome.

Viral Gastroenteritis. This is "stomach flu" with nausea, vomiting, diarrhea, and crampy abdominal pain. It may be incapacitating and can mimic a variety of other more serious conditions, including appendicitis.

Hay Fever

Allergic rhinitis is commonly called "hay fever" even though it's not a fever and

TABLE 6: Viral, Bacterial, or Allergic?	Viral	Bacterial	Allergic
Runny nose?	Often	Rare	Often
Aching muscles?	Usual	Rare	Never
Headache (nonsinus)?	Often	Rare	Never
Dizzy?	Often	Rare	Rare
Fever?	Often	Often	Never
Cough?	Often	Sometimes	Rare
Dry cough?	Often	Rare	Sometimes
Raising sputum?	Rare	Often	Rare
Hoarseness?	Often	Rare	Sometimes
Recurs in a particular season?	No	No	Often
Only a single complaint? (sore throat, earache, sinus pain, or cough)	Unusual	Usual	Unusual
Do antibiotics help?	No	Yes	No
Can the doctor help?	Seldom	Yes	Sometimes

Remember, viral infections and allergies **do not** improve with treatment by penicillin or other antibiotics.

not caused by hay. It is, however, the most common problem caused by allergies. A stuffy, runny nose, watering itchy eyes, headache, and sneezing are all common symptoms. Hay fever seems to run in families. Patients usually diagnose this condition accurately themselves.

As with viruses, hay fever is treated simply to relieve symptoms. Given enough time, the condition runs its course without doing any permanent harm. Avoiding the offending allergen is often the best preventive action. The cause in infants is often dust or food; in adults, it's dust or pollen.

Antihistamines block the action of histamine, a substance released during allergic reactions. They also have a drying effect on the runny nose. Their most common side effect is drowsiness. Decongestants (pseudoephedrine, etc.) can help with the runny nose and open up nasal passages, as well as combat the sleepiness (page 62).

Sinusitis

Inflammation of the sinuses is often associated with hay fever and asthma. Symptoms include a sense of heaviness behind the nose and eyes, often resulting in a "sinus headache." If the sinuses are infected, there may be fever and nasal discharge. Antihistamines and decongestants (page 62) may be helpful in cases of sinusitis that accompany colds or hay fever. Don't use nasal sprays (page 63) for more than three days. For recurring or chronic sinusitis, consult a doctor to determine the cause and treatment; antibiotics are controversial, but corticosteroids usually provide relief.

Strep Throat

Bacterial infections tend to localize at a single point. Involvement of the respiratory tract by strep is usually limited to the throat. However, symptoms outside the respiratory tract can occur, most commonly fever and swollen lymph glands (from draining the infection) in the neck. A scarlet fever rash sometimes may help to distinguish a streptococcal (strep) infection from a viral infection. In children, abdominal pain may be associated with a strep throat. The point of diagnosing and treating strep is to pre-vent a complication, rheumatic fever; treatment has very little effect on the throat itself. Unfortunately, wrong diagnosis of strep and unreasonable fear of strep are widespread and major causes of the overuse of antibiotics.

Other Conditions

Factors other than diseases may cause or contribute to upper respiratory symptoms. Smoking is probably the largest single cause of coughs and sore throats. Pollution (smog) can produce the same problems. Tumors and other frightening conditions account for only a very small number. Complaints lasting beyond two weeks without one of the common diseases as the obvious cause aren't alarming but should be investigated by the doctor.

Colds and Flu

The common cold and the different kinds of flu account for more unnecessary visits to the doctor than any other illness.

Because viruses cause colds and the flu, an antibiotic won't work. You can care for yourself as well as the doctor can. Nonprescription drugs—pain relievers, decongestants, and antihistamines—can relieve your symptoms while your body recovers.

Read the appropriate pages for information about specific symptoms, such as Ear Pain and Stuffiness (page 130), Sore Throat (page 128), Cough (page 138), Nausea and Vomiting (page 266), and Diarrhea (page 268). The doctor can help if you develop an ear infection (page 130) or bacterial pneumonia. A very young child with a viral infection needs medical attention.

A runny nose is an important sign that the body is trying to rid itself of cold or flu viruses. Sneezes are one way that the nose removes germs and other irritants. Unfortunately, sneezes also help viruses pass from person to person. Cover your nose and mouth with a tissue or handkerchief when you sneeze. Wash your hands often when you have a runny nose or sneeze; cold and flu viruses are spread most often by direct contact.

Complications from a runny nose are due to the excess mucus, which can run into the throat (postnasal drip) and cause a sore throat or a cough. Mucus drip can block the eustachian tube, resulting in ear infection and pain. It can also lead to infection and sinus pain.

A runny nose can also be a sign of:

▲ **Allergies.** Hay fever (allergic rhinitis) can cause the nose to run clear, very thin mucus. People with hay fever will often have other symptoms, including sneezing and itching, and watery eyes. Hay fever lasts longer than a viral infection, often for weeks or months. Allergies are more common in the spring and fall, when pollen and other allergens are in the air. Other substances that can cause allergic rhinitis include house dust, mold, and animal dander.

▲ **Nose Sprays.** Prolonged use of nose sprays or drops can lead to a runny nose. Nose drops containing substances like ephedrine should never be used for more than three consecutive days. You can avoid this problem by switching to saline nose drops for a few days.

▲ **Head Injury.** Head injury is a rare but serious cause of a runny nose (page 108). If a person has a clear discharge that began after a head injury, he or she needs immediate medical attention.

Home Treatment

You can take acetaminophen, aspirin, ibuprofen, or naproxen remedies (page 54) for the fever and aches of

Chicken Soup

A word about chicken soup: People with colds often feel dizzy when standing up, and this condition is helped by drinking salty liquids. Bouillon and chicken soup are excellent.

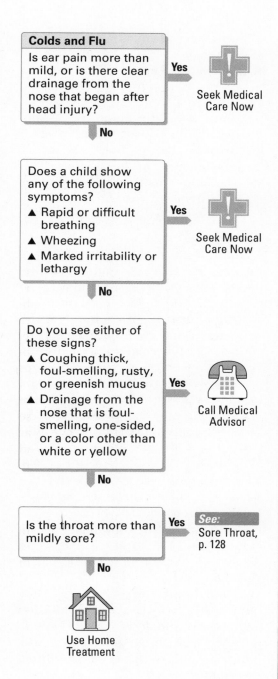

Colds and Flu

Is ear pain more than mild, or is there clear drainage from the nose that began after head injury? → **Yes** → **Seek Medical Care Now**

↓ **No**

Does a child show any of the following symptoms?
▲ Rapid or difficult breathing
▲ Wheezing
▲ Marked irritability or lethargy
→ **Yes** → **Seek Medical Care Now**

↓ **No**

Do you see either of these signs?
▲ Coughing thick, foul-smelling, rusty, or greenish mucus
▲ Drainage from the nose that is foul-smelling, one-sided, or a color other than white or yellow
→ **Yes** → **Call Medical Advisor**

↓ **No**

Is the throat more than mildly sore? → **Yes** → *See:* Sore Throat, p. 128

↓ **No**

Use Home Treatment

the common cold. These symptoms are usually worse in the afternoon and evening, so take medications regularly during this time. Don't give aspirin to children or teenagers; give them acetaminophen instead.

There are two basic kinds of cold symptom remedies. Save money and have fewer side effects by matching the remedy to your symptoms.

▲ Decongestants that shrink the nasal membranes and open the passages
▲ Antihistamines that reduce secretions in the nose

Drink a lot of liquid. The body requires more fluid when you have a fever. Fluids help to keep the mucus more liquid and to prevent complications such as bronchitis and ear infection. A vaporizer, particularly in the winter, can help as well.

Blowing your nose makes you feel better and offers the advantage of safely moving mucus, virus particles, and allergens outside the body. Sniffing a runny nose increases your risk of ear infection. Wash your hands often.

Call the doctor if symptoms last more than two weeks.

What to Expect at the Doctor's Office

The doctor will take the history and do a physical examination. He or she may order a chest X-ray or swab the nose or throat for laboratory analysis.

The doctor may prescribe a decongestant or antihistamine. If you have a bacterial infection, the doctor may prescribe an antibiotic. If you suffer from allergies, the doctor may advise you how to reduce your exposure to pollen and other triggers.

Sore Throat

Sore throat can affect a person of any age but is most common among children 5 to 10 years old. One cause is breathing through the mouth, which can dry and irritate the air passages; this irritation improves quickly when moist air is breathed. The most common causes of sore throat, however, are viruses and bacteria.

Antibiotics are useless against viral infections. A sore throat caused by a virus must improve on its own. Pain relievers, throat lozenges, anesthetic sprays, and other medications may relieve symptoms.

Infectious mononucleosis, also called "mono" or "the kissing disease," is a viral sore throat common among older children and adolescents. The person with mono may have a severe sore throat for more than a week and feel particularly weak.

"Strep throat" is what we commonly call sore throat caused by a streptococcal bacterium. Strep throat is more common in children than adults. If one child in a family has strep throat, other children with a sore throat are also likely to be infected with strep.

A sore throat is unlikely to be strep if the person has several other cold symptoms: runny nose, stuffy ears, cough, and so on.

A strep throat diagnosed and treated with antibiotics may help to avoid rare but serious complications, such as:

▲ **Throat Abscess.** Suspect a throat abscess if a child drools excessively or has great difficulty in swallowing or opening his or her mouth.

▲ **Rheumatic Fever.** This condition appears one to four weeks after the sore throat and results in painful joints, skin rashes, and heart damage. Antibiotic treatment of strep throat can prevent rheumatic fever.

▲ **Inflammation of the Kidney.** This condition also comes one to four weeks after the sore throat.

Home Treatment

You can ease the symptoms of sore throat with nonprescription pain relievers. Fever and sore throat pain can be relieved by cold remedies, acetaminophen, aspirin, ibuprofen, and naproxen. Don't give aspirin or aspirin-containing cold remedies to children or teenagers.

A vaporizer will moisten the air and ease dry air passages. Saltwater gargles or tea with honey or lemon also may help. Your symptoms will improve over time.

What to Expect at the Doctor's Office

The doctor may do a "quick test" for strep or swab the throat for lab tests. Some doctors delay prescribing an antibiotic until they know the results of culture tests. A delay of treatment by a day or two doesn't increase the risk of rheumatic fever.

The doctor may prescribe antibiotics; these treat a bacterial infection and prevent complications but don't do much to ease throat discomfort. Antibiotics are useless against a sore throat caused by a virus.

Sore Throat

Does a child show any of these signs?
- ▲ Severe difficulty in swallowing
- ▲ Difficulty in breathing
- ▲ Excessive drooling

Yes → Seek Medical Care Now

No

Do you see any of the following signs?
- ▲ Temperature of 101°F (38°C) or more
- ▲ Yellowish pus in back of throat
- ▲ Red rash on skin that feels like sandpaper, redness in skin creases, and fever

Yes → Call Medical Advisor

No

Is person less than 30 years of age?

No → Use Home Treatment

Yes

Are the tonsils swollen?

No → Use Home Treatment

Yes

See doctor: for strep throat test.

Tonsils

Children between the ages of 5 and 10 commonly have sore throats. There is no evidence that removing the tonsils lowers their frequency. Doctors now agree that children very seldom need the tonsillectomy operation.

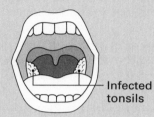

Infected tonsils

Ear Pain and Stuffiness

Ear pain often is caused by a buildup of fluid and pressure in the middle ear (the portion of the ear behind the ear-drum). Under normal circumstances, the middle ear is drained by a short nar-row tube, the eustachian tube, into the nasal passages. Often during a cold or allergy, the mucous membranes lining the eustachian tube will swell, closing off the tube. This occurs most easily in small children in whom the tube is smaller. When the tube closes, the nor-mal flow of fluid from the middle ear is prevented, and the fluid begins to accu-mulate. This causes stuffiness and de-creased hearing.

The stagnant fluid provides a good place for the start of a bacterial in-fection. A bacterial infection usually results in pain and fever, often in one ear only.

Ear pain and ear stuffiness may occur when going from low to high altitudes, such as when going up in an airplane. Here again the mechanism for the stuffiness or pain is a clog in the eustachian tube. Swallowing will fre-quently relieve this pressure. Closing the mouth and holding the nose closed while pretending to blow your nose is another way to open the eustachian tube. Using a decongestant may help prevent this problem.

Ear Infection in Children

The symptoms of an ear infection in children may include fever, ear pain, fussiness, increased crying, irritability, or pulling at the ears. Because infants can't tell you that their ears hurt, increased irritability or ear pulling should make a parent suspicious of ear infection.

Parents are often concerned about whether their children will lose hearing after ear infections. Most children will have a temporary and minor hearing loss during and immediately follow-ing an ear infection, but with adequate treatment, there is seldom any perma-nent hearing loss.

Home Treatment

Antihistamines, decongestants, and nose drops are used to decrease the amount of fluid flowing from the middle ear and shrink the mucous membranes in order to open the eustachian tube. See page 62 for more information on these drugs. Fluid in the ear will often respond to home treatment alone.

Over-the-counter pain relievers will provide partial relief (page 54). Although ear pain isn't usually a part of chicken pox or the flu, avoid the use of aspirin in teenagers or children because of the association with Reye's syndrome, a seri-ous problem of the brain and liver.

Moisture and humidity are import-ant in keeping the mucus thin that flows from the middle ear. Use a vapor-izer if you have one. If symptoms con-tinue beyond two weeks, or if there is a decrease in your hearing, see the doctor.

What to Expect at the Doctor's Office

The doctor will examine the ear, nose, and throat as well as the bony portion of the skull behind the ears, known as the mastoid. Pain, tenderness, or redness of the mastoid means a serious infection.

Therapy will generally consist of an antibiotic and an attempt to open the eustachian tube by medication. Nose

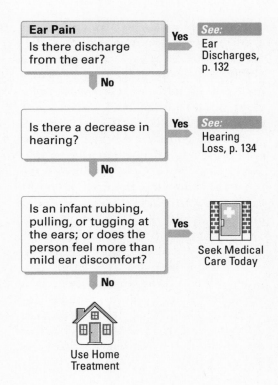

Ear Pain

Is there discharge from the ear?

Yes → See: Ear Discharges, p. 132

No ↓

Is there a decrease in hearing?

Yes → See: Hearing Loss, p. 134

No ↓

Is an infant rubbing, pulling, or tugging at the ears; or does the person feel more than mild ear discomfort?

Yes → Seek Medical Care Today

No ↓

Use Home Treatment

drops, decongestants, and antihistamines can be used for this purpose. Antibiotic therapy generally will be prescribed for at least a week, while other treatments will usually be given for a shorter period. Be sure to take all of the antibiotic prescribed, and do so on schedule.

Occasionally, fluid in the middle ear will persist for a long period without infection. In this case, there may be a slight decrease in hearing. This condition, known as "serous otitis media," is usually treated by trying to open the eustachian tube to allow the fluids to drain; it isn't treated with antibiotics. If this condition persists, the doctor may resort to insertion of ear tubes in order to reestablish proper functioning of the middle ear. Inserting ear tubes sounds frightening, but this is actually a simple and very effective procedure.

Ear Discharges

Ear discharges are usually just wax but may be caused by minor irritation or infection. Ear wax is almost never a problem unless attempts are made to "clean" the ear canal, the opening that leads from the external part of the ear to the internal parts. Earwax functions as a protective lining for the ear canal. Taking warm showers or washing the external ears with a washcloth dipped in warm water usually provides enough vapor to prevent the buildup of wax. Children often like to push things in their ear canals, and they may pack the wax tightly. Adults armed with a cotton swab (for example, Q-tips) often accomplish the same awkward result.

Swimmer's Ear

In the summertime, ear discharges are commonly caused by swimmer's ear, an irritation of the ear canal, not a problem of the inner ear or eardrum. A tug on the ear that causes pain can be a helpful clue to an inflammation of the outer ear and canal, such as swimmer's ear. Children with such inflammation will often complain that their ears are itchy. The urge to scratch inside the ear is very tempting but must be resisted. We especially caution against the use of hairpins or other instruments because injury to the eardrum can result.

Ruptured Eardrum

In a child who has been complaining of ear pain, relief of pain accompanied by a white or yellow discharge— sometimes bloody—may be the sign of a ruptured eardrum. Sometimes parents will find dry crusted material on the child's pillow; here again, a ruptured eardrum should be suspected. The child should be taken to a doctor for evaluation. Don't be unduly alarmed. A ruptured eardrum is actually the first stage of a natural healing process that the antibiotics will help. Children have remarkable healing powers, and most eardrums will heal completely within a matter of weeks.

A very rare, but very serious, cause of ear discharge is a head injury (page 108). If a person has clear discharge that began after a head injury, there is a possibility that a serious injury has occurred and spinal fluid is leaking through the ear. Treat the possibility of this situation as an urgent need for the doctor's help.

Home Treatment

Packed-down earwax can be removed by using warm water flushed in gently with a syringe available at drugstores. A water jet (Waterpik, etc.) that is set at the lowest setting can also be useful, but it can be frightening to young children and is dangerous at higher settings. We don't advise that parents try to remove impacted earwax unless they are dealing with an older child and can see the impacted, blackened ear wax.

Wax softeners such as ordinary olive oil, Debrox, or Cerumenex are useful; however, all commercial products may be irritating, especially if not used properly. Cerumenex, for example, must be flushed out of the ear, using warm water, within 30 minutes.

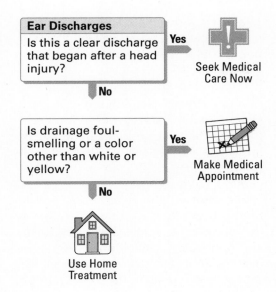

Ear Discharges

Is this a clear discharge that began after a head injury?

Yes → Seek Medical Care Now

No ↓

Is drainage foul-smelling or a color other than white or yellow?

Yes → Make Medical Appointment

No ↓

Use Home Treatment

Two warnings:

▲ The water must be as close to body temperature as possible; the use of cold water may result in dizziness and vomiting.

▲ Washing should never be tried if there is any question about the condition of the eardrum; it must be intact and undamaged.

Although swimmer's ear (or other causes of similar "otitis externa") is often caused by a bacterial infection, the infection is very shallow and doesn't often require antibiotic treatment. The infection can be effectively treated by placing a cotton wick soaked in Burow's Solution in the ear canal overnight, followed by a brief washing out with 3% hydrogen peroxide and then warm water. Success has also been reported with Merthiolate mixed with mineral oil (enough to make it pink), followed by the hydrogen peroxide and warm water rinse. For particularly severe or itching cases or persistence beyond five days, a doctor's visit is advisable.

What to Expect at the Doctor's Office

A thorough examination of the ear will be performed. In severe cases, a culture for bacteria may be taken. Corticosteroid and antibiotic preparations that are placed in the ear canal may be prescribed, or one of the regimens described above under Home Treatment may be advised. Oral antibiotics will usually be given if a perforated eardrum is causing the discharge.

Hearing Loss

Problems with hearing may be divided into two broad categories: sudden and slow. When a child of age five or older complains of difficulty in hearing that has developed over a short period, the problem is usually a blockage in the ear. On the outside of the eardrum, such a blockage may be due to the accumulation of wax, a foreign object that the child has put in the ear canal, or an infection of the ear canal. On the inside of the eardrum, a blockage may occur when fluid accumulates because of an ear infection or allergy.

Hearing problems in children may be present from birth. Hearing can now be tested in a child of any age through the use of computers that analyze changes in brain waves in response to sounds. More simply, an infant with normal hearing will react to a noise such as a hand clap, horn, or whistle. Normal speech development relies on hearing. A child whose speech is developing slowly or not at all may, in fact, have hearing problems.

Some decrease in hearing, especially of the higher frequencies, is normal after the age of 20. If this decrease becomes a problem in later life, it is time to visit the doctor. Occasionally, hearing problems will mimic problems with thinking or understanding, so people will wrongly suspect senility, Alzheimer's disease, or other neurological problems.

Sudden loss of hearing in one ear in an adult may be due to autoimmune or infectious causes and may need immediate treatment. Slow loss of hearing in one ear in an adult, severe or associated with dizziness, can be a sign of an acoustic neuroma, a small benign tumor, which needs medical attention.

Home Treatment

An accurate ear examination requires a trip to the doctor. However, if you know for sure that the problem is caused by too much ear wax, you may treat it at home. (See Home Treatment in Ear Discharges, page 132.)

Be cautious about removing foreign bodies from ears. Don't try to remove the object unless it is easily accessible and removing it clearly poses no threat of damage to ear structures. Never use sharp instruments to remove foreign bodies. Many times, trying to remove an object pushes it farther into the ear or damages the eardrum.

What to Expect at the Doctor's Office

A thorough examination of both ears often reveals the cause of the hearing loss. If it doesn't, the doctor may recommend audiometry (an electronic hearing test) or other tests. Hearing can often be improved by a variety of methods, including hearing aids.

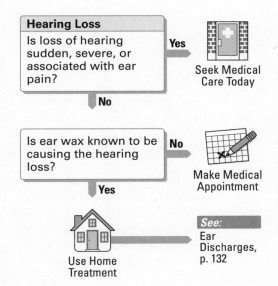

Hearing Loss

Is loss of hearing sudden, severe, or associated with ear pain?

Yes → Seek Medical Care Today

No ↓

Is ear wax known to be causing the hearing loss?

No → Make Medical Appointment

Yes ↓

Use Home Treatment →

See:
Ear Discharges, p. 132

Runny Nose

The hallmark of the common cold is a runny nose. It helps the body fight the viral infection. Nasal secretions contain antibodies against viruses. A runny nose means these secretions are carrying the virus outside the body.

Allergy is also a common cause of runny noses. People whose runny noses are due to an allergy have allergic rhinitis (hay fever). The nasal secretions are often clear and very thin. People with hay fever often have other symptoms, including sneezing, itching, and watery eyes. This problem often lasts for weeks or months, and occurs most commonly during the spring and fall when pollen particles or other allergens are in the air. Other substances may cause allergic rhinitis, including house dust, mold, and animal dander.

Another common cause of stuffy noses is prolonged use of nose drops. This problem is known as "rhinitis medicamentosum." Nose drops containing substances like pseudoephedrine should never be used for longer than three days. This problem can be cured by switching to saline nose drops for a few days (page 63).

Complications from a runny nose are due to the excess mucus. The mucus can run into the throat (postnasal drip) and cause a sore throat or a cough that is most obvious at night. The mucus drip may plug the eustachian tube between the nasal passages and the ear, resulting in ear infection and pain (page 130). It may plug the sinus passages, resulting in sinus infection.

A very rare, but very serious, cause of a runny nose is a head injury (page 108). If a person has a clear discharge that began after a head injury, there is a possibility that a serious injury has occurred and spinal fluid is draining through the nose. Treat the possibility of this situation as an urgent need for the doctor's help.

Home Treatment

Using handkerchiefs or tissues to blow your nose has the great advantage of safely moving mucus, virus particles, and allergens outside the body. A facial tissue has no side effects and costs less than drugs.

If drugs must be used, there are two types:

▲ **Decongestants** such as pseudoephedrine shrink the mucous membranes and open the nasal passages.
▲ **Antihistamines** block allergic reactions and decrease the amount of secretion.

Decongestants make some children overly active. Some antihistamines may cause drowsiness and interfere with sleep (page 62).

Gesundheit!

Sneezes are healthy. They remove germs, allergens, or dust from the nose. The only danger is infecting other people with the germ or virus that makes you sneeze. Cover your nose and mouth with a tissue or handkerchief. Wash your hands frequently. And let people say "Bless you."

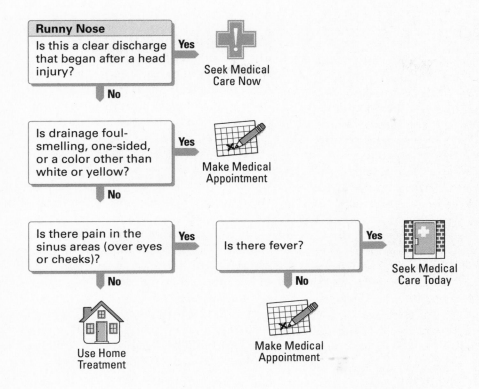

Runny Nose

Is this a clear discharge that began after a head injury? — **Yes** → Seek Medical Care Now

No ↓

Is drainage foul-smelling, one-sided, or a color other than white or yellow? — **Yes** → Make Medical Appointment

No ↓

Is there pain in the sinus areas (over eyes or cheeks)? — **Yes** → Is there fever? — **Yes** → Seek Medical Care Today

No ↓ (Use Home Treatment)

No ↓ (Make Medical Appointment)

If you choose to treat a runny nose with medication, nose drops are suitable. Saline nose drops are fine for young children. Older children and adults may use drops containing decongestants (page 63).

Complications such as ear and sinus infections may often be prevented by ensuring that the mucus is thin rather than thick and sticky. This helps prevent plugging of the nasal passages. Increasing the humidity in the air with a vaporizer or humidifier helps liquefy the mucus. Heated air inside a house is often very dry; cooler air contains more moisture. Drinking a large amount of liquid will also help liquefy the secretions. If symptoms persist beyond three weeks, consult your doctor.

What to Expect at the Doctor's Office

The doctor will thoroughly examine the ears, nose, and throat and will check for tenderness over the sinuses. Often a swab of the nasal secretions will be taken and examined under a microscope for certain types of cells, known as eosinophils, which indicate hay fever (allergic rhinitis). For allergic rhinitis, antihistamines may be prescribed, and a program of avoidance of dust, mold, dander, and pollen suggested.

Cough

The cough reflex is one of the body's best defenses. The violent rush of air clears foreign material from the air passages. Smoke, air pollutants, accidentally inhaled food, or any other airway irritation can trigger a cough.

When you have a cold, mucus from the nasal passages may drain into the airway (postnasal drip) and trigger the cough reflex. You can treat this with a cough suppressant.

If your lungs are congested, coughing may expel pus and mucus. This type of "productive" cough is helpful in clearing the lungs. You should not suppress a productive cough with drugs.

Here are some of the common causes of cough:

▲ **Smoking** kills the cells lining the airway so that you can't expel mucus normally. The smoker's chronic cough is evidence of the continual irritation of the air passages.

▲ **Viral infections** can cause a cough that usually produces yellow or white mucus. Antibiotics are useless to treat a viral infection. The illness runs its course within a few days.

▲ **Bacterial infections** can cause a cough that usually produces rusty or green mucus. The mucus looks like it contains pus. Your doctor can prescribe an antibiotic to treat a bacterial infection. Doctors use the term "pneumonia" most often to mean a bacterial infection of the lung, but the same label can be applied to other lung infections, more or less serious. Don't panic if you hear that word.

For very young infants, coughing is unusual and may suggest a serious lung problem. Older infants are prone to swallow things and can get a foreign object lodged in the airway. Young children tend to inhale bits of peanut and popcorn, which can cause coughing.

Home Treatment

Increase humidity by using a cold-steam vaporizer or running a steamy shower. Drinking large quantities of fluids also is helpful.

In addition to moisture, guaifenesin (e.g., Robitussin, Naldecon-Cx), available without a prescription, may help thin mucus and relieve a cough (page 66). Cough lozenges or hard candy may relieve a dry, tickling cough.

Dextromethorphan (e.g., Romilar, Vicks Formula 44, Robitussin-DM) helps suppress a dry, hacking cough that is not removing mucus (page 66).

Decongestants and/or antihistamines can help if postnasal drip is causing the cough. Otherwise, avoid antihistamines because they dry and thicken secretions.

Hiccups

Hiccups, which are caused by irregular contractions of the diaphragm muscle, may occasionally prove troublesome. Although there have been many home remedies recommended over the years, including drinking large amounts of water and startling the sufferer, research suggests that one-half teaspoon (3 ml) of dry sugar placed on the back of the tongue is the most effective treatment.

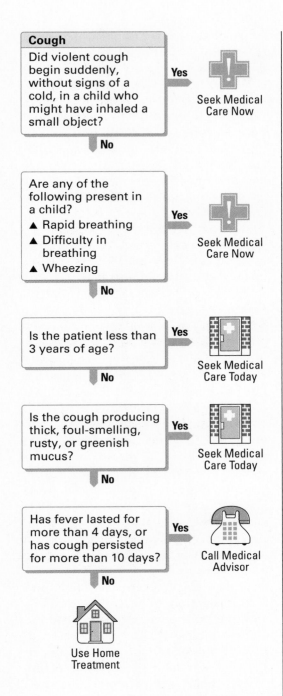

Cough

Did violent cough begin suddenly, without signs of a cold, in a child who might have inhaled a small object? → **Yes** → Seek Medical Care Now

↓ **No**

Are any of the following present in a child?
▲ Rapid breathing
▲ Difficulty in breathing
▲ Wheezing → **Yes** → Seek Medical Care Now

↓ **No**

Is the patient less than 3 years of age? → **Yes** → Seek Medical Care Today

↓ **No**

Is the cough producing thick, foul-smelling, rusty, or greenish mucus? → **Yes** → Seek Medical Care Today

↓ **No**

Has fever lasted for more than 4 days, or has cough persisted for more than 10 days? → **Yes** → Call Medical Advisor

↓ **No**

Use Home Treatment

Unless a cold or other illness causes it, hoarseness may be difficult to treat. Rest the vocal cords; crying or shouting makes them worse. Humidifying the air can help. Healing may take several days as nature takes its course.

What to Expect at the Doctor's Office

The doctor will take the history and do a physical exam. He or she may order a chest X-ray or blood tests. In some cases of hoarseness, the doctor may look at the vocal cords with the help of a small mirror.

If you have a cough that over-the-counter remedies have not helped, the doctor may prescribe medication. Doctors don't usually prescribe antibiotics for a cough or hoarseness.

Croup

Croup may be the most frightening of the common illnesses that parents encounter. It generally occurs in children under the age of three or four. In the middle of the night, a child may sit up in bed gasping for air. Often there will be an accompanying cough from the area of the voice box in the neck that sounds like the barking of a seal. The child's symptoms are so frightening that panic is often the response. However, the most severe problems with croup usually can be relieved safely, simply, and quickly at home.

Croup is caused by one of several viruses. The viral infection causes a swelling and outpouring of secretions in the larynx (voice box), trachea (windpipe), and bronchi (the larger airways going to the lungs). The air passages of the young child are narrowed by the swelling and further aggravated by the secretions, which may become dry and caked, making it difficult to breathe. There may also be a considerable amount of spasm of the airway passages, further complicating the problem. Treatment is aimed at dissolving the dried secretions.

In some children, croup is a recurring problem. These children may have three or four bouts of croup. This seldom represents a serious underlying problem, but you should seek a doctor's advice. Croup will be outgrown as the airway passages grow larger. It is unusual after the age of seven.

Epiglottitis

Occasionally, a more serious obstruction caused by a bacterial infection known as epiglottitis can be confused with croup. Epiglottitis is more common in children over the age of three, but there is considerable overlap in the ages of children affected by these two conditions. Children with epiglottitis often have more serious difficulty in breathing. They may have an extremely difficult time swallowing all of their saliva and may drool. Often they will gasp for air with the head tilted forward and the jaw pointed out.

Epiglottitis won't be relieved by the simple measures that bring prompt relief of croup. It must be brought to medical attention immediately.

Home Treatment

Mist is the backbone of therapy for croup and can be supplied efficiently by a cold-steam vaporizer. Cold-steam vaporizers are preferable to hot-steam ones because the possibility of scalding from hot water is eliminated.

If breathing is very difficult, you can obtain faster results by taking the child to the bathroom and turning on the hot shower to make thick clouds of steam. (Don't put the child in the hot shower!) Steam can be created more efficiently if there is some cold air in the room. Remember that steam rises, so the child won't benefit from the steam by sitting on the floor.

Relief usually occurs promptly and should be noticeable within the first 15 minutes. It is important to keep the child calm and not become alarmed; holding the child may comfort him or her and may help relieve some of the airway spasm. If the child doesn't show significant improvement within 15 minutes, contact your doctor or the local

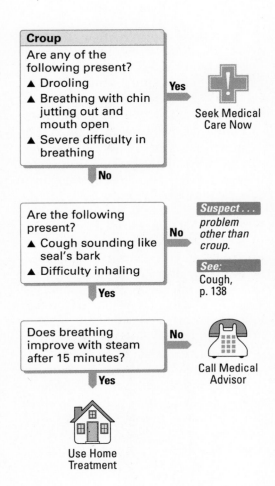

Croup

Are any of the following present?
▲ Drooling
▲ Breathing with chin jutting out and mouth open
▲ Severe difficulty in breathing

Yes → Seek Medical Care Now

No ↓

Are the following present?
▲ Cough sounding like seal's bark
▲ Difficulty inhaling

No → *Suspect...* problem other than croup.
See: Cough, p. 138

Yes ↓

Does breathing improve with steam after 15 minutes?

No → Call Medical Advisor

Yes ↓

Use Home Treatment

emergency room immediately. They'll want to see the child and will make arrangements in advance while you are in transit. Unfortunately, few emergency rooms can provide steam as easily as the home shower.

If the child shows significant improvement but the problem persists for more than an hour, call the doctor.

What to Expect at the Doctor's Office

If the doctor feels confident that this is croup, further use of mist will be tried. In difficult cases, X-rays of the neck are a reliable way of differentiating croup from epiglottitis. A swollen epiglottis often can be seen in the back of the throat. If epiglottitis is diagnosed, the child will be admitted to the hospital; an airway will be placed in the child's trachea to enable the child to breathe, and intravenous antibiotics directed at curing the bacterial infection will be started. In the case of croup, the trip to the doctor often cures the problem that was resistant to steam at home.

Wheezing

Wheezing is the high-pitched whistling sound produced by air flowing through narrowed breathing tubes (bronchi and bronchioles). It's most obvious when the person breathes out but may be present when breathing both in and out. Wheezing comes from the breathing tubes deep in the chest, in contrast to the croupy, crowing, or whooping sounds that come from the area of the voice box in the neck (see Croup, page 140). Most often, a narrowing of the breathing tubes is due to a viral infection or an allergic reaction, as in asthma.

In infants younger than age two, the smallest air passages may narrow because of a viral infection. Pneumonia may also produce wheezing. Occasionally, a foreign body may be lodged in a breathing tube, causing a localized wheezing that's difficult to hear without a stethoscope.

Wheezing is commonly associated with emphysema (chronic obstructive pulmonary disease, or COPD), and asthma often exacerbates this problem. The irritation of smoking by itself is sufficient to cause wheezing, although almost all smokers have some degree of emphysema and bronchitis as well.

Asthma

Asthma is an obstructive lung disease that's most common in children and adolescents. It is becoming more frequent. The wheezing in asthma is caused by spasm of the muscles in the walls of the smaller air passages in the lungs. An excess amount of mucus production further narrows the air passages and can aggravate the difficulty in getting the air out.

An asthma attack can be triggered by an infection, an emotionally upsetting event, cold air, air pollution, or exposure to an allergen. Common allergens include house dust, pollen, mold, food, and animal dander. Wheezing can follow an insect sting or the use of a medicine; some individuals even wheeze after taking aspirin. Most often, however, there's no clear reason for a particular asthmatic attack.

Wheezing Together with Fever

In a child with a respiratory infection, wheezing may occur before shortness of breath is obvious. Therefore, when wheezing appears in the presence of a fever—a sign of possible respiratory infection—early consultation with a doctor is advisable, even though the illness seldom turns out to be serious.

Home treatment is an important part of the approach. However, the doctor's help is needed so that drugs that widen the breathing passages can be used. Intravenous fluids may be required on some occasions.

Home Treatment

All wheezing in children is potentially serious and should be evaluated by a medical professional, at least for the first few occurrences. Asthma tends to occur in families where other members have asthma, hay fever, or eczema (page 188).

Drinking fluids is very important. Water is best, but use fruit juices or soft drinks if the person will swallow more. The doctor will recommend hydration (drinking more water), so you may begin even before you visit the doctor.

The use of a vaporizer, preferably one that produces a cold mist, may sometimes

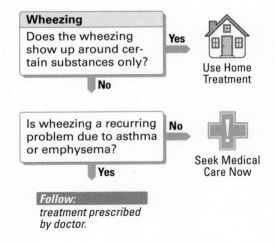

Wheezing
Does the wheezing show up around certain substances only? **Yes** → Use Home Treatment

No ↓

Is wheezing a recurring problem due to asthma or emphysema? **No** → Seek Medical Care Now

Yes ↓

Follow:
treatment prescribed by doctor.

help. If a vaporizer isn't available, you can use the shower to produce a mist.

A relatively clean and dust-free house is essential for a person whose allergies cause asthma. Regularly vacuum rugs, furniture, drapes, bedspreads, and other items that are particular dust-catchers, especially in an asthmatic's bedroom. Keep toy animals clean; washable ones are best. Avoid products that may be stuffed with animal hair. Finally, don't forget to change heating filters and air conditioner filters regularly.

Asthmatics *can* participate in athletics. Athletes with asthma have won numerous gold medals in Olympic swimming. Swimming appears to be far and away the best exercise and the best sport for the asthmatic.

What to Expect at the Doctor's Office
Physical examination will focus on the chest and neck. The doctor will ask questions not only about the current illness but also about a past history of allergies in either the patient or the family. The possibility that a foreign body has been swallowed may also be investigated in small children. Infections can trigger asthma, but the doctor shouldn't give antibiotics unless an infection is definitely present.

Drugs to open the breathing tube, such as epinephrine or theophylline, may be given by injection, by mouth, or by rectal suppository. Occasionally, the patient will need to stay in a hospital to receive replacement fluids through a vein and to breathe humidified air. Most important, in a hospital, the patient can be closely watched to prevent the condition from getting worse before it gets better.

After the crisis has passed, the doctor will work with you to prevent future asthma attacks. This should include working on environmental and emotional causes. More than half of the children diagnosed with asthma never have an asthma attack as an adult, and another 10% will have only occasional attacks during adult life.

Drug Treatments for Asthma
There are many medications that may produce symptomatic relief of asthma. Your doctor will determine which combination makes sense for you and it will be up to you to use them as directed.

Learn to administer inhaled drugs correctly. If you feel the medicine hit your tongue or the back of your throat, it's not going into your airways where it belongs.

Antihistamines aren't useful in the treatment of asthma. In fact, by drying nasal secretions, antihistamines may actually cause airways to plug up.

Hoarseness

Hoarseness is usually caused by a problem in the vocal cords.

Children

In infants under three months of age, this can be due to a serious problem, such as a birth defect or thyroid disorder. In young children, hoarseness is more often due to prolonged or excessive crying, which puts a strain on the vocal cords.

In older children, viral infections are the most common cause of hoarseness. If the hoarseness is accompanied by difficulty in breathing or a cough that sounds like a barking seal, the hoarseness is considered a symptom of croup (page 140). Croup is characteristic in children under age three or four, while the symptom of hoarseness by itself is more common in older children.

If hoarseness is accompanied by difficulty in breathing or swallowing, drooling, gasping for air, or breathing with the mouth wide open and the chin jutting forward, a doctor must be seen immediately. This is a medical emergency. This problem is known as epiglottitis (page 140) and is a bacterial infection that affects the entrance to the airway.

Adults

In adults, a virus is most often responsible for the development of hoarseness or laryngitis when no other symptoms are present. As with any symptom of an upper respiratory tract infection, hoarseness may linger after other symptoms disappear.

When hoarseness is mild, the most common cause is cigarette smoke. If persistent hoarseness is not associated with either a viral infection or smoking, it should be investigated by a doctor. The amount of time to wait before seeing a doctor is controversial; we suggest one month. If you are a smoker, stop smoking and wait one month.

Persistent hoarseness has many causes. The most common are cysts or polyps on the vocal cords. Cancer is also a cause but is relatively rare. Overuse of the voice may result in hoarseness and requires voice rest.

Home Treatment

Hoarseness not associated with other symptoms is resistant to medical therapy. Nature must heal the inflamed area. Humidifying the air with a vaporizer or taking in fluids can offer some relief; however, healing may not occur for several days. Resting the vocal cords is sensible; crying or shouting makes the situation worse. For the treatment of hoarseness associated with coughs, see Cough (page 138).

What to Expect at the Doctor's Office

If a child has severe difficulty in breathing, the first priority is to ensure that the air passage is adequate. This may require the placement of a breathing tube in the child's air passageway at the emergency room, hospital, or doctor's office. If X-rays of the neck are taken, a doctor should accompany the child at all times in case emergency care is needed.

For uncomplicated hoarseness that has persisted for a long time, a doctor will look at the vocal cords with the aid of a small mirror. Occasionally a more extensive physical examination and blood tests will be performed.

Hoarseness

Are any of the following present in a small child?

▲ Difficulty in breathing

▲ Difficulty in swallowing

▲ Drooling

Yes →

Seek Medical Care Now

No ↓

Is the child less than 3 months of age?

Yes →

Call Medical Advisor

No ↓

Has hoarseness persisted for more than a week in a child or more than a month in an adult?

Yes →

Make Medical Appointment

No ↓

Use Home Treatment

Swollen Glands

The most common types of swollen glands are lymph glands and salivary glands. The biggest salivary glands are located below and in front of the ears. When they swell, the characteristic swollen jaw appearance of mumps is the result (page 212).

Lymph glands play a part in the body's defense against infection. They may become swollen even if the infection is trivial or not apparent, although you can usually identify the infection that is causing the swelling.

The locations of the lymph glands are shown on page 113.

▲ Swollen neck glands frequently accompany sore throats or ear infections. The swelling of a gland simply indicates that it is taking part in the fight against infection.

▲ Lymph glands in the groin are enlarged when there is infection in the feet, legs, or genital region. These glands are often swollen when no obvious infection can be found.

▲ Swollen glands behind the ears are often the result of an infection in the scalp. If there is no scalp infection, it is possible that the person currently has or recently had rubella (page 218). Infectious mononucleosis (mono) can also cause swelling of the glands behind the ears (see Sore Throat, page 128).

If a swollen gland is red and tender, there may be a bacterial infection within the gland itself that requires antibiotic treatment. Swollen glands otherwise require no treatment because they are merely fighting infections elsewhere. If there is an accompanying sore throat or earache, these should be treated as described on pages 128 and 130, respectively. However, swollen glands are usually the result of viral infections that require no treatment.

If you have noticed one or several glands progressively enlarging over a period of three weeks, a doctor should be consulted. On very rare occasions, swollen glands can signal serious underlying problems.

Home Treatment

Observe the glands over several weeks to see if they are continuing to enlarge or if other glands become swollen. The vast majority of swollen glands that persist beyond three weeks aren't serious, but a doctor should be consulted if the glands show no tendency to become smaller. Soreness in the glands will usually disappear in a couple of days; the pain results from the rapid enlargement of the gland in the early stages of fighting the infection. The gland takes much longer to return to normal size than it does to swell up.

What to Expect at the Doctor's Office

The doctor will examine the glands and search for infections or other causes of the swelling. Other glands that may not have been noticed by the patient will be examined. The doctor will inquire about fever, weight loss, or other symptoms associated with the swelling of the glands. The doctor may decide that blood tests are indicated or may simply observe the glands for a period of time. In rare cases, it might be necessary to remove (biopsy) a small piece of the gland for examination under a microscope.

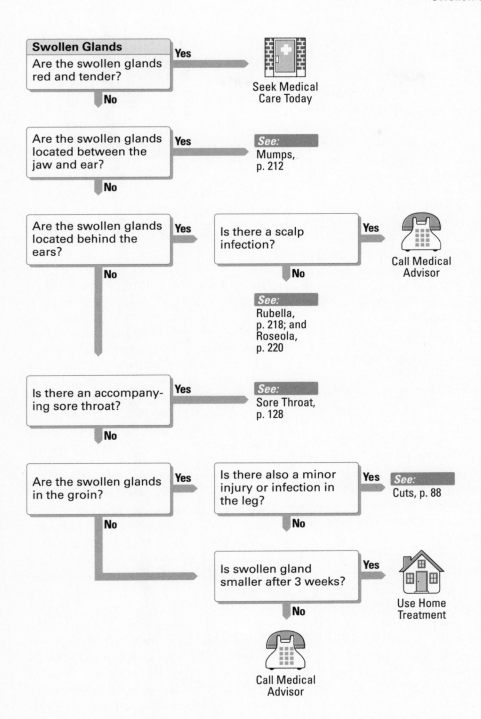

Swollen Glands

Are the swollen glands red and tender? — **Yes** → Seek Medical Care Today

No ↓

Are the swollen glands located between the jaw and ear? — **Yes** → *See:* Mumps, p. 212

No ↓

Are the swollen glands located behind the ears? — **Yes** → Is there a scalp infection? — **Yes** → Call Medical Advisor

No ↓ (scalp infection) → *See:* Rubella, p. 218; and Roseola, p. 220

No ↓

Is there an accompanying sore throat? — **Yes** → *See:* Sore Throat, p. 128

No ↓

Are the swollen glands in the groin? — **Yes** → Is there also a minor injury or infection in the leg? — **Yes** → *See:* Cuts, p. 88

No ↓ (injury/infection) → Is swollen gland smaller after 3 weeks? — **Yes** → Use Home Treatment

No → Call Medical Advisor

Nosebleeds

The blood vessels within the nose lie very near the surface, and bleeding may occur with the slightest injury. In children, picking the nose is a common cause. Keeping their fingernails cut and discouraging the habit are good preventive medicine.

Nosebleeds are frequently due to irritation by a cold virus or to vigorous nose blowing. The main problem in this case is the cold, and treatment of cold symptoms will reduce the probability of a nosebleed. If the mucous membrane of the nose is dry, cracking and bleeding are more likely.

Remember these key points:

▲ You can almost always stop the bleeding yourself.
▲ The majority of nosebleeds are associated with colds or minor injury to the nose.
▲ Treatment such as packing the nose with gauze has significant drawbacks and should be avoided if possible.
▲ Investigation into the cause of recurrent nosebleeds is not urgent and is best accomplished when the nose isn't bleeding.

Home Treatment

The nose consists of a bony part and a cartilaginous part: a "hard" portion and a "soft" portion. The area of the nose that usually bleeds lies within the soft portion, and compression will control the nosebleed. Simply squeeze the nose between thumb and forefinger just below the hard portion of the nose. Pressure should be applied

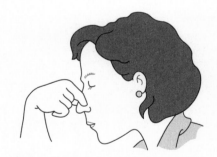

To stop a nosebleed. Sit down and squeeze just below the hard portion of the nose. Hold for five minutes. It isn't necessary to tilt the head back.

for at least five minutes. The patient should be seated. Holding the head back isn't necessary. It merely directs the blood flow backward rather than forward. Cold compresses or ice applied across the bridge of the nose may help. Almost all nosebleeds can be controlled in this manner if sufficient time is allowed for the bleeding to stop. If it just won't stop and bleeding is major, of course you should go to the emergency room.

Nosebleeds are more common in the winter when viruses and dry, heated interiors are common. A cooler house and a cold-steam vaporizer to return humidity to the air help many people. Hot-steam vaporizers work fast, but there are many accidental burns that result from their use.

If nosebleeds are a recurrent problem, are becoming more frequent, and aren't associated with a cold or other minor irritation, a doctor should be consulted. A doctor need not be seen immediately after the nosebleed because examination at that time may simply restart the nosebleed.

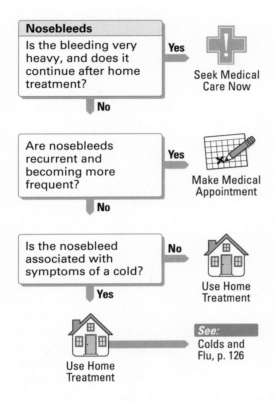

Nosebleeds

Is the bleeding very heavy, and does it continue after home treatment? — **Yes** → Seek Medical Care Now

No ↓

Are nosebleeds recurrent and becoming more frequent? — **Yes** → Make Medical Appointment

No ↓

Is the nosebleed associated with symptoms of a cold? — **No** → Use Home Treatment

Yes ↓

Use Home Treatment → *See:* Colds and Flu, p. 126

What to Expect at the Doctor's Office

To stop the bleeding, the doctor will seat the patient and compress the nostrils. This will be done even if the patient has tried this at home, and it will usually work.

If the nosebleed can't be stopped, the doctor will try to find the bleeding point in the nose. If a bleeding point is visible, the doctor may try to make the blood clot by searing the bleeding point with either electrical or chemical cauterization. If this isn't successful, packing of the nose may be unavoidable. Such packing is uncomfortable and may lead to infection; thus, the patient must be carefully observed.

If a doctor is visited because of recurrent nosebleeds, questions about events preceding the nosebleeds and a careful examination of the nose itself should be expected. Depending on the history and the physical examination, blood-clotting tests may be ordered on rare occasions.

High Blood Pressure

Medical opinion is divided about whether high blood pressure causes nosebleeds, but most doctors believe that the two conditions are seldom related. As a precaution, an individual with high blood pressure who experiences a nosebleed may want to have his or her blood pressure taken within a few days.

Foreign Body in Eye

Eye injuries must be taken seriously. If there's any question, visit the doctor. A foreign body in the eye must be removed to avoid the threat of infection and loss of sight. Be particularly careful if the foreign body was caused by metal striking metal; a small metal particle can strike the eye with great force and penetrate the eyeball.

Under certain circumstances, you may treat this problem at home. If the foreign particle was minor, such as sand, and didn't strike the eye with great velocity, it is easily removed. Small round particles like sand rarely stick behind the upper eyelid for long.

In fact, the foreign body may not even be in the eye anymore; it may simply feel as if it is. This feeling indicates that there has been a scrape or cut on the cornea, the clear membrane that covers the colored portion of the eye. A minor corneal injury will usually heal quickly without problems, but a major one requires medical attention.

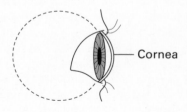
Cornea

Even if you think the injury is minor, run through the decision chart daily. If any symptoms at all are present after 48 hours and aren't clearly resolving, see a doctor. Minor problems will heal within 48 hours; the eye repairs injury quickly.

Home Treatment

Be gentle. Wash the eye out. Water is good; a weak solution of boric acid is better, if available (follow label directions).

Inspect the eye yourself and have someone else check it as well. Use a good light and shine it from both the front and the side. Pay particular attention to the cornea.

Don't rub the eye; if a foreign body is present, you will scratch the cornea.

Check vision each day; compare the two eyes by reading different sizes of newspaper type from across the room, first with one eye, then with the other. If you aren't sure all is going well, see a doctor.

What to Expect at the Doctor's Office

The doctor will check your vision and inspect the eye, including under the upper lid—this isn't painful. Usually he or she will drop a fluorescent stain into the eye and then examine it under ultraviolet light—this isn't painful or hazardous. An ophthalmologist (surgeon specializing in diseases of the eye) will examine the eye with a special microscope.

The doctor will remove any foreign body in the eye. In the office, the doctor may use a cotton swab, an eyewash solution, or a small needle or "eye spud." He or she sometimes will apply an antibiotic ointment or provide an eye patch. Eye drops that dilate the pupil may be employed. The doctor may have X-rays taken if a foreign body may be inside the globe of the eye.

Foreign Body in Eye

Do any of the following apply?

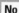 Can the foreign body be seen, and does it remain after gentle washing?

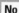 Could the injury have penetrated the globe of the eye?

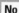 Can you see blood in the eye?

Yes →

Seek Medical Care Now

No ↓

Is there any problem with vision, or does it feel as if a foreign body might be trapped behind the upper lid?

Yes →

Seek Medical Care Now

No ↓

Use Home Treatment

Blood in the Eye

Sometimes a blood vessel in the white of the eye will break, causing an ugly red spot. This blood in the eye is called a subconjunctival hemorrhage and will go away in a few weeks. If you have no visual problems or pain and the problem is only in the white part of the eye, you can wait it out without a doctor. If you're taking blood-thinning medications, call your doctor and report the problem. If the blood can be seen inside the eye at the bottom of the cornea, the physician should be visited.

Eye Pain

Pain in the eye can be an important symptom and can't be safely ignored for long. Fortunately it is an unusual complaint. Itching and burning (page 156) are more common. Eye pain may be due to injury, infection, or an underlying disease.

An important disease that can cause eye pain is glaucoma. Glaucoma may slowly lead to blindness if not treated. In glaucoma, the fluid inside the eye is under abnormally high pressure, and the globe of the eye is tense, causing discomfort. Vision to the sides is the first to be lost. Gradually and almost imperceptibly, the field of vision narrows until the individual has "tunnel vision." In addition, a person often will see "halos" around lights. Unfortunately, this sequence can occur even when there is no associated pain.

Eye pain is a nonspecific complaint, and questions relating to the pain are often better answered under the more specific headings in this chapter.

A feeling of tiredness in the eyes or some discomfort after a long period of fine work (eyestrain) is generally a minor problem and doesn't really qualify as eye pain. Severe pain behind the eye may result from migraine headaches, and pain either above or below the eye may suggest sinus problems.

Pain in both eyes, particularly upon exposure to bright light, "photophobia," is common with many viral infections such as the flu and will go away as the infection improves. More severe photophobia, particularly when only one eye is involved, may indicate inflammation of the deeper layers of the eye and requires a doctor.

Home Treatment

Except for eye pain associated with a viral illness or eyestrain, or minor discomfort that is more tiredness than pain, we don't recommend home treatment. In these instances, resting the eyes, taking a few acetaminophen, and avoiding bright light may help. Follow the decision chart to the discussion of other problems where appropriate. When symptoms persist, check them out in a routine appointment with your doctor.

What to Expect at the Doctor's Office

The doctor will check vision, eye movements, and the back of the eye with an ophthalmoscope. An ophthalmologist (surgeon specializing in diseases of the eye) may look at the eye through a microscope or a device called a slit lamp. If glaucoma is possible, the doctor may check the pressure of the globe. This is simple, quick, and painless. Many doctors commonly refer patients with eye symptoms to an ophthalmologist. You may wish to go directly to an ophthalmologist if you have a major concern.

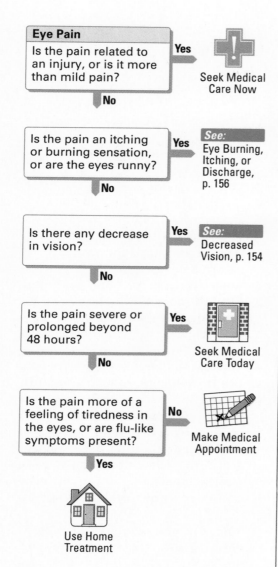

Eye Pain

Is the pain related to an injury, or is it more than mild pain? — **Yes** → Seek Medical Care Now

No ↓

Is the pain an itching or burning sensation, or are the eyes runny? — **Yes** → *See:* Eye Burning, Itching, or Discharge, p. 156

No ↓

Is there any decrease in vision? — **Yes** → *See:* Decreased Vision, p. 154

No ↓

Is the pain severe or prolonged beyond 48 hours? — **Yes** → Seek Medical Care Today

No ↓

Is the pain more of a feeling of tiredness in the eyes, or are flu-like symptoms present? — **No** → Make Medical Appointment

Yes ↓

Use Home Treatment

Computer Problems

Staring at a computer screen for a long time can cause eyestrain, irritation, blurred vision, and headaches. However, several studies conclude that these problems are temporary. To make them less likely:

▲ Blink often, rest your eyes with momentary glances away from the screen, and use eye drops if necessary. Staring at the screen tends to reduce your blinking and thus dry out your eyes.

▲ Avoid glare from the screen by using indirect lighting, repositioning the screen, or using an antiglare filter over it.

▲ Make sure your monitor produces sharp, crisp images. Fuzzy screen images increase eyestrain.

▲ Get special glasses for your computer work if necessary. If you wear bifocals, you may be tilting your head at an uncomfortable angle to see the screen through the lower portion of your glasses.

For more information about working at your computer, see Wrist Pain (page 236).

Decreased Vision

Few people need urging to protect their sight. Decreased vision is a major threat to the quality of life. Usually, professional help is needed.

A few situations don't require a visit to a health professional. When small, single "floaters" drift across the eye from time to time and don't affect vision, they aren't a matter for concern. Slight, reversible blurring of vision may occur after outdoor exposure or with overall fatigue. In young people, sudden blindness in both eyes is commonly a hysterical reaction and isn't a permanent threat to sight; such patients need a doctor but not necessarily an eye doctor.

Usually the question is not whether to see a health professional but, rather, which one to see. Opticians dispense glasses; they aren't medical doctors and don't diagnose eye problems.

The optometrist evaluates the need for glasses, screens for eye diseases, and determines what prescription lens gives the best vision. Conditions usually treated by an optometrist are nearsightedness (myopia), farsightedness (hyperopia), and crooked-sightedness (astigmatism). Although optometrists aren't medical doctors, in some states they can prescribe medicine.

If another problem is suspected, the optometrist may refer you to an ophthalmologist, who is a medical doctor and a surgical specialist. The ophthalmologist is the final authority on eye diseases. Sometimes an eye problem is part of a general health problem; in these cases, the primary physician may be appropriate.

Try to find the right health professional on the first attempt; this will save you time and money. The following examples may help you in your decision-making:

▲ **School nurse detects decreased vision in child.** Visit ophthalmologist or optometrist; possible myopia (nearsightedness).

▲ **Sudden blindness in one eye in an elderly person.** Visit ophthalmologist or internist now; possible stroke or temporal arteritis.

▲ **Halos around lights and eye pain.** Visit ophthalmologist; possible acute glaucoma (increased pressure in the eye).

▲ **Gradual decrease in vision in an adult who wears glasses.** Visit ophthalmologist or optometrist; change in refraction of the eye.

▲ **Sudden blindness in both eyes in a healthy young person.** Visit internist or ophthalmologist now; possible hysterical reaction.

▲ **Gradual blurring of vision in an older person, with no improvement by moving closer or farther away.** Visit ophthalmologist; possible cataract (scar tissue forming in the lens of the eye).

▲ **Older person who sees far objects best.** Visit optometrist or ophthalmologist; possible presbyopia (condition that diminishes the eye's ability to focus on near objects).

▲ **Visual change while taking a medicine.** Call the prescribing doctor; the drug may be responsible.

▲ **Decreased vision in one eye, with a "shadow" or "flap" in the visual field.** Visit ophthalmologist now; possible retinal detachment.

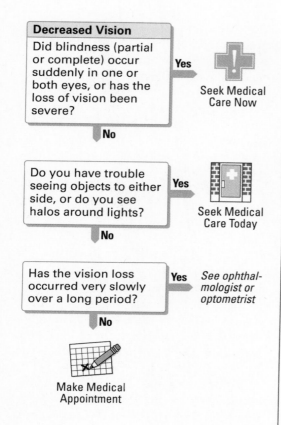

Decreased Vision

Did blindness (partial or complete) occur suddenly in one or both eyes, or has the loss of vision been severe?

Yes → Seek Medical Care Now

No

Do you have trouble seeing objects to either side, or do you see halos around lights?

Yes → Seek Medical Care Today

No

Has the vision loss occurred very slowly over a long period?

Yes → *See ophthalmologist or optometrist*

No

Make Medical Appointment

What to Expect at the Doctor's Office

The doctor will check vision, eye movements, pupils, back of the eye, and eye pressure when appropriate; a slit-lamp examination may be done. A general medical evaluation will be done as required. Testing for eyeglasses may be needed; busy ophthalmologists will sometimes refer this procedure to an optometrist. Surgery may be recommended for some conditions. Laser surgery is increasingly an option instead of changing glasses or contact lens prescriptions.

Eye Burning, Itching, or Discharge

These symptoms usually mean conjunctivitis, or "pinkeye," with inflammation of the membrane that lines the eye and the inner surface of the eyelids. The inflammation may be due to an irritant in the air, an allergy to something in the air, a viral infection, or a bacterial infection. The bacterial infections and some of the viral infections (particularly herpes) are potentially serious but are least common.

Chemicals and particles in smog can produce burning and itching that sometimes seem as severe as the symptoms experienced in a tear-gas attack. These symptoms represent a chemical conjunctivitis and affect anyone exposed to enough of the chemical. The smoke-filled room, the chlorinated swimming pool, the desert sandstorm, sun glare on a ski slope, or exposure to a welder's arc can provoke similar physical or chemical irritation.

In contrast, allergic conjunctivitis affects only those people who have allergies. Almost always, the allergen (what causes the body's reaction) is in the air. This problem may occur in spring, summer, or fall, depending on the offending pollen, and usually lasts two to three weeks. Grass pollens are probably the most frequent offenders.

A minor conjunctivitis frequently accompanies a viral cold, triggering the well-known symptoms and lasting only a few days. Some viruses, such as herpes, cause deep ulcers in the cornea and interfere with vision.

Bacterial infections cause pus to form, and a thick, plentiful discharge runs from the eyes. Often the eyelids are crusted over and "glued" shut upon wakening. These infections can cause ulceration of the cornea and are serious.

Some major diseases affect the deeper layers of the eye, those layers that control the operation of the lens and the size of the pupil. This condition is termed "iritis" or "uveitis" and may cause irregularity of the pupil or pain when the pupil reacts to light. Medical attention is required. For Eye Pain, see page 152.

Home Treatment

If a physical, chemical, or allergic exposure is the cause of the symptoms, the most important thing is avoiding exposure. Dark glasses, goggles at work, houses and cars with air-conditioning to filter the air, avoidance of chlorinated swimming pools, and other such measures are appropriate.

Antihistamines, either over the counter or by prescription, may help slightly if the problem is an allergy, but don't expect total relief without a good deal of drowsiness from the medication. Similarly, a viral infection related to a cold or flu will run its course in a few days, and it is best to be patient.

If the eye irritation doesn't clear up, if the discharge gets thicker, or if you have eye pain or a problem with vision, see your doctor. Don't expect a fever with a bacterial infection of the eye; it may be absent. Because the infection is superficial, washing the eye gently with a boric acid solution (follow directions on the label) will help remove some of the bacteria, but you should still see a doctor. Eye drops (Murine, Visine, etc.) may soothe minor conjunctivitis but won't cure it (page 69).

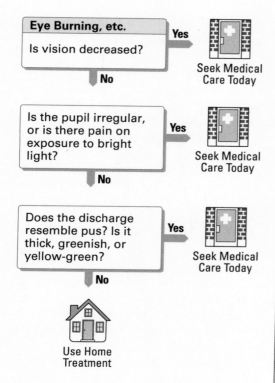

Eye Burning, etc.

Is vision decreased?

Yes → Seek Medical Care Today

No ↓

Is the pupil irregular, or is there pain on exposure to bright light?

Yes → Seek Medical Care Today

No ↓

Does the discharge resemble pus? Is it thick, greenish, or yellow-green?

Yes → Seek Medical Care Today

No ↓

Use Home Treatment

Burning eyes may be a call to social action. If the smoking of others around you is annoying, say so. If an industrial plant in your area is polluting, get the company to clean up its act.

What to Expect at the Doctor's Office

The doctor will check vision, eye motion, eyelids, and the reaction of the pupil to light. An ophthalmologist (surgeon specializing in eye diseases) may perform a slit-lamp examination. Antihistamines may be prescribed, and general advice may be given. Antibiotic eye drops or ointments are frequently given. Cortisone-like eye ointments should be prescribed infrequently; certain infections (herpes) may get worse with these medicines. If herpes is diagnosed—usually by an ophthalmologist—special eye drops and other medicines will be needed.

Styes and Blocked Tear Ducts

We might have called this problem "bumps around the eyes" because that is how they appear.

Styes are infections (usually with staphylococcal bacteria) of the tiny glands in the eyelids. They are really small abscesses, and the bumps are red and tender. They grow to full size over a day or so.

Another type of bump in the eyelid, called a chalazion, appears over many days or even weeks and isn't red or tender. A chalazion often requires drainage by a doctor, whereas most styes will respond to home treatment. However, there is no urgency in the treatment of a chalazion.

Tears are the lubricating system of the eye. They are continually produced by the tear glands and then drained away into the nose by the tear ducts. These tear ducts are often incompletely developed at birth so that the drainage of tears is blocked. When this happens, the tears may collect in the tear duct and cause it to swell, appearing as a bump along the side of the nose just below the inner corner of the eye. This bump isn't red or tender unless it has become infected. Most blocked tear ducts will open by themselves in the first month of life, and most of the remainder will respond to home treatment. Tears running down the cheeks are seldom noted in the first month of life because the infant produces only a small volume of tears.

The eyeball itself isn't involved in a stye or a blocked tear duct. Problems with the eyeball, and especially with vision, should not be attributed to these two relatively minor problems.

Home Treatment

For styes, apply warm, moist compresses for 10 to 15 minutes at least three times a day. As with all abscesses, the objective is to drain the abscess. The compresses help the abscess to "point." This means that the tissue over the abscess becomes quite thin and the pus in the abscess is very close to the surface. After an abscess points, it often will drain spontaneously. If this doesn't happen, the abscess may need to be lanced by the doctor. Most styes will drain spontaneously even without home treatment. They may drain inward toward the eye or outward onto the skin. Sometimes the stye goes away without coming to a point and draining.

Chalazions usually don't respond to warm compresses, but they won't be harmed by them. If no improvement is noted with home treatment after 48 hours, see the doctor.

For blockage of the tear ducts, simply massage the bump downward with warm, moist compresses several times a day. If the bump is not red and tender (indicating infection), this may be continued for up to several months. If the problem exists for this long, discuss it with your doctor. If the bump becomes red and swollen, antibiotic drops will be needed.

What to Expect at the Doctor's Office

If the stye is pointing and ready to be drained, the doctor will open it with a small needle. If it isn't pointing, compresses will usually be advised, and antibiotic eye drops sometimes will be

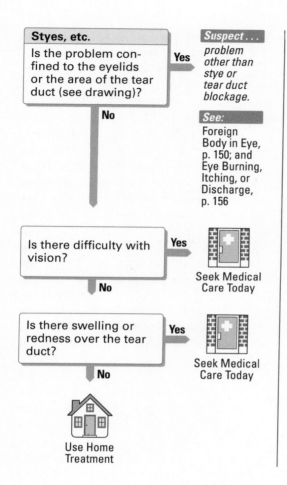

Styes, etc.

Is the problem confined to the eyelids or the area of the tear duct (see drawing)? — **Yes** → *Suspect...* problem other than stye or tear duct blockage. *See:* Foreign Body in Eye, p. 150; and Eye Burning, Itching, or Discharge, p. 156

No ↓

Is there difficulty with vision? — **Yes** → Seek Medical Care Today

No ↓

Is there swelling or redness over the tear duct? — **Yes** → Seek Medical Care Today

No ↓

Use Home Treatment

added. Trying to drain a stye that isn't pointing is usually not very satisfactory.

A chalazion may be removed with minor surgery. Whether to have the surgery will be up to you. Chalazions aren't dangerous and usually don't require removal.

If a child is over six months of age and is still having problems with blocked tear ducts, the ducts can be opened in almost all cases with a very fine probe. This probing is successful on the first try in about 75% of all cases and on subsequent attempts in the remainder. Only rarely is a surgical procedure necessary to open a tear duct. For red and swollen ducts, antibiotic drops as well as warm compresses will usually be recommended.

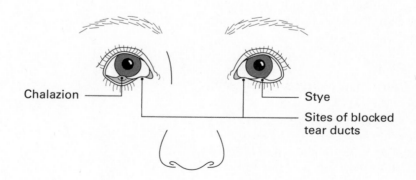

Chalazion ——— Stye

Sites of blocked tear ducts

Bad Breath

Poor dental hygiene and smoking cause most cases of bad breath in adults. Infections of the mouth and sore throat infections may also cause bad breath. Recently it has been suggested that bad breath is occasionally due to gases absorbed from the intestine and released through the lungs. Unfortunately, even if this is correct, it isn't clear what can be done about it.

Finally, unusual problems such as abscesses of the lung or heavy worm infestations have been reported to cause bad breath, although we haven't seen these in our practices.

Smoker's Breath

The bad breath of smoking comes from the lungs as well as the mouth. Thus, mouthwashes and breath fresheners do little to help smoker's breath. Getting rid of this problem is another benefit of giving up cigarettes.

Morning Breath

Bad breath in the morning is very common in adults. Flossing and regular toothbrushing should eliminate this problem.

In Children

A rare cause of prolonged bad breath in a child is a foreign body in the nose. This is especially common in toddlers who have inserted some small object that remains unnoticed. Often, but not always, there is a white, yellowish, or bloody discharge from one nostril.

Home Treatment

Proper dental hygiene, especially flossing, and avoiding smoking will prevent most cases of bad breath. If this doesn't eliminate the odor, a visit to the doctor or dentist may be helpful.

Mouthwashes are of questionable value. Don't use mouthwashes that simply perfume the breath. These cover up but don't treat the underlying problem. If you smoke, bad breath is another good reason to quit.

What to Expect at the Doctor's Office

The doctor will thoroughly examine the mouth and the nose. A culture may be taken if the patient has a sore throat or mouth sores. Antibiotics may be prescribed. If there is an object in the nose, the doctor will use a special instrument to remove it.

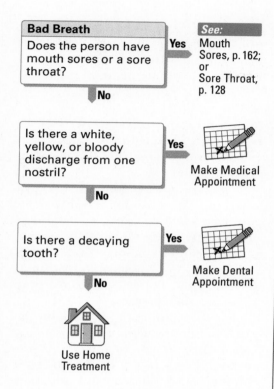

Bad Breath

Does the person have mouth sores or a sore throat?

Yes → *See:* Mouth Sores, p. 162; or Sore Throat, p. 128

No ↓

Is there a white, yellow, or bloody discharge from one nostril?

Yes → Make Medical Appointment

No ↓

Is there a decaying tooth?

Yes → Make Dental Appointment

No ↓

Use Home Treatment

Mouth Sores

Fever blisters or cold sores are a familiar problem caused by the herpes virus. They are usually found on the lips, although they can sometimes appear inside the mouth. Often the blisters have ruptured and only the remaining sore is seen. Fever is usually but not always present. Herpes viruses often live in the body for years, causing trouble only when another illness causes a rise in body temperature. Generally, fever blisters heal by themselves several days after the fever diminishes.

A canker sore is a painful ulcer that often follows an injury, such as accidentally biting the inside of the lip or the tongue, or it may appear without obvious cause. Eventually, it heals by itself.

In Children

Large white spots on the roof of the mouth are a sign of thrush, a yeast infection. It often disappears without treatment.

A virus that can cause mouth lesions in children is the Coxsackie virus. These lesions are often accompanied by spots on the hands and feet—hence the name "hand-foot-mouth syndrome." The child feels well and there is no fever. Again, this problem will go away by itself.

Other Causes

Drugs sometimes cause mouth ulcers. In such cases, a skin rash may be present on other parts of the body as well, and a doctor must be contacted. You will have to stop the drug.

A cancer of the lip or gum is rare except in smokers. It must be treated but is not an emergency. Syphilis transmitted by oral sexual contact may produce a mouth sore. Both of these problems are usually painless. Other conditions that may cause mouth ulcers may also involve eyes, joints, or other organs.

Home Treatment

Mouth sores caused by viruses heal by themselves. The goal of treatment is to reduce fever, relieve pain, and maintain adequate fluid intake.

Children will seldom want to eat when they have painful mouth lesions. Although children can go several days without taking solid foods, it is very important that they maintain an adequate liquid diet. Cold liquids are the most soothing, and Popsicles or iced frozen juices are often helpful.

For sores inside the lip and on the gums, a nonprescription preparation called Orabase may be applied for protection. For canker sores and fever blisters, one of the phenol and camphor preparations (Blistex, Campho-Phenique, etc.) may provide relief, especially if applied early. If one of these preparations appears to cause further irritation, discontinue its use.

Mouth sores usually resolve in one to two weeks. Any sore that persists beyond three weeks should be examined by the doctor.

What to Expect at the Doctor's Office

A thorough examination of the mouth will be carried out. A prescription will usually be given for thrush. For viral infections, doctors have no more to offer than home remedies. We caution against the use of oral anesthetics, such as viscous Xylocaine, for children. This anesthetic can interfere with proper swallowing and can lead to inhalation of food into the lungs.

Mouth Sores

Could this problem be due to medication?

Yes →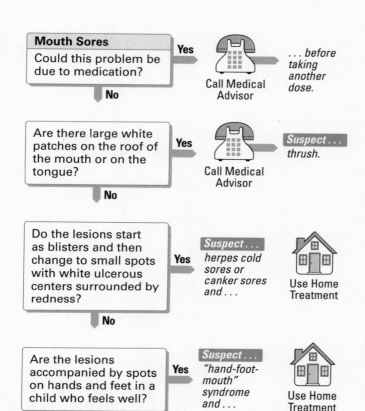

Call Medical Advisor

. . . before taking another dose.

No ↓

Are there large white patches on the roof of the mouth or on the tongue?

Yes →

Call Medical Advisor

Suspect . . . thrush.

No ↓

Do the lesions start as blisters and then change to small spots with white ulcerous centers surrounded by redness?

Yes →

Suspect . . . herpes cold sores or canker sores and . . .

Use Home Treatment

No ↓

Are the lesions accompanied by spots on hands and feet in a child who feels well?

Yes →

Suspect . . . "hand-foot-mouth" syndrome and . . .

Use Home Treatment

No ↓

Use Home Treatment

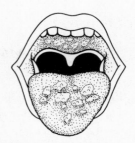

Thrush. Suspect thrush if there are large white patches on the roof of the mouth or on the tongue.

Toothaches

A toothache is often the sad result of poor dental hygiene. Although resistance to tooth decay is partly inherited, the majority of dental problems are preventable through flossing, brushing with a fluoride toothpaste, and professional cleaning. Sealants and fluoride applications by the dentist may be especially important for children.

Certainly, if you can see a decayed tooth or an area of redness surrounding a tooth, a diseased tooth is most likely the cause of pain. Tapping an infected tooth will often accentuate the pain, even though the tooth appears normal.

If the person appears ill, has a fever, and has swelling of the jaw or redness surrounding the tooth, a tooth abscess—a pocket of pus inside the gum—is likely. The person will need antibiotics in addition to proper dental care.

Other Possibilities

Occasionally it is difficult to distinguish a toothache from other sources of pain. Earaches, sore throats, mumps, sinusitis, and injury to the joint that attaches the jaw to the skull (temporomandibular joint or TMJ) may all be confused with a toothache. A call to the doctor may clarify the situation.

If pain occurs every time the patient opens his or her mouth wide, it is likely that the joint of the jaw has been injured. This can occur from a blow or just by trying to eat too big a sandwich. A call to the doctor will help you decide what, if anything, should be done.

Home Treatment

Acetaminophen, aspirin, ibuprofen, or naproxen may be used for pain when a toothache is suspected and while the dental appointment is being arranged. They are also helpful for problems in the joint of the jaw. We recommend acetaminophen for children and teenagers.

What to Expect at the Dentist's Office

The dentist will fill cavities, extract teeth, or do other procedures. For problems with baby teeth, an extraction will be the most likely course. Root canals are generally performed on permanent teeth if the problem is severe. If there is fever or swelling of the jaw, the dentist will usually prescribe an antibiotic.

Toothaches

Are any of the
following present?

▲ Fever

▲ Earache

▲ Pain upon opening
the mouth wide

Yes

Call Medical
Advisor

No

*See dentist
today*

CHAPTER 6

Skin Problems

Skin problems must be approached somewhat differently from other medical problems. Decision charts that proceed from complaints such as "red bumps" are complicated and somewhat unsatisfactory because most people, including doctors, identify skin diseases by recognizing a particular pattern. This pattern is composed of not only what the skin problem looks like at a particular time but also how it began, where it spread, and whether it is associated with other symptoms such as itching or fever. Also important are elements of the medical history that may suggest an illness to which the patient has been exposed.

Fortunately, many times the patient already has a good idea how the problem developed, and it is possible to proceed immediately with the question of whether this is poison ivy, ringworm, or something else.

The decision chart for each section in this chapter begins with the question of whether the problem follows the pattern for the skin disease being discussed. (A longer description of the pattern is given in the text that accompanies each decision chart.) If it doesn't, the chart often directs you to reconsider the problem and to consult Table 7 on pages 168–169.

Most cases of a particular skin disease do not look exactly as a textbook says they should. We have tried to allow for a reasonable amount of variation in the descriptions. Don't be afraid to ask for other opinions. Grandparents and others have seen a lot of skin problems over the years and know what they look like. We have listed some of the more common problems, but by no means all. If your problem doesn't seem to fit any of the descriptions and you think the problem could be serious, call the doctor.

Finally, because every case is at least a little bit different, even the best doctors won't be able to identify all skin problems immediately. Simple office laboratory methods can help sort out the possibilities. Fortunately, the vast majority of skin problems are minor, get better by themselves, and pose no major threat to health. Usually it is reasonable for you to wait quite some time to see if the problem goes away by itself.

If you are confused about where to start, we have provided a decision chart on page 167 to help point you in the right direction. This chart and Table 7 on pages 168–169 allow you to quickly review the major symptoms of common skin problems.

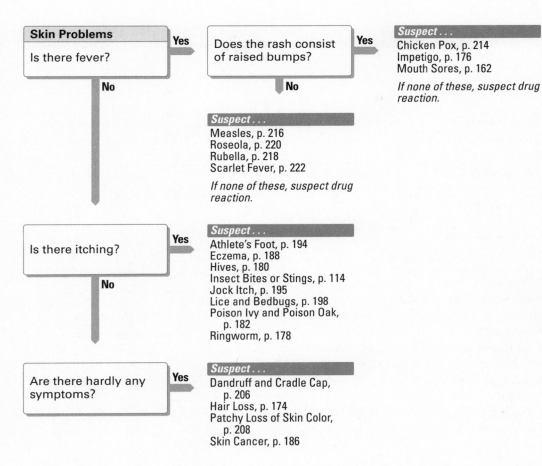

Skin Problems

Is there fever? — **Yes** → Does the rash consist of raised bumps? — **Yes** →

Suspect...
Chicken Pox, p. 214
Impetigo, p. 176
Mouth Sores, p. 162

If none of these, suspect drug reaction.

No ↓

Suspect...
Measles, p. 216
Roseola, p. 220
Rubella, p. 218
Scarlet Fever, p. 222

If none of these, suspect drug reaction.

No ↓

Is there itching? — **Yes** →

Suspect...
Athlete's Foot, p. 194
Eczema, p. 188
Hives, p. 180
Insect Bites or Stings, p. 114
Jock Itch, p. 195
Lice and Bedbugs, p. 198
Poison Ivy and Poison Oak, p. 182
Ringworm, p. 178

No ↓

Are there hardly any symptoms? — **Yes** →

Suspect...
Dandruff and Cradle Cap, p. 206
Hair Loss, p. 174
Patchy Loss of Skin Color, p. 208
Skin Cancer, p. 186

Table 7: Skin Problems and Childhood Diseases

	Fever	Itching	Elevation
Baby Rashes (p. 170)	No	Sometimes	Slightly raised dots
Diaper Rash (p. 172)	No	No	Only if infected
Impetigo (p. 176)	Sometimes	Occasionally	Crusts on sores
Ringworm (p. 178)	No	Occasionally	Slightly raised rings
Hives (p. 180)	No	Intense	Raised with flat tops
Poison Ivy (p. 182)	No	Intense	Blisters are elevated
Rashes Caused by Chemicals (p. 184)	No	Moderate to intense	Sometimes blisters
Eczema (p. 188)	No	Moderate to intense	Occasional blisters when infected
Acne (p. 192)	No	No	Pimples, cysts
Athlete's Foot (p. 194)	No	Mild to intense	No
Dandruff and Cradle Cap (p. 206)	No	Occasionally	Some crusting
Chicken Pox (p. 214)	Yes	Intense during pustular stage	Flat, then raised, then blisters, then crusts
Measles (p. 216)	Yes	None to mild	Flat
Rubella (p. 218)	Yes	No	Flat or slightly raised
Roseola (p. 220)	Yes	No	Flat, occasionally with a few bumps
Scarlet Fever (p. 222)	Yes	No	Flat, feels like sandpaper
Fifth Disease (p. 224)	No	No	Flat, lacy appearance

Color	Location	Duration of Problem	Other Symptoms
White or red dots; surrounding skin may be red	Trunk, neck, skin folds on arms and legs	Until controlled	
Red	Under diaper	Until controlled	
Golden crusts on red sores	Arms, legs, face first, then most of body	Until controlled	
Red	Anywhere, including scalp and nails	Until controlled	
Pale raised lesions surrounded by red	Anywhere	Minutes to days	
Red	Exposed areas	7 to 14 days	Oozing; some swelling
Red	Areas exposed to chemicals	Until exposure to chemical stopped	Some oozing and/or swelling
Red	Elbows, wrists, knees, cheeks	Until controlled	Moist; oozing
Red	Face, back, chest	Until controlled	Blackheads
Colorless to red	Between toes	Until controlled	Cracks; scaling; oozing blisters
White to yellow to red	Scalp, eyebrows, behind ears, groin	Until controlled	Fine, oily scales
Red	May start anywhere; most prominent on trunk and face	4 to 10 days	Lesions progress from flat to tiny blisters, then become crusted
Pink, then red	First face, then chest and abdomen, then arms and legs	4 to 7 days	Preceded by fever, cough, red eyes
Red	First face, then trunk, then extremities	2 to 4 days	Swollen glands behind ears; occasional joint pains in older children and adults
Pink	First trunk, then arms and neck; very little on face and legs	1 to 2 days	High fever for 3 days that disappears with rash
Red	First face, then elbows; spreads rapidly to entire body in 24 hours	5 to 7 days	Sore throat; skin peeling afterward, especially palms
Red	First face, then arms and legs, then rest of body	3 to 7 days	"Slapped-cheek" appearance, rash comes and goes

Baby Rashes

The skin of the newborn child may exhibit a wide variety of bumps and blotches. Fortunately, almost all of these are harmless and clear up by themselves. Only one, heat rash, requires any treatment. If the baby was delivered in a hospital, many of these conditions may occur before discharge so that advice will be readily available from nurses or doctors.

Heat Rash

Heat rash is caused by blockage of the pores that lead to the sweat glands. It actually can occur at any age but is most common in the very young child whose sweat glands are still developing. When heat and humidity rise, these glands attempt to secrete sweat as they would normally. But because of the blockage, sweat is held within the skin and forms little red bumps. It is also known as "prickly heat" or "miliaria."

Milia

The little white bumps of milia appear when too many normal skin cells accumulate in spots. As many as 40% of children have these bumps at birth. Eventually the bumps break open, the trapped material escapes, and the bumps disappear without treatment.

Erythema Toxicum

Erythema toxicum is an unnecessarily long and frightening term for the flat red splotches that appear in up to 50% of all babies. These seldom appear after five days of age and usually disappear by seven days. Children who exhibit these splotches are otherwise normal.

Acne

Because the baby is exposed to the mother's adult hormones, a mild case of acne may develop. (The little white dots often seen on a newborn's nose represent "sebaceous gland hyperplasia," an excess amount of normal skin oil that has been produced by the hormones.) Acne usually becomes evident at between two and four weeks of age and clears up within six months to a year. It virtually never requires treatment.

Home Treatment

Heat Rash

Heat rash is effectively treated simply by providing a cooler and less humid environment. Powders carefully applied do no harm but are unlikely to help. Avoid ointments and creams because they tend to keep the skin warmer and block the pores.

Milia, Erythema Toxicum, and Acne

Milia and erythema toxicum should require no treatment. They will go away by themselves.

Acne in babies should not be treated with the medicines used by adolescents and adults. Normal washing is usually all that is required.

These problems are not associated with fever and, with the exception of minor discomfort in heat rash, should be painless. If any questions arise about these conditions, a telephone call to the doctor's office will often provide answers.

What to Expect at the Doctor's Office

Discussion of these problems can usually wait until the regularly scheduled well-baby visit. The doctor then can confirm your diagnosis.

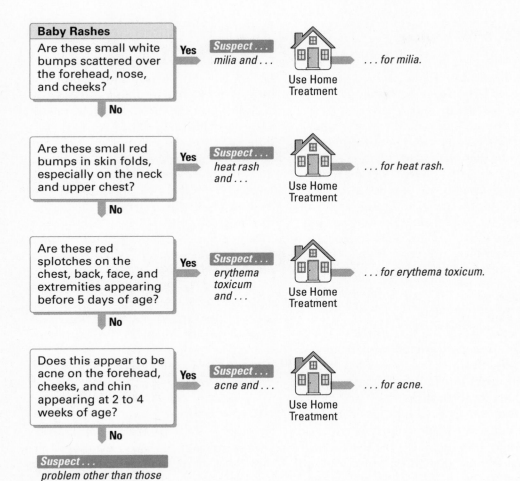

Baby Rashes

Are these small white bumps scattered over the forehead, nose, and cheeks? — **Yes** → *Suspect... milia and ...* → Use Home Treatment → *... for milia.*

No ↓

Are these small red bumps in skin folds, especially on the neck and upper chest? — **Yes** → *Suspect... heat rash and ...* → Use Home Treatment → *... for heat rash.*

No ↓

Are these red splotches on the chest, back, face, and extremities appearing before 5 days of age? — **Yes** → *Suspect... erythema toxicum and ...* → Use Home Treatment → *... for erythema toxicum.*

No ↓

Does this appear to be acne on the forehead, cheeks, and chin appearing at 2 to 4 weeks of age? — **Yes** → *Suspect... acne and ...* → Use Home Treatment → *... for acne.*

No ↓

Suspect... problem other than those listed. Call physician.

Diaper Rash

The only children who never have diaper rash are those who never wear diapers. An infant's skin is particularly sensitive and likely to develop diaper rash. Diaper rash is basically an irritation caused by dampness and the interaction of urine, feces, and skin. An additional factor is thought to be the ammonia produced from urine, and often its odor is unmistakably present. Factors that tend to keep the baby's skin wet and exposed to the irritant promote diaper rash. These are:

▲ Constantly wet or infrequently changed diapers
▲ Using plastic pants

For the most part, treatment consists of reversing these factors.

The irritation of simple diaper rash may become complicated by an infection due to yeast (candida) or bacteria. When yeast is the culprit, small red spots may be seen. Also, small patches of the rash may appear outside the area covered by the diaper, as far away as the chest. Infection with bacteria leads to development of large fluid-filled blisters. If the rash is worse in the skin creases (a condition called intertrigo), a mild underlying skin problem known as seborrhea may be present. This skin condition is also responsible for dandruff and cradle cap (page 206).

Occasionally, parents may notice blood or what appears to be blood spots when boys have diaper rash. This is due to a rash at the urinary opening at the end of the penis. This problem will clear up when the diaper rash clears up.

Home Treatment

Treatment of diaper rash is aimed at keeping the skin dry and exposed to air. As implied previously, the first things to do are to change diapers frequently and stop using plastic pants. Leaving diapers off altogether for as long as possible will also help. Cloth diapers should be washed in a mild soap and rinsed thoroughly. Occasionally, the soap residues left in diapers will act as an irritant. Adding a half cup (120 ml) of vinegar to the last rinse cycle may help counter the irritating ammonia. Avoid using baby wipes with alcohol or cornstarch-based powders.

While the rash will take at least several days to completely clear, you should see definite improvement within the first 48 to 72 hours. If the rash does not start clearing up by that time or if it is extraordinarily severe, consult your doctor.

To prevent diaper rash, some parents use zinc oxide ointments, petroleum jelly, or other protective ointments. Others use baby powders. (**Caution:** Talc dust can injure babies' lungs if they breathe it in.) Always place powder in your hand first and then pat on the baby's bottom. Caldesene powder is helpful in preventing seborrhea and monilial rashes. We do not feel that all babies need powders and creams. If a rash has begun, avoid ointments and creams because they may delay healing.

What to Expect at the Doctor's Office

All of the baby's skin should be inspected to determine the true extent of the rash. Occasionally, a scraping from the involved skin will be examined under the microscope. If a yeast (monilial)

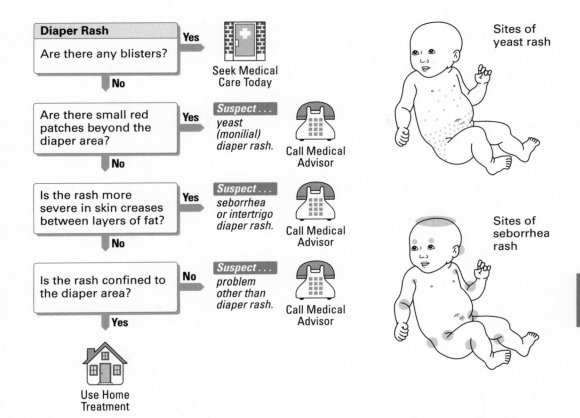

Diaper Rash

Are there any blisters? — **Yes** → **Seek Medical Care Today**

↓ **No**

Are there small red patches beyond the diaper area? — **Yes** → *Suspect...* yeast (monilial) diaper rash. → **Call Medical Advisor**

↓ **No**

Is the rash more severe in skin creases between layers of fat? — **Yes** → *Suspect...* seborrhea or intertrigo diaper rash. → **Call Medical Advisor**

↓ **No**

Is the rash confined to the diaper area? — **No** → *Suspect...* problem other than diaper rash. → **Call Medical Advisor**

↓ **Yes**

Use Home Treatment

Sites of yeast rash

Sites of seborrhea rash

infection has complicated a simple diaper rash, the doctor will prescribe home treatment plus a medication to kill the yeast. If a bacterial infection has occurred, then an antibiotic to be taken orally will be recommended. If the rash is very severe or seborrhea is suspected, then a steroid cream (sometimes stronger than the hydrocortisone available without prescription) may be advised. In any case, home therapy may be safely started before seeing the doctor.

Hair Loss

This section is not about the normal hair loss that most men and many women experience as they get older. (See Aging Spots, Wrinkles, and Baldness, page 210.) Baldness isn't the only kind of hair loss.

Sometimes all the hair in one small area is lost, but the scalp is normal. This problem is called alopecia areata, and its cause is unknown. Usually, the hair will come back completely within 12 months, although about 40% of patients will have a similar loss within the next four to five years. This problem also resolves by itself. Corticosteroid injections sometimes make the hair grow back faster.

Hair loss that may require a doctor's treatment is characterized by abnormalities in the scalp skin or the hairs themselves. The most frequent problem in this category is ringworm (page 178). Ringworm may be red and scaly, or there may be oozing pustules. The ringworm fungus infects the hairs so they become thickened and break easily. Whenever the scalp skin or hairs appear abnormal, the doctor may be able to help.

Hair pulling by children is often responsible for hair loss. Tight braids or ponytails may also cause some hair loss. If a child constantly pulls out his or her hair, you should discuss the problem with a doctor.

Home Treatment

In this instance, home treatment is reserved for presumed alopecia areata and consists of watchful waiting unless it is particularly disturbing to you and you would like to consider the treatments your doctor can offer. Remember, the skin in the area involved must be completely normal for a diagnosis of alopecia areata. If the appearance of scalp or hairs becomes abnormal, the doctor should be consulted.

What to Expect at the Doctor's Office

An examination of the hair and scalp is usually sufficient to determine the nature of the problem. Occasionally, the hairs may be examined under a microscope. Certain types of ringworm of the scalp can be identified because they fluoresce (glow) under an ultraviolet lamp. Ringworm of the scalp will require the use of an oral drug, usually griseofulvin, because creams and lotions applied to the affected area won't penetrate the hair follicles to kill the fungus.

We hope that no doctor would recommend the use of X-rays today as some did decades ago. If X-ray treatment is offered, you should flatly reject it and find another doctor.

There has been much discussion about medical treatments to prevent baldness. Hair transplants can help in some instances but are usually not fully satisfactory. The creams (minoxidil) work only a little and only early on; a lot of people are disappointed by this treatment.

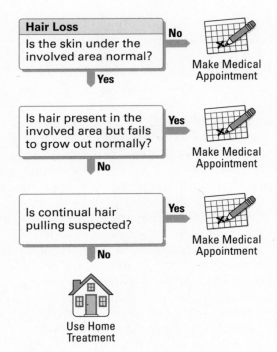

Hair Loss

Is the skin under the involved area normal?

No → Make Medical Appointment

Yes ↓

Is hair present in the involved area but fails to grow out normally?

Yes → Make Medical Appointment

No ↓

Is continual hair pulling suspected?

Yes → Make Medical Appointment

No ↓

Use Home Treatment

Impetigo

Impetigo can be recognized by the characteristic rash that begins as small red spots and progresses to tiny blisters that eventually rupture, producing an oozing, sticky, honey-colored crust. This rash usually spreads very quickly with scratching and is particularly troublesome in the summer, especially in warm, moist climates.

Impetigo is a skin infection caused by streptococcal bacteria; occasionally, other bacteria may also be found. If it spreads, impetigo can be a very uncomfortable problem. There is usually a great deal of itching. After the sores heal, there may be a slight decrease in skin color at the site. Skin color usually returns to normal, so this need not concern you.

Complication in the Kidneys

Of greatest concern is a rare reaction to streptococcal infection, a kidney problem known as glomerulonephritis. Glomerulonephritis will cause the urine to turn a dark brown (cola) color and is often accompanied by headache and elevated blood pressure. Although this complication has a formidable name, it is short-lived and heals completely in most people.

Unfortunately, antibiotics won't prevent glomerulonephritis but may help prevent the impetigo from spreading to other people, thus protecting them from both conditions. Antibiotics are effective in healing the impetigo.

Although there is some debate on this matter, many doctors believe that if only one or two lesions are present and the lesions are not progressing, home treatment may be used for impetigo. The exception to this rule is if an epidemic of glomerulonephritis is occurring within your community.

Home Treatment

Crusts may be soaked off with either warm water or Burow's Solution (Domeboro, Bluboro, etc.). The lesions should be washed with soap and water after the crusts have been soaked off. An antibiotic ointment (Bacitracin, Neosporin, etc.) may prevent the spread of impetigo to others. If lesions do not show prompt improvement or if they seem to be spreading, see the doctor without delay.

What to Expect at the Doctor's Office

After examining the sores and taking an appropriate medical history, the doctor will usually prescribe an oral antibiotic or a special antibiotic (mupirocin) cream. Some doctors may check the blood pressure or urine in order to look for early signs of glomerulonephritis.

Impetigo

Does the person have small, crusted, yellow sores with or without a tiny surrounding area of redness?

No →

Suspect . . .
problem other than impetigo. Check Table 7 on pp. 168–169.

↓ **Yes**

Has anyone in your neighborhood had glomerulonephritis recently?

Yes →

Call Medical Advisor

↓ **No**

Is there fever?

Yes →

Call Medical Advisor

↓ **No**

Are there only 1 or 2 lesions?

No →

Call Medical Advisor

↓ **Yes**

Are the lesions healing and not spreading to other family members?

No →

Call Medical Advisor

↓ **Yes**

Use Home Treatment

Ringworm

Worms have nothing whatsoever to do with this condition. Ringworm is a shallow fungal infection of the skin. The designation "ringworm" is derived from the characteristic red ring that appears on the skin.

Ringworm can generally be recognized by its pattern of development. The lesions begin as small, round, red spots and get progressively larger. When they are about the size of a pea, the center begins to clear. When the lesions are about the size of a dime, they will have the appearance of a ring. The border will be red, elevated, and scaly. Often there are groups of infections so close to one another that it is difficult to recognize them as individual rings.

Ringworm may also affect the scalp or nails. These infections are more difficult to treat but, fortunately, are not seen very often. Ringworm epidemics of the scalp were common many years ago.

Home Treatment

Topical antifungals (page 71) applied to the skin are effective treatments for ringworm. They are available in cream, solution, and powder and can be purchased over the counter. Either the cream or the solution should be applied two or three times a day. Only a small amount is required for each application.

Resolving this problem may take several weeks, but you should see improvement within one week. Ringworm that either shows no improvement after a week of therapy or continues to spread should be checked by a doctor.

What to Expect at the Doctor's Office

The diagnosis of ringworm can be confirmed by scraping the scales, soaking them in a potassium hydroxide solution, and viewing them under a microscope. Some doctors may culture the scrapings.

For ringworm of the skin, oral medicines are used if topical antifungals have failed, but this is unusual.

In infections involving the scalp, an ultraviolet light (called a Wood's lamp) will cause affected hairs to become fluorescent. The Wood's lamp is used to make the diagnosis; it does not treat ringworm. Ringworm of the scalp must be treated by medicines taken orally, usually for at least a month. These medicines are also effective for fungal infections of the nails. Ringworm of the scalp should never be treated with X-rays.

Ringworm. Lesions begin as small, round, red spots. When they are about the size of a dime, they will have the appearance of a ring.

Ringworm

Are all of the following conditions present?

▲ Rash begins as a small red, colorless, or depigmented circle that becomes progressively larger.

▲ The circular border is elevated and perhaps scaly.

▲ The center of the circle begins healing as the circle becomes larger.

No →

Suspect ...

problem other than ringworm. Check Table 7 on pp. 168–169.

↓ **Yes**

Is the scalp infected? **Yes** →

Make Medical Appointment

↓ **No**

Use Home Treatment

Hives

Hives, also called urticaria, are an allergic reaction. Unfortunately, the reaction can be to almost anything, including cold, heat, and even emotional tension. Unless you already have a good idea what is causing the hives or you have just taken a new drug, the doctor is unlikely to be able to determine the cause. Most often, searching for a cause is fruitless.

Here is a list of some of the things that are frequently mentioned as causes:

▲ Drugs
▲ Eggs
▲ Dairy products
▲ Wheat
▲ Pork
▲ Shellfish
▲ Freshwater fish
▲ Berries
▲ Nuts
▲ Pollen
▲ Animal dander
▲ Insect bites

The only sure way to know whether one of these is the culprit is to expose the patient to it. The problem with this approach is that if an allergy does exist, the allergic reaction may include not only hives but also a general reaction causing difficulty with breathing or circulation.

As indicated by the decision chart, a systemic reaction is a potentially dangerous situation, and a doctor should be consulted immediately. This is an **emergency.** Avoid exposure to a suspected cause to see if the attacks cease. Such a test is difficult to interpret because attacks of hives are often separated by long periods of time. Actually, most people suffer only one attack, lasting from a period of minutes to weeks.

Finally, an occasional single hive on the arm or trunk is so common that it is considered of no significance.

Home Treatment

Determine whether there has been any pattern to the appearance of the hives. Do they appear after meals? After exposure to cold? During a particular season of the year? If there seem to be likely causes, eliminate them and see what happens.

If the reactions seem to be related to foods, an alternative is available. Lamb and rice virtually never cause allergic reactions. The person with hives may be placed on a diet consisting only of lamb and rice until completely free of hives. Foods are then added back to the diet one at a time, and the person is observed for a recurrence of hives. This is referred to as an elimination diet.

Itching may be relieved by applying cold compresses, taking an over-the-counter pain medicine (page 54), or antihistamine (page 62).

What to Expect at the Doctor's Office

If the patient is suffering a systemic reaction with difficulty breathing or dizziness, injections of adrenalin and other drugs may be given. In the more usual case of hives alone, the doctor may do two things. First, the doctor may prescribe an antihistamine or use adrenalin injections to relieve swelling and itching. Second, the doctor can review the history of the reaction to try to find an offending agent and advise home

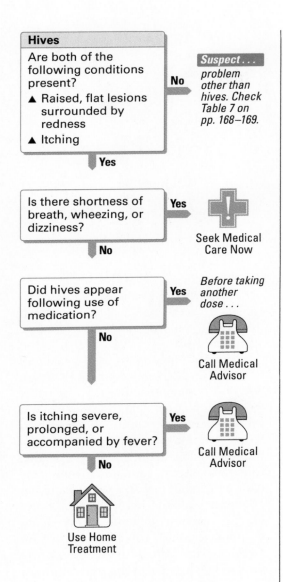

Hives

Are both of the following conditions present?

▲ Raised, flat lesions surrounded by redness

▲ Itching

No → *Suspect...* problem other than hives. Check Table 7 on pp. 168–169.

Yes ↓

Is there shortness of breath, wheezing, or dizziness?

Yes → **Seek Medical Care Now**

No ↓

Did hives appear following use of medication?

Yes → *Before taking another dose...* **Call Medical Advisor**

No ↓

Is itching severe, prolonged, or accompanied by fever?

Yes → **Call Medical Advisor**

No ↓

Use Home Treatment

treatment. Remember that most often the cause of hives goes undetected, and they stop occurring without any therapy.

If the problem is severe and chronic, the doctor may prescribe strong medicines such as corticosteroids (prednisone), but only very rarely is this required. If the problem is severe or systemic, the doctor may prescribe an emergency kit so that you can inject yourself if you have another attack.

Poison Ivy and Poison Oak

Poison ivy and poison oak need little introduction. The itching skin lesions that follow contact with the plant oil of these and other members of the Rhus plant category are the most common example of a larger category of skin problems known as contact dermatitis. Contact dermatitis simply means that something that has touched the skin has caused the skin to react. An initial exposure is necessary to "sensitize" the person; a subsequent exposure will result in an allergic reaction if the plant oil remains in contact with skin for several hours. The resulting rash begins after a delay of 12 to 48 hours and persists for about two weeks.

You do not have to come into direct contact with plants to get poison ivy. The plant oil may be spread by pets, contaminated clothing, or the smoke from burning *Rhus* plants. It can occur during any season.

Home Treatment

The best approach is learning to recognize and avoid these plants, which are hazardous even in the winter, when they have dropped their leaves.

Next best is to remove the plant oil from the skin as soon as possible. If the oil has been on the skin for less than six hours, thorough cleansing with ordinary soap, repeated three times, will often prevent a reaction. Alcohol-based cleansing tissues, available in prepackaged form (such as Alco Wipes), are much more effective. Rubbing alcohol on a washcloth is even better and is our favorite remedy. Soap

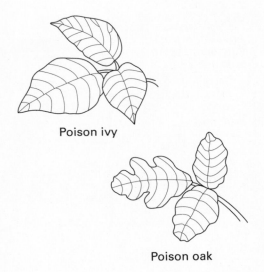

Poison ivy

Poison oak

first, then rubbing alcohol, then soap again and rinse.

To relieve itching, many doctors recommend cool compresses of Burow's Solution (Domeboro, Bluboro) or baths with Aveeno or oatmeal (one cup to a tub full of water). Acetaminophen, aspirin, ibuprofen, and naproxen are also effective in reducing itching. The old standby, calamine lotion, sometimes helps for early lesions but may spread the plant oil. (**Caution:** Caladryl is reported to cause allergic reactions in some people. Plain calamine lotion is probably best.) Be sure to cleanse the skin, as above, even if you are too late to prevent the rash entirely.

Another method of obtaining symptomatic relief is a hot bath or shower. Heat releases histamine, the substance in skin cells that causes the intense itching. A hot shower or bath will cause intense itching as the histamine is released. The heat should be gradually increased to the maximum tolerable and continued until the itching has

Poison Ivy

Are all of the following
conditions present?

▲ Itching

▲ Redness, minor
swelling, blisters, or
oozing

▲ Probable exposure
to poison ivy,
poison oak, or
poison sumac

No →

Suspect ...

*problem
other than
poison ivy or
poison oak.
Check
Table 7 on
pp. 168–169.*

↓ **Yes**

Use Home
Treatment

subsided, in just a few minutes. This process will deplete the cells of histamine,
and the person will obtain up to eight
hours of relief from the itching. This
method has the advantage of not requiring frequent applications of ointments
to the lesions and is a good way to get
some sleep at night.

The itching may be treated with an
antihistamine (page 62) and/or an over-
the-counter pain medicine (page 54).

Hydrocortisone creams (Cortaid or
Lanacort, for example) are available
without a prescription. They will decrease inflammation and itching, but
relief is not immediate. The cream must
be applied often (four to six times a
day). Do not use these creams for more
than a week or two (page 71).

Poison ivy and poison oak will persist
for the same length of time with or without medication. If secondary bacterial
infection occurs, healing will be delayed; hence, scratching is not helpful.

(Just in case you can't avoid the urge to
scratch, cut your nails to avoid damage
to the skin.)

Poison ivy and poison oak are not
contagious. They can't be spread once
the oil has been either absorbed by the
skin or removed.

If the lesions are too extensive to be
easily treated, if home treatment is ineffective, or if the itching is so severe that
it can't be tolerated, a call to the doctor
may be necessary.

What to Expect at the Doctor's Office

After a history and physical examination,
the doctor may prescribe a corticosteroid
cream stronger than hydrocortisone to
be applied to the lesions four to six times
a day. This often helps only moderately.
An alternative is to give a steroid (such
as prednisone) by mouth for a short
period. A rather large dose is given the
first day, and the dose is then gradually
reduced. We don't recommend oral
steroids except when there have been
previous severe reactions or extensive
exposure to poison ivy or poison oak.

Rashes Caused by Chemicals

Chemicals may cause a rash in two ways. The chemical may have a direct caustic effect that irritates the skin—a minor "chemical burn." Or, more often, the chemical may cause an allergic reaction of the skin, resulting in a rash.

The most common allergic skin irritation is poison ivy (page 182). If you see a rash that looks like poison ivy but contact with poison ivy or poison oak seems impossible, consider other chemicals that might cause "contact dermatitis" and produce an identical rash.

The chemicals most frequently found to cause contact dermatitis are dyes and other chemicals found in clothing, chemicals used in elastic and rubber products, cosmetics, and deodorants (including "feminine" deodorants).

Usually the tip-off to the cause of the rash is its location and shape. Sometimes this is very striking, as when the rash leaves a perfect outline of a bra or the elastic bands of underwear or some other article of clothing. More often the rash is not so distinct, but its location suggests the possible cause.

Home Treatment

If you have had difficulty with particular types of clothing, cosmetics, deodorants, and so on, then avoiding contact is the best way to avoid a problem. Changing brands may also help. For example, some cosmetics are manufactured so that they are less likely to cause an allergic reaction (hypoallergenic products). Rashes caused by deodorants are often relieved by using a milder preparation less often.

Once the rash has occurred, eliminating contact with the chemical is essential. Washing thoroughly with soap and water may remove chemicals on the skin and is especially important with materials such as cement dust. Oily substances may best be removed with rubbing alcohol, or use paint thinner, quickly followed by soap and water to prevent contact dermatitis from the thinner itself.

The rest of the home treatment is identical to that for poison ivy (page 182) and consists of using Burow's Solution, hot water, and hydrocortisone cream to achieve relief from itching. If the lesions are too extensive to be treated easily, if home treatment is ineffective, or if the itching is so severe that it can't be tolerated, a call to the doctor may be necessary.

What to Expect at the Doctor's Office

The doctor will examine the rash. A review of the patient's history will focus on possible exposure to substances such as those mentioned above. A corticosteroid cream stronger than hydrocortisone may be prescribed. Another alternative is to give a corticosteroid (such as prednisone) for a short time; a rather large dose is given the first day, and the dose is then gradually reduced.

Itching may be treated with either an antihistamine (page 62) and/or over-the-counter pain reliever (page 54).

Rashes Caused by Chemicals

Is this a red rash (sometimes with bumps or blisters and usually itchy or burning) that by its shape and location suggests contact with articles of clothing, cosmetics, deodorant, or other chemicals?

No → *Suspect...* problem other than contact dermatitis. Check Table 7 on pp. 168–169.

Yes

Use Home Treatment

Skin Cancer

There is no easy, sure way to identify skin cancer. The guidelines here are those that doctors use in confronting this dilemma. When in doubt, they will remove the lesion for testing (biopsy). You can do no better, so when in doubt, see a doctor.

Prevention is the best approach to skin cancer. Sun exposure is the cause of all three of these types of cancer, and prevention means sun avoidance. You first, and your spouse. Then the kids, and the grandkids, and their friends. Let's face it, sun is no good for your skin. Sunscreens, hats with wide brims, and long sleeves will lower the risk of skin cancer and keep your skin younger looking. Use a good sunscreen (page 72). See also "Sunburn," page 196.

Decisions about when to see a doctor are easier if you know common noncancerous skin lesions:

▲ Plain old freckles (flat, uniform, tan to dark brown color, regular border, usually less than one-quarter inch, or 6 mm, in diameter)
▲ Warts (skin-colored, raised, rounded, rough or flat surface)

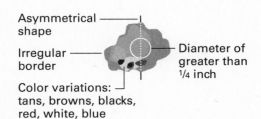

Asymmetrical shape
Irregular border
Diameter of greater than 1/4 inch
Color variations: tans, browns, blacks, red, white, blue

Characteristics of skin cancer. Look for changes in size, color, surface, or border. It is not necessary for all of these characteristics to be present for a spot to be regarded as suspicious.

▲ Skin tags (wobbly tags of skin)
▲ Seborrheic keratoses (greasy, dirty tan to brown, raised, flat lesions that first appear in midlife on face, chest, and back and increase in number with the passing years)

Types of Skin Cancer

The vast majority of skin cancers fall into three categories.

Malignant Melanoma. Malignant melanoma is by far the most dangerous. Though described as moles that have undergone cancerous change, melanomas often do not look like moles—they may be flat.

Doctors look for three characteristics in judging the likelihood of a melanoma:

▲ Changes in size, color, surface, shape, or border appearance. The more rapid, unusual, and irregular, the higher the suspicion.
▲ Variation in color (tans, browns, or blacks) is unusual for a benign lesion. Hues of red, white, and blue may signal melanomas.
▲ An irregular border suggests the spread of abnormal cells; a benign lesion usually has a regular border.

Squamous Cell Cancers. Squamous cell cancers are raised, usually somewhat bumpy lesions with rough, scaly surfaces on a reddish base, and they often bleed. The border is usually irregular. These lesions grow slowly and usually do not spread to other parts of the body. Most often, they are recognized as sores that don't heal. Solar keratoses appear similar to squamous cell carcinoma, but they are not bumps and rarely bleed. Although solar keratoses are not malignant, they are considered to be a precur-

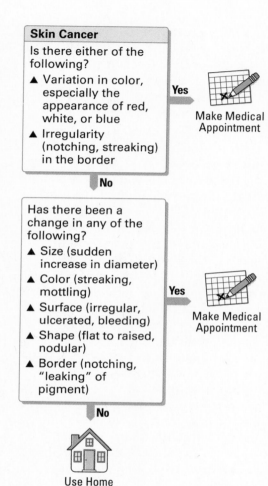

Skin Cancer

Is there either of the following?

▲ Variation in color, especially the appearance of red, white, or blue

▲ Irregularity (notching, streaking) in the border

Yes → Make Medical Appointment

No ↓

Has there been a change in any of the following?

▲ Size (sudden increase in diameter)

▲ Color (streaking, mottling)

▲ Surface (irregular, ulcerated, bleeding)

▲ Shape (flat to raised, nodular)

▲ Border (notching, "leaking" of pigment)

Yes → Make Medical Appointment

No ↓

Use Home Treatment

sor of cancer and are often treated to avoid the development of cancer.

Basal Cell Cancers. Basal cell cancers appear as pearly or waxy nodules with central depressions or craters. As this cancer enlarges, the center usually becomes more ulcerated, giving it the appearance of having been gnawed. Hence, the term "rodent ulcer" is sometimes applied. This type of cancer grows slowly and only by direct extension so

that it never spreads (metastasizes) to other organs of the body.

All these cancers are related to sun exposure. Squamous cell and basal cell cancers appear almost exclusively on the areas of skin most exposed to sun (head, neck, hands). Melanoma is also common in these areas but may appear on the chest or back. Melanoma is most common in people who have had one or more severe blistering sunburns before the age of 18.

Home Treatment

Home treatment consists of watchful waiting and prevention. If the lesion has none of the characteristics that raise suspicion, then closely watching for change makes sense. But if you are in doubt, ask questions at your next doctor visit.

What to Expect at the Doctor's Office

Dermatologists (skin specialists) can usually offer the best advice about skin lesions. Successful treatment may sometimes be done on the initial visit.

A reminder: If you get one of these cancers, you are likely to get another. So, once you've had the first one cured, it is a good idea to have regular examinations to make sure that nothing new has developed. Avoid further damage to the skin from the sun.

Warts

Warts can be treated successfully at home using nonprescription preparations such as Compound W (page 72). They usually go away by themselves anyway. You should see a doctor only for plantar warts appearing on the sole of the foot (see Foot Pain, page 257).

Eczema

Eczema, or atopic dermatitis, is commonly found in people with a family history of eczema, hay fever, or asthma. As with asthma, a variety of conditions can aggravate eczema: infection, emotional stress, food allergy, and sweating.

The underlying problem is the inability of the skin to retain adequate amounts of water. The skin of people with eczema is consequently very dry, which causes the skin to itch. Most of the manifestations of eczema are a result of scratching. The scratching produces weeping, infected skin. Dried weepings lead to crusting. Sufficient scratching will produce a thickened, rough skin, which is characteristic of long-standing atopic dermatitis.

In young infants who can't scratch, the most common manifestation is red, dry, mildly scaling cheeks, caused when the child rubs them against the bedsheets. In infants, eczema may also be found in the area where plastic pants meet the skin. The tightness of the elastic produces the characteristic red, scaling lesion. In older children, it's very common for eczema to involve the area behind the knees and inside the elbows. Adults often have problems with their hands, especially if they're in frequent contact with water.

If there's a large amount of weeping or crusting, the eczema may be infected with bacteria, and a call to the doctor will most likely be required.

The course of eczema is quite variable. Some people will have only a brief, mild problem; others have mild to severe manifestations throughout life. Bouts of eczema are often related to emotional factors; identifying and dealing with such emotional triggers may be the key to successful therapy.

Home Treatment

Therapy is based on good skin care and, if the eczema is allergic in nature, avoiding allergens.

Try to keep the skin from becoming too dry. Frequent bathing actually makes the skin drier. Although the person will feel comfortable in the bath, the itching will become more intense afterward. Avoid bathing with soap and water because these tend to dry the skin. Instead use "nonlipid" cleansers, such as those with cetyl alcohol (Cetaphil, etc.). Use rubber gloves to protect the hands when washing dishes or the car. Freshwater or pool swimming can aggravate eczema, but ocean swimming doesn't.

Sweating aggravates eczema. Avoid overdressing. Lightweight night clothing is important. Cotton clothing is suggested; contact with wool and silk seems to aggravate eczema and should be avoided. Avoid synthetic fabrics that don't "breathe."

Avoid all oil or grease preparations; they clog the skin, increasing sweat retention and itching. Keep nails trimmed short to minimize the effects of scratching, especially with children.

Itching is often worse at bedtime. Over-the-counter pain medications (page 54) and antihistamines may reduce itching (page 62).

Avoiding cow's milk is often suggested, particularly for children. Make sure this really works for your child before permanently changing to more expensive foods. When trying any

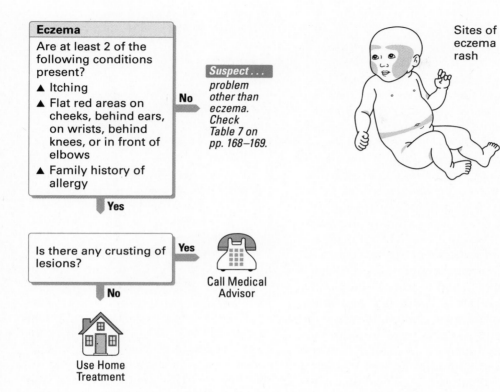

Eczema

Are at least 2 of the following conditions present?

▲ Itching

▲ Flat red areas on cheeks, behind ears, on wrists, behind knees, or in front of elbows

▲ Family history of allergy

No → *Suspect...* problem other than eczema. Check Table 7 on pp. 168–169.

Yes ↓

Is there any crusting of lesions?

Yes → Call Medical Advisor

No ↓

Use Home Treatment

Sites of eczema rash

milk-avoidance diet, make no other changes in food or other care for a full two weeks unless absolutely necessary, in order to see if it works.

What to Expect at the Doctor's Office

By gathering the patient's history and examining the lesions, the doctor can determine whether the problem is eczema. If crusted or weeping lesions are present, bacterial infection is likely and an oral antibiotic will be prescribed. There has been no benefit demonstrated from either skin testing or hyposensitization (allergy shots).

If home treatment hasn't improved the problem, the doctor may prescribe corticosteroid creams and lotions. While these are effective, they aren't curative; eczema is characterized by repeated occurrences. Furthermore, because of their potential side effects, corticosteroid creams should be used only for a short period.

Boils

A familiar term, "painful as a boil," emphasizes the severe discomfort that can arise from this common skin problem.

A boil is a localized infection, usually due to staphylococcus bacteria. Often a particularly savage strain of the bacteria is responsible. When this particular germ inhabits the skin, recurrent problems with boils may persist for months or years. Often, several family members will be affected at about the same time.

Boils may be single or multiple, and they may occur anywhere on the body. They range from the size of a pea to the size of a walnut or larger. The surrounding red, thickened, and tender tissue increases the problem even further. The infection begins in the tissues beneath the skin and develops into an abscess—a pocket filled with pus. Eventually the pus pocket "points" toward the skin surface and finally ruptures and drains. Then it heals.

Boils often begin as infections around hair follicles; hence, the term folliculitis for minor infections. Areas under pressure (such as the buttocks) are often likely spots for boils to begin. A boil that extends into the deeper layers of the skin is called a carbuncle.

Special consideration should be given to boils on the face because they are more likely to lead to serious complicating infections.

Home Treatment

The goal of treatment is to let it all out—the pus, that is. Boils are handled gently, because rough treatment can force the infection deeper inside the body. Warm, moist compresses are applied gently several times each day to speed the development of a pocket of pus and to soften the skin for the eventual rupture and drainage. Once drainage begins, the compresses will help keep the opening in the skin clear. The more drainage, the better. Frequent, thorough soaping of the entire skin area helps prevent reinfection. Ignore all temptation to squeeze the boil.

What to Expect at the Doctor's Office

If there is fever or a facial boil, the doctor will usually prescribe an antibiotic. Otherwise, antibiotics may not be used. They are of limited help in abscess-like infections.

If the boil feels as if fluid is contained in a pocket but has not yet drained, the doctor may lance the boil. In this procedure, a small incision is made to allow the pus to drain. After drainage, the pain is reduced, and healing is quite prompt. While this is not a complicated procedure, it is tricky enough that you should not attempt it yourself.

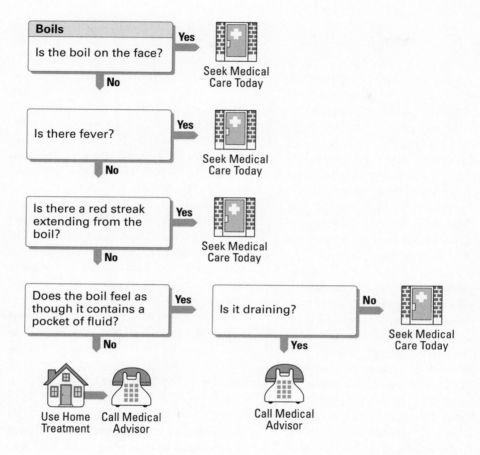

Boils

Is the boil on the face? — **Yes** → Seek Medical Care Today

No ↓

Is there fever? — **Yes** → Seek Medical Care Today

No ↓

Is there a red streak extending from the boil? — **Yes** → Seek Medical Care Today

No ↓

Does the boil feel as though it contains a pocket of fluid? — **Yes** → Is it draining? — **No** → Seek Medical Care Today

No ↓

Use Home Treatment   Call Medical Advisor

Yes ↓

Call Medical Advisor

Acne

Acne begins before puberty with the accumulation of skin cells (keratinocytes) and oil (sebum) in skin follicles. The accumulation can plug the skin follicle and form what is called a microcomedo. Why this process occurs is not known.

As puberty approaches, an increase in male hormones from the adrenal gland causes more sebum to be produced. This distends the follicle and converts a microcomedo into a whitehead or closed comedo. As sebum continues to accumulate, the follicle opens, forming a blackhead or open comedo. Densely packed keratinocytes, oxidized sebum, and melanin all contribute to the dark color of the blackhead.

Inflammation occurs when the comedo becomes infected with a bacterium called *P. acne,* one of the bacteria that are normally found on the skin. Inflammation causes the follicle to rupture into the surrounding skin with the formation of pustules, papules, nodules, and/or cysts.

Cosmetics may contribute to the development of acne. Oils, greases, and dyes in hair products and cosmetics can make acne worse, while water-based products are less likely to be a problem.

Any kind of rough treatment that promotes rupture of follicles into skin can make acne much worse. While scrubbing with soaps, detergents, and astringents will remove sebum from the skin surface, it actually may make things worse by promoting inflammation. Anything that rubs the skin—turtlenecks, bra straps, shoulder pads, orthopedic casts, sports helmets—can have the same effect.

Humidity and heavy sweating also can exacerbate acne, so avoiding occlusive clothing and hot, humid conditions can help.

Medications that can sometimes cause acne include ACTH, androgens, azathioprine, barbiturates, bromides, corticosteroids, cyclosporine, disulfiram, halogens, iodides, isoniazid, lithium, phenytoin, psoralens, thiourea, and vitamins B2, B6, and B12.

A rare type of acne, chloracne, is caused by exposure to halogenated hydrocarbons. These chemicals are found in industrial products such as cutting oils and herbicides, in contaminated food products, and in chemical warfare.

Diet does not influence production of sebum; research has not identified a link between diet and acne. Diet modification, such as avoiding chocolate, usually has been unsuccessful.

Home Treatment

The first step is to avoid those things that can make acne worse (see above).

Benzoyl peroxide, a topical antibiotic, is the active ingredient in most nonprescription acne preparations. It reduces inflammation by combating the *P. acne* infection. It also helps to open and drain comedos. There are many such preparations. Choosing among them is largely a matter of personal preference and price.

A few nonprescription preparations (Pernox, etc.) contain salicylic acid, a chemical that is effective in opening comedos.

If nonprescription medications fail to control the problem, make an appointment with the doctor.

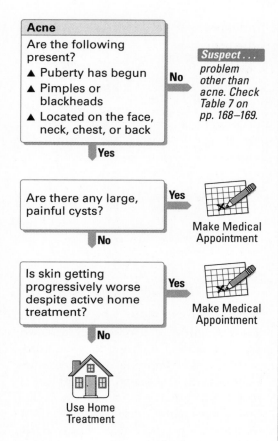

Acne

Are the following present?

▲ Puberty has begun

▲ Pimples or blackheads

▲ Located on the face, neck, chest, or back

No → *Suspect...* problem other than acne. Check Table 7 on pp. 168–169.

Yes ↓

Are there any large, painful cysts?

Yes → Make Medical Appointment

No ↓

Is skin getting progressively worse despite active home treatment?

Yes → Make Medical Appointment

No ↓

Use Home Treatment

What to Expect at the Doctor's Office

The doctor will reinforce the need to avoid factors that make acne worse. Use of benzoyl peroxide and/or salicylic acid preparations likely will be continued.

Many medicines are available for the treatment of acne; often the same medicine may be used topically or given orally. The choice of medicines will depend on the type and severity of acne.

Topical retinoids (tretinoin, isotretinoin, adapaline) are usually the first choice for treating comedos. These drugs can have significant side effects, so be sure you understand their use before leaving the doctor's office. Although topical isotretinoin does not pose the same threat to pregnancy as does oral isotretinoin, it is contraindicated when pregnancy is possible.

Oral isotretinoin (Accutane) is very useful in severe acne, but it is a powerful drug that can cause serious side effects. If taken by a pregnant woman, there's a very high risk that the baby will be harmed. **Women who might be pregnant should not take isotretinoin.**

Antibiotics, either topically or orally or both, are almost always prescribed. Combinations of antibiotics are often used in topical preparations to increase effectiveness and to decrease the development of resistant strains of *P. acne.*

Hormones (estrogens or antiandrogens) maybe an alternative to oral isotretinoin in women with acne that does not respond to other treatments. Glucocorticoids are sometimes used when there is excessive adrenal androgen production.

In addition to drugs, there are other therapies that may help some individuals. Comedo extraction is a simple office procedure. Chemical peels with glycolic acid or other chemicals may be used to decrease acne papules. Blue light therapy (ClearLight) is expensive and only works in about one-third of cases. Pulsed dye laser (PDL) treatment may help and is being studied.

Athlete's Foot

Athlete's foot is very common during and after adolescence, and relatively uncommon before. It is the most common of the fungal infections and is often persistent. When it involves toenails, it can be difficult to treat.

Moisture contributes significantly to the development of this problem. Some doctors believe bacteria and moisture cause most of the problem and that the fungus is responsible only for keeping things going. When many people share locker room and shower facilities, exposure to this fungus is impossible to prevent; infection is the rule rather than the exception. But you don't have to participate in sports to contract this fungus; it's all around.

Home Treatment

Scrupulous hygiene, without resorting to drugs, is often effective. Twice a day, wash the space between the toes with soap, water, and a cloth. Dry the entire area carefully with a towel, particularly between the toes (despite the pain) and put on clean socks.

Use shoes that allow evaporation of moisture. Avoid shoes with plastic linings. Sandals or canvas sneakers are best. Changing shoes every other day to allow them to dry out is a good idea.

Keeping the feet dry with the use of a powder is helpful in preventing reinfection. Over-the-counter drugs such as Desenex powder or cream may be used. The powder has the virtue of helping keep the toes dry. Topical antifungals (page 71) are effective.

Athlete's Foot

Are both of the following conditions present?

▲ Redness and scaling between toes (may have cracks and small blisters)

▲ Itching

No → *Suspect...* problem other than athlete's foot. Check Table 7 on pp. 168–169.

Yes ↓

Use Home Treatment

What to Expect at the Doctor's Office

Through history, physical examination, and, possibly, microscopic examination of a skin scraping, the doctor will establish the diagnosis. Several other problems, notably a condition called dyshydrosis, may mimic athlete's foot. Oral antifungals may be used in resistant cases. Oral drugs are also used for the nails but cure the problem only about 30% of the time.

Jock Itch

We might wish for a less graphic name for this condition, but the medical term, *tinea cruris*, is understood by few. Jock itch is a fungal infection of the pubic region. It is aggravated by friction and moisture. It usually doesn't involve the scrotum or penis, nor does it spread beyond the groin area. (For the most part, this is a male disease.) Frequently, the fungus grows in an athletic supporter turned old and moldy in a locker room far from a washing machine. The preventive measure for such a problem is obvious.

Home Treatment

The problem should be treated by removing the contributing factors: friction and moisture. This is done by wearing boxer shorts rather than closer-fitting shorts or jockey briefs, by applying a powder to dry the area after bathing, and by frequently changing soiled or sweaty underclothes. It may take up to two weeks to completely clear up the problem, and it may recur. The "powder-air-and-clean-shorts" treatment will usually be successful without any medication. Topical antifungals will usually eliminate the fungus if the problem persists (page 71).

What to Expect at the Doctor's Office

Occasionally, a yeast infection will mimic jock itch. By examining the area and asking questions, the doctor will try to establish the diagnosis and may also make a scraping in order to identify yeast. Medicines for this problem are virtually always applied to the affected skin; oral drugs are rarely used.

Jock Itch

Are all of the following conditions present?

▲ Involves only the groin and thighs

▲ Redness, oozing, or some peripheral scaling

▲ Itching

No → *Suspect...* problem other than jock itch. Check Table 7 on pp. 168–169.

Yes

Use Home Treatment

Sunburn

Sunburn is common, painful, and avoidable. It is better prevented than treated. Effective sunscreens are available in a wide variety of strengths, as indicated by their sun protection factor, or SPF. An SPF of 4 offers little protection, whereas 15 or above offers substantial protection. Use a waterproof product if you are going to get wet, and don't forget the long sleeves and the hat.

Regardless of what you have heard, there are no sun rays that tan but don't burn. Tanning salons can fry you just as surely as the sun can.

The pain of sunburn is worst between 6 and 48 hours after sun exposure. Peeling of injured layers of skin occurs later—between 3 and 10 days after the burn.

Very rarely, people with sunburn have difficulty with vision. If so, they should see a doctor. Otherwise, a visit to the doctor is unnecessary unless the pain is extraordinarily severe or extensive blistering (not peeling) has occurred. Blistering indicates a second-degree burn and only rarely follows sun exposure.

The worst consequence of sunburn is malignant melanoma, a potentially fatal cancer. It is the result of sun exposure, most usually the exposure in the teenage years, and doctors often cite the danger of "three or more blistering sunburns before the age of 18" as a possible cause. It is usually completely preventable with the timely interventions of "high number" sunscreens and avoidance of direct sun exposure with clothing and hats, avoidance of tanning salons, and seeking shade. The good doctor will take the time to remind you that sunburn causes skin cancer and that skin cancer can be fatal.

Home Treatment

Cool compresses or cool oatmeal baths (Aveeno, etc.) may be useful. Ordinary baking soda (one-half cup to a tub) is nearly as effective. Lubricants such as Vaseline feel good to some people, but they retain heat and shouldn't be used the first day. Be careful with products that contain benzocaine. These may give temporary relief but can irritate the skin and may actually delay healing. Pain-relieving medication may ease pain and thus help the person sleep (page 54). Hydrocortisone creams may decrease inflammation and decrease pain.

What to Expect at the Doctor's Office

The doctor will direct the history and physical examination toward determining the extent of the burn and the possibility of other heat-related injuries like sunstroke. If only first-degree burns are found, a prescription corticosteroid lotion may be prescribed. This isn't particularly beneficial. The rare second-degree burns may be treated with antibiotics in addition to analgesics (pain relievers).

Sunburn

Are any of these conditions present following prolonged exposure to sun?

▲ Fever
▲ Fluid-filled blisters
▲ Dizziness
▲ Visual difficulties

Yes

Call Medical Advisor

No

Use Home Treatment

Frostbite

Minor frostbite is surprisingly common among skiers and others indulging in winter sports. Prevention is the key. Wear warm clothing. When your torso is warm, the blood flow to the fingers and toes is better. Don't forget a face mask. Use mittens instead of gloves when it is very cold. If there is wind, be sure that you have windproof outer garments.

If your fingers or nose or toes start to hurt despite these precautions, it's a warning to get out of the cold. If they begin to numb, you are starting to get frostbite. It used to be said that you should warm up a frostbitten limb slowly. Not so. Warm it up as quickly as possible. Dip the limb in warm water—100° to 104°F (38° to 40°C)—if you can. Do not rub the affected area. As the blood flow resumes, the frostbitten part will begin to hurt, sometimes a lot. This is a good sign, since the tissues are obviously still alive.

You may have leftover numbness for several months after minor frostbite, but this doesn't require medical attention. However, if tissues turn black, see a doctor so that the threatened tissues can be preserved.

Lice and Bedbugs

Lice and bedbugs are found in the best of families. Lack of prejudice with respect to social class is as close as these insects come to having a virtue. At best, they are a nuisance, and at worst, they can cause real disability.

Lice

Lice themselves are very small and are seldom seen without the aid of a magnifying glass. Usually it is easier to find the "nits," which are clusters of louse eggs. Without magnification, nits will appear as tiny white lumps on hair strands.

The louse bite leaves only a pinpoint red spot, but scratching makes things worse. Itching and occasional small, shallow sores at the bases of hairs are clues to the disease.

Pubic lice aren't a venereal disease, although they may be spread from person to person during sexual contact. Unlike syphilis and gonorrhea, lice may be spread by toilet seats, infected linen, and other sources. Pubic lice bear some resemblance to crabs. Hence, the term "crabs" is used to indicate a lice infestation of the pubic hair. A different species of louse may inhabit the scalp or other body hair.

Lice like to be close to a warm body all the time and won't stay for long in clothing that isn't being worn, or in bedding or other places.

Bedbugs

Although related to lice, bedbugs present a considerably different picture. The adult is flat, wingless, reddish in color, oval in shape, and about one-quarter inch (6 mm) in length. Like lice, they stay alive by sucking blood. Unlike lice, they feed for only 10 to 15 minutes at a time and spend the rest of the time hiding in crevices and crannies.

Bedbugs feed almost entirely at night, because that is when bodies are in bed and because bedbugs strongly dislike light. They have such a keen sense of the nearness of a warm body that the army has used them to detect the approach of an enemy at ranges of several hundred feet! Catching these pests out in the open is very difficult and may require some curious behavior. One technique is to dash into the bedroom at bedtime, flip on the lights, and pull back the bedcovers in an effort to catch them anticipating their next meal.

The bite of the bedbug leaves a firm bump. Usually, there are two or three bumps clustered together. Occasionally, sensitivity develops to these bites, in which case, itching may be severe and blisters may form.

Home Treatment

Over-the-counter preparations containing permethrin or pyrethrins are effective against lice. (RID has the advantage of supplying a fine-tooth comb, a rare item these days.) Instructions that come with these drugs must be followed carefully. Linen and clothing must be changed simultaneously. Sexual partners should be treated at the same time.

Because bedbugs don't hide on the body or in clothes, it is the bed and the room that should be treated. Contact your local health department for information and help in doing this. Chemical sprays may be useful, but simply getting

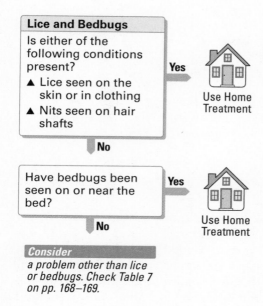

Lice and Bedbugs

Is either of the following conditions present?
▲ Lice seen on the skin or in clothing
▲ Nits seen on hair shafts

Yes → Use Home Treatment

No ↓

Have bedbugs been seen on or near the bed?

Yes → Use Home Treatment

No ↓

Consider
a problem other than lice or bedbugs. Check Table 7 on pp. 168–169.

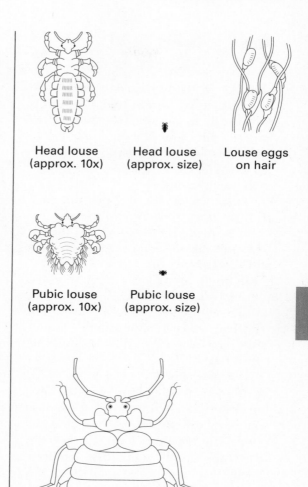

Head louse
(approx. 10x)

Head louse
(approx. size)

Louse eggs
on hair

Pubic louse
(approx. 10x)

Pubic louse
(approx. size)

Bedbug
(approx. 10x)

Bedbug
(approx. size)

the infested bedding outdoors and exposed to sun and air for several days works, too.

What to Expect at the Doctor's Office

If lice are the suspected problem, the doctor will make a careful inspection to find nits or the lice themselves. Doctors often use the same compounds used in the over-the-counter preparations (permethrin, pyrethrins). Malathion is available by prescription and is sometimes used.

The doctor will be hard-pressed to make a certain diagnosis of bedbug bites without information from you that bedbugs have been seen in the house. However, the bumps may be suggestive, and initially it may be decided to assume that the problem is bedbugs. If this is the case, treatment with an insecticide as discussed under Home Treatment will be recommended.

Ticks

Outdoor living has its dangers. While bears, mountain lions, and steep cliffs can usually be avoided, shrubs and tall grasses hide tiny insects eager for a blood meal from a passing animal or person. Ticks are the most common of these small hazards.

Ticks are about one-quarter inch (6 mm) long and are easily seen. The tick that made the tick bite can usually be found sticking out of it, head buried and legs kicking.

In some areas, ticks carry diseases, such as Rocky Mountain spotted fever and Lyme disease. If a fever, rash, joint pains, or headache follows a tick bite by a few days or weeks, a doctor should be consulted.

If a pregnant female tick is allowed to remain feeding for several days, under certain circumstances, a peculiar condition called tick paralysis may develop. The female tick secretes a toxin that can cause temporary paralysis, which clears up shortly after the tick is removed. This complication is quite rare and can happen only if the tick stays in place many days.

In tick-infested areas, check yourself, your children, and your pets several times a day. You may be able to catch the ticks before they become embedded.

Home Treatment

Ticks should be removed, although they will eventually "fester out"; complications are unusual. The trick is to get the tick to "let go" and not to squeeze the tick before getting it out. If the mouthparts and the pincers remain under the skin, heal-

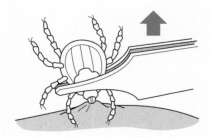

Removing a tick

ing may require several weeks. Rocky Mountain spotted fever and Lyme disease are somewhat more likely if mouthparts are left in or the tick is squeezed during removal. Make the tick uncomfortable: for example, put a lighted match an inch or so away from the tick and move it toward the tick slowly until the tick starts to kick its legs around and, at the same time, disengages its mouth parts. Then, grasp the tick with tweezers or with gloved fingers as close to the skin as possible, and pull straight out with slow, even pressure. If the head is inadvertently left under the skin, soak gently with warm water twice daily until healing is complete. Call the doctor at once if the person gets a fever, rash, or headache within three weeks. If the tick has been left attached for more than a day, Lyme disease is more likely, so remove the tick as soon as possible.

What to Expect at the Doctor's Office

The doctor can remove the tick but can't prevent any illness that might have been transmitted except Lyme disease. Early antibiotics can blunt or prevent Lyme disease. However, Lyme disease occurs only in localized areas where deer ticks may be infected with the spirochete that

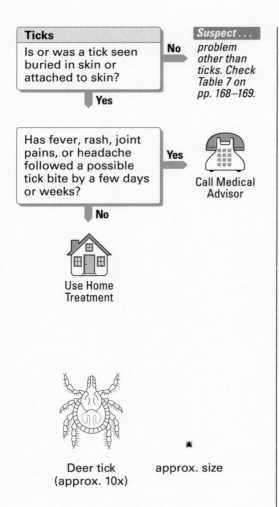

Ticks

Is or was a tick seen buried in skin or attached to skin?

No → *Suspect...* problem other than ticks. Check Table 7 on pp. 168–169.

Yes ↓

Has fever, rash, joint pains, or headache followed a possible tick bite by a few days or weeks?

Yes → Call Medical Advisor

No ↓

Use Home Treatment

Deer tick (approx. 10x)   approx. size

causes the illness. Your doctor may know where that is. Otherwise, you can do just as well with the tweezers. Ticks are often removed from unusual places, such as armpits and belly buttons, but the scalp is the most common location. The technique is exactly the same no matter where the tick is.

Chiggers

Chiggers, like ticks, are a small hazard of nature. Anyone who grew up in areas where they are common can testify to how excruciating the itch from chiggers' bites can be.

Chiggers are small red mites, sometimes called "redbugs," that live on grasses and shrubs. Their bite contains a chemical that eats away at the skin, causing a tremendous itch. Usually, the small red sores are around the belt line or other openings in clothes. Careful inspection may reveal the tiny red larvae in the center of the itching sore.

Home Treatment

Chiggers are better avoided than treated. Using insect repellents, wearing appropriate clothing, and bathing after exposure help to cut down on the frequency of bites. Once you get them, they itch, often for several weeks. Keep the sores clean and soak them with warm water twice daily. Anti-lice medications (page 198) applied immediately may help kill the larvae, but the itch will persist.

Corticosteroid creams (Cortaid, Lanacort, etc.) may be tried but are usually not much help. Don't use these creams for more than a week or two without a doctor's advice (page 71).

Nail polish is said to give relief from itching, but we aren't aware of scientific studies of its effect.

Antihistamines (page 62) aren't often used unless intense itching persists despite home treatment with over-the-counter pain relievers (page 54), warm baths, oatmeal soaks (Aveeno, etc.), and calamine lotion.

What to Expect at the Doctor's Office

Doctors may use either a topical cream or a pill. These are probably more effective than anti-lice medicines for killing the larvae, but they don't stop the itching either. So, most often, doctors use home treatment too.

Chiggers

Are any of the following present?

- ▲ Itching red sores around the belt line or other opening in clothes
- ▲ Itching red sores following contact with grass or shrubs
- ▲ Small red mites seen on the skin or red spot in center of sore

No →

Suspect... *problem other than chiggers. Check Table 7 on pp. 168–169.*

↓ **Yes**

Use Home Treatment

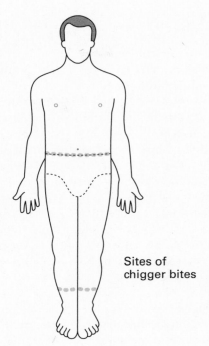

Sites of chigger bites

Scabies

Scabies is an irritation of the skin caused by a tiny mite related to the chigger. No one knows why, but scabies seems to be on the rise in the United States. As with lice, it is no longer true that scabies is related to hygiene. It occurs in the best of families and in the cleanest of neighborhoods. The mite easily spreads from person to person or by contact with items such as clothing and bedding that may harbor the mite. Epidemics often spread through schools despite strict precautions against contact with known cases.

The mite burrows into the skin to lay eggs; its favorite locations are given in the decision chart. These burrows may be evident, especially at the beginning of the problem. However, the mite soon causes the skin to have a reaction so that redness, swelling, and blisters follow within a short period. Intense itching causes scratching, so there are plenty of scratch marks. These may become infected from the bacteria on the skin. Thus, the telltale burrows are often obscured by scratch marks, blisters, and secondary infection.

If you can locate something that looks like a burrow, you might be able to see the mite with the aid of a magnifying lens. This is the only way to be absolutely sure that the problem is scabies, but it is often not possible. The diagnosis is most often made based on symptoms and history that are consistent with scabies, as well as the fact that scabies is known to be in the community.

Home Treatment

Benzyl benzoate (25% solution) is effective against scabies and doesn't require a prescription. Unfortunately, it isn't widely available. If you are able to find it, apply it once to the entire body except for the face and around the urinary opening of the penis or the vaginal opening. Wash it off 24 hours later. This medicine does have an odor that some find unpleasant. If you can't find benzyl benzoate, you'll have to get a prescription from your doctor.

For itching, we recommend cool soaks, calamine lotion, and/or over-the-counter pain medicines (page 54). Antihistamines may help (page 62); follow the directions on the package. As in the case of poison ivy, warmth makes the itching worse by releasing histamine, but if all the histamine is released, relief may be obtained for several hours (see Poison Ivy and Poison Oak, page 182).

It will take some time before the skin becomes normal, even with effective treatment, but at least some improvement should be noted within 72 hours. If this isn't the case, visit the doctor.

What to Expect at the Doctor's Office

The doctor should examine the entire skin surface for signs of the problem and may examine an area with a magnifying lens in an attempt to identify the mite. A scraping of a lesion may be taken for examination under a microscope. Most of the time, the doctor will be forced to make a decision based on the probability of various kinds of diseases and then treat it much as you would at home. The proof will be whether or not the treatment is successful.

Scabies

Are all of the following conditions present?

▲ Intense itching
▲ Raised red skin in a line (represents a burrow) and possibly blisters or pustules
▲ Located on the hands, especially between the fingers, in the elbow crease, armpit, groin crease, or behind the knees
▲ Exposure to scabies

No →

Suspect . . .
problem other than scabies. Check Table 7 on pp. 168–169.

Yes

Use Home Treatment

A prescription cream or oral medicine will be prescribed depending on how widespread the problem is. Often the advice will be to use hydrocortisol cream (1%) for several days, several times a day. This cream is readily available without a prescription. Prolonged use, perhaps a month or more, can result in thinning of the skin. It is very helpful, but use it cautiously.

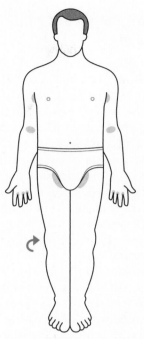

Sites of scabies bites

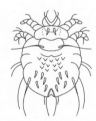

Scabies mite, greatly enlarged (approx. size: ·)

Dandruff and Cradle Cap

Although they look different, cradle cap and dandruff are really part of the same problem; its medical term is seborrhea. Oil glands in the skin become stimulated by adult hormones, leading to oiliness and flaking of the scalp. This occurs in infants because of exposure to the mother's hormones and in older children when they begin to make their own adult hormones. The problem also occurs between infancy and puberty, and once a child has the problem, it tends to recur.

Seborrhea itself is a somewhat ugly but relatively harmless condition. However, it may make the skin more susceptible to infection with yeast or bacteria. Children with seborrhea frequently have redness and scaling of the eyebrows and behind the ears as well.

Look-alike Problems
Occasionally this condition is mistaken for ringworm of the scalp. Careful attention to the conditions listed in the decision chart will usually avoid this confusion. Remember also that ringworm would be unusual in the newborn and very young child. See Ringworm (page 178).

Another potentially confusing problem is psoriasis. This condition resembles seborrhea somewhat but often stops at the hairline. The scales of psoriasis are on top of raised lesions called "plaques," which isn't the case in seborrhea. Home treatment is unlikely to be helpful for psoriasis, so the help of a doctor is needed.

Home Treatment
Many widely available antidandruff shampoos are helpful in mild to moderate cases of dandruff. For severe and more stubborn cases, there are some less well known but effective over-the-counter shampoos that contain selenium sulfide. Selsun (available by prescription only) and Selsun Blue are examples of such shampoos. Over-the-counter preparations, while weaker, are just as good if you apply them more liberally and frequently. When using these shampoos, it is important that you follow the directions carefully because oiliness and yellowish discoloration of the hair may occur. Sebulex, Sebucare, and Ionil are effective and must be used strictly according to directions also.

Cradle cap is best treated with a soft scrub brush. If cradle cap is thick, rub in warm baby oil, cover with a warm towel, and leave for 15 minutes. Use a fine-tooth comb or scrub brush to help remove the scales. Then shampoo with Sebulex or one of the other preparations listed above. Be careful to avoid getting shampoo in the eyes.

No matter what you do, the problem will often return, and you may have to repeat the treatment. If the problem gets worse despite home treatment over several weeks, see the doctor.

What to Expect at the Doctor's Office
Severe cases of seborrhea may require more than the medications mentioned above; a cortisone cream is most often prescribed. Usually a trip to the doctor clears up any question concerning the diagnosis. The doctor generally makes the diagnosis on the basis of the appearance of the rash.

Dandruff

In an infant, are all of the following conditions present?

▲ Thick, adherent, oily, yellowish scaling or crusting patches

▲ Located on the scalp, behind the ears, in the eyebrows, or (less frequently) in the skin creases of the groin

▲ Only mild redness in involved areas

No →

Suspect . . .
problem other than cradle cap. Check Table 7 on pp. 168–169.

In an older child (or adult), are all of the following conditions present?

▲ Fine, white, oily scales

▲ Confined to scalp and/or eyebrows

▲ Only mild redness in involved areas

No →

Suspect . . .
problem other than dandruff. Check Table 7 on pp. 168–169.

↓ **Yes**

Use Home Treatment

Occasionally, scrapings from the involved areas will be looked at under the microscope. Drugs by mouth or by injection aren't indicated for seborrhea unless bacterial infection has complicated the problem.

Patchy Loss of Skin Color

Seeing patches of paler skin on yourself or your child can be unnerving. Luckily, this condition is usually temporary and harmless.

Children are constantly getting minor cuts, scrapes, insect bites, and minor skin infections. During the healing process, it is common for the skin to lose some of its color. With time, the skin coloring generally returns.

Occasionally ringworm, a fungal infection, will begin as a small round area of scaling with associated loss of skin color (page 178).

In the summertime, many children have small round spots on the face in which there is little color. The spots have probably been present for some time, but skin doesn't tan in these areas, thus making them visible. This condition is known as pityriasis alba. The cause is unknown, but it is a mild condition of cosmetic concern only. It may take many months to disappear and may recur, but there are virtually never any long-term effects.

If there are slightly scaly, tan, pink, or white patches on the neck or back, the problem is most likely due to a fungal infection known as tinea versicolor. This is a very minor and superficial fungal infection.

Home Treatment

Waiting is the most effective home treatment for loss of skin color. Topical antifungal lotions and creams are effective (page 71). Unfortunately, tinea versicolor often comes back no matter what type of treatment is used.

What to Expect at the Doctor's Office

A history and careful examination of the skin will be performed. Scrapings of the lesions may be taken because tinea versicolor can be identified from them. Pityriasis alba should be distinguished from more severe fungal infections that may occur on the face. Again, scrapings will help to identify the fungus.

Patchy Skin Color

Are the following conditions present?
- ▲ Scaling edges
- ▲ Circular enlarging areas
- ▲ Clearing of center

Yes → *See:* Ringworm, p. 178

No ↓

Are the following conditions present?
- ▲ Lightly scaled, tan, pink, or white confluent patches
- ▲ Confined to the neck and upper back

Yes → *Suspect...* *tinea versicolor and...*

Use Home Treatment

No ↓

Are the following conditions present?
- ▲ White scaly patches on face
- ▲ More noticeable with suntan
- ▲ No signs of infection (crusting, redness, oozing, or fever)

Yes → *Suspect...* *pityriasis alba and...*

Use Home Treatment

No ↓

Did loss of skin color follow cut or infection?

Yes →

Use Home Treatment

No ↓

Call Medical Advisor

Aging Spots, Wrinkles, and Baldness

Our aging skin presents a lot of superficial problems. The problems result from a combination of two factors:

▲ As we age, the skin loses its elasticity. It develops more scar tissue and doesn't spring back as quickly into a smooth contour.

▲ Damage from the sun accumulates over a lifetime and causes additional problems in the sun-exposed areas of the body.

The aging skin lets air leak into the hair follicles so that the hair turns white. Some or all hair follicles lose the ability to produce hairs at all, and the hair thins or disappears. The loss of elasticity means that skin tends to sag, and crinkles in the face turn into deeper, fixed wrinkles.

In general, don't worry about these problems. The aging face is expressive of character. Thinning hair and baldness aren't diseases, nor are aging spots.

Aging spots are pigmentary changes in the skin without any medical significance. Some cells lose the ability to produce the pigment melanin, whereas others produce a bit too much of it. These changes can be thought of as an adult form of freckles. As such, they are flat, are uniformly brown or tan in color, and have regular borders. If they are raised, are irregular in outline, or have multiple colors in one spot (especially shades of red, white, and blue), see Skin Cancer (page 186).

Home Treatment

Stay out of the sun and use a sunscreen. This is particularly important if you are fair-skinned because such skin is far more prone to sun damage. Outside of these precautions, there isn't much you can do at home for these problems except not to worry about them. And that is all that is really needed.

For baldness, minoxidil (Rogaine) is now available without prescription. It is an effective medication for improving hair growth and can cause new hair to grow over previously bald spots. Unfortunately, the new minoxidil hair isn't usually everything that you would want; it is unusual that very much hair grows back, and the older you are, the less effective this treatment is.

What to Expect at the Doctor's Office

There are good medical approaches to these "problems," but they are entirely optional. Many people prefer their natural aging appearance to artificial cosmetic devices. Others, who can afford it, elect to fight the aging stereotype by a variety of measures that preserve a more youthful appearance. Alternatives currently available have low risk but high cost. The choices range all the way from wrinkle creams to an elaborate series of plastic surgery operations.

If you want to go the expensive route, you probably should see a dermatologist first and then, perhaps, a plastic surgeon. The dermatologist is likely to be more familiar with the effective cosmetic interventions than a family physician or internist. The dermatologist is also the key person to take care of any lumps and bumps about which you are concerned.

Retin-A is the first wrinkle cream that actually works. Unfortunately, Retin-A doesn't seem to work very well with old,

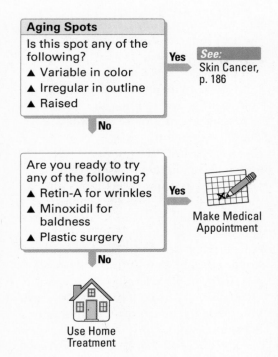

Aging Spots

Is this spot any of the following?
▲ Variable in color
▲ Irregular in outline
▲ Raised

Yes → *See:* Skin Cancer, p. 186

No ↓

Are you ready to try any of the following?
▲ Retin-A for wrinkles
▲ Minoxidil for baldness
▲ Plastic surgery

Yes → Make Medical Appointment

No ↓

Use Home Treatment

---

fixed wrinkles, it may cause heat rashes in skin exposed to the sun, and it dries out the skin.

Plastic Surgery

The plastic surgeon can take out wrinkles by removing skin and stretching the remaining skin tighter. Many procedures are available. Wrinkles around the eyes can be taken out, as can bags under the eyes. A full facelift tightens the skin over the entire face. Sagging breasts can be reduced in size and lifted. Tucks can be taken in the tummy. Liposuction can remove fat, although the result is usually a little lumpy. Hair transplants can be partially effective in some people. Again, in good hands, done by a surgeon who performs the procedure often, these operations have low risk. However, they are expensive. There is pain and discomfort involved. There is an occasional serious complication. With some of the procedures, you won't want to be seen in public for a week or so after the operation.

CHAPTER 7

Childhood Diseases

Mumps

Mumps is a viral infection of the salivary glands. The major salivary glands are located directly below and in front of the ear. Before any swelling is noticeable, there may be a low fever, headache, earache, or weakness. Fever is variable. It may be only slightly above normal or as high as 104°F (40°C). After several days of these symptoms, one or both salivary glands (parotid glands) may swell.

It is sometimes difficult to distinguish mumps from swollen lymph glands in the neck (page 146). In mumps, you won't be able to feel the edge of the jaw that is located beneath the ear. Chewing and swallowing may produce pain behind the ear. Sour substances such as lemons and pickles may make the pain worse. When swelling occurs on both sides, people take on the appearance of chipmunks! Other salivary glands besides the parotid may be involved, including those under the jaw and tongue. The openings of these glands into the mouth may become red and puffy.

Approximately one-third of all patients who have mumps don't demonstrate any swelling of glands whatsoever. Therefore, many people concerned about exposure to mumps will already have had the disease without realizing it.

Mumps is quite contagious during the period from two days before the first symptoms to the complete disappearance of the parotid gland swelling, usually about a week after the swelling has begun. Mumps will develop in a susceptible exposed person approximately 16 to 18 days after exposure to the virus. In children, it is generally a mild illness.

The decision chart is directed toward detection of rare complications. These include encephalitis (viral infection of the brain), pancreatitis (viral infection of the pancreas), kidney disease, deafness, and involvement of the testicles or the ovaries. Complications are more frequent in adults than in children.

Home Treatment

Over-the-counter pain relievers are important (page 54). (**Caution:** Aspirin never should be given to children or teenagers if the possibility of a viral infection exists.) There may be difficulty in eating, but adequate fluid intake is important. Sour foods should be avoided, including orange juice. Adults who haven't had mumps should avoid exposure to the patient until the swelling disappears completely.

Many adults who don't recall having mumps as a child may have had an

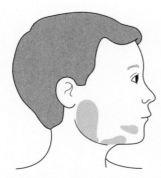

Sites of swelling in mumps

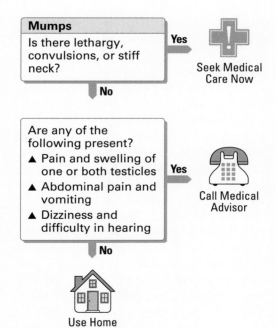

Mumps

Is there lethargy, convulsions, or stiff neck? — **Yes** → Seek Medical Care Now

No ↓

Are any of the following present?
▲ Pain and swelling of one or both testicles
▲ Abdominal pain and vomiting
▲ Dizziness and difficulty in hearing — **Yes** → Call Medical Advisor

No ↓

Use Home Treatment

extremely mild case and consequently aren't at risk of developing mumps.

If swelling hasn't gone down within three weeks, call the doctor.

What to Expect at the Doctor's Office

If a complication is suspected, a visit to the doctor's office may be necessary. The history and physical examination will be directed at confirming the diagnosis or the presence of a complication. The rare complication of an ovarian mumps infection on the right side may be confused with appendicitis, and blood tests may be required. Because mumps is a viral disease, there is no medicine that will directly kill the virus. Supportive measures may be necessary for some of the complications. Fortunately, complications are rare, and permanent damage to hearing or other functions is unusual. Mumps very rarely produces sterility in men or women even when the testes or ovaries are involved.

The mumps vaccination is listed on page 30. Infants should be immunized at 15 months. Adolescents who have never had mumps or the immunization should be vaccinated because of the potential for testicular or ovarian inflammation.

Chicken Pox

Because chicken pox spreads quickly and because taking aspirin during this disease is associated with Reye's syndrome, it is valuable to know its signs.

Signs of Chicken Pox

Before the Rash. Occasionally, there is fatigue and some fever 24 hours before.

The Rash. The typical rash goes through the following stages:

1. It appears as flat red splotches.

2. The splotches become raised and may resemble small pimples.

3. They develop into small fragile blisters, called vesicles. They may look like drops of water on a red base. The tops are easily scratched off.

4. As the vesicles break, the sores become pustular and form a crust. This is dried serum and not true pus. Itching is often severe. This stage may be reached in the first several hours of the rash.

5. The crust falls away between the ninth and thirteenth day.

The vesicles tend to appear in crops (multiple sores appearing at the same time), with two to four crops appearing within two to six days. The rashes often appear first on the scalp and then spread to the rest of the body, but they may begin anywhere. They are most numerous over the shoulders, chest, and back. They are seldom found on the palms of the hands or the soles of the feet. There may be only a few sores or hundreds.

Fever. After most of the sores have formed crusts, the fever usually subsides.

How Chicken Pox Spreads

Chicken pox spreads very easily—over 90% of brothers and sisters catch it. It may be transmitted from 24 hours before the rash up to about 6 days after. It is spread by droplets from the mouth or throat or by direct contact with contaminated articles of clothing. It isn't spread by dry scabs. The incubation period is from 14 to 17 days. Having chicken pox once leads to lifelong immunity, with rare exceptions.

Most of the time, chicken pox should be treated at home. Complications are rare. Two severe complications may require medical treatment: encephalitis (viral infection of the brain) and bacterial infection of the lesions. Encephalitis is rare.

Home Treatment

The major problems in dealing with chicken pox are control of the intense itching and reduction of the fever. Over-the-counter pain and fever medications can help (page 54). Warm baths containing baking soda (one-half cup to a tubful of water) frequently help. Antihistamines may help (page 62).

Caution: Because recent information indicates an association among aspirin, chicken pox, and a rare but serious problem of the liver and brain known as Reye's syndrome, aspirin should never be given to children or teenagers who may have chicken pox or influenza.

Cut the fingernails or use gloves to prevent skin damage from intense scratching. When lesions occur in the mouth, gargling with salt water may help give comfort: add one-half teaspoon

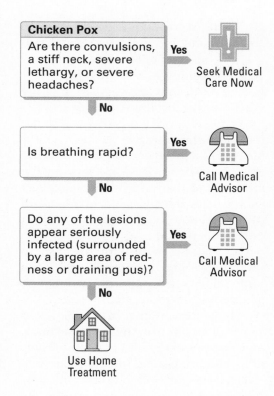

Chicken Pox

Are there convulsions, a stiff neck, severe lethargy, or severe headaches? → **Yes** → Seek Medical Care Now

↓ **No**

Is breathing rapid? → **Yes** → Call Medical Advisor

↓ **No**

Do any of the lesions appear seriously infected (surrounded by a large area of redness or draining pus)? → **Yes** → Call Medical Advisor

↓ **No**

Use Home Treatment

(3 ml) salt to an eight-ounce (150 ml) glass of water. Hands should be washed at least three times a day, and all of the skin should be kept gently but scrupulously clean. Scratching and infection can result in permanent scars.

If itching can't be controlled or the problem persists beyond three weeks, call the doctor. Using the phone or email for questions to the doctor will avoid exposing others to the disease. Call the doctor if a child has been exposed who has an immunity problem or is taking steroids, or if a woman is pregnant.

What to Expect at the Doctor's Office

Don't be surprised if the doctor is willing and even anxious to treat the case over

Shingles

The same herpes virus that causes chicken pox also causes shingles, and the individual who has had chicken pox may develop shingles (herpes zoster) later in life. Shingles is usually limited to one side of the body in a broad stripe, representing the skin area of a single nerve. Because it is limited to the nerve in which the virus is living, there is seldom fever, although there may be pain. Follow the same treatment as you do for chicken pox.

Senior citizens are the most likely to develop shingles and to have persistent pain afterward. Talk to your doctor about the pros and cons of having the shingles vaccine. It prevents most cases of the shingles.

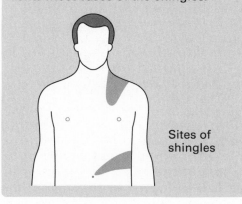

Sites of shingles

the phone. If it is necessary to go to the doctor's office, attempts should be made to keep the patient separate from others. In healthy children, chicken pox has few lasting ill effects, but in people with other serious illnesses, it can be a devastating or even fatal disease. A visit to the doctor's office may not be necessary unless a complication seems possible.

Measles

This type of measles is also called red measles, seven-day measles, and ten-day measles, as opposed to rubella, also called German or three-day measles (page 218). It is a preventable disease but, unlike some of the other childhood illnesses, can be quite severe. It is tragic that decades after the licensing of the measles vaccine, thousands of people still contract this disease annually, and some of them die. We would like to be able to eliminate this section in the next edition of this book. Only immunization of everyone can make this possible. Some parents and even groups of parents believe that the measles vaccine causes autism. This possibility has been completely disproved.

How to Recognize Measles

Early Signs. Measles is a viral illness that begins with fever, weakness, a dry "brassy" cough, and inflamed eyes that are itchy, red, and sensitive to light. These symptoms begin three to five days before the appearance of the rash.

Another early sign of measles is the appearance of fine white spots on a red base inside the mouth opposite the molar teeth (Koplik's spots). These fade as the skin rash appears.

The Rash. The rash begins on about the fifth day as a pink, blotchy, flat rash. The rash first appears around the hairline, on the face, on the neck, and behind the ears. The spots, which fade early in the illness when pressure is applied, become somewhat darker and tend to merge into larger red patches as they mature.

The rash spreads from head to chest to abdomen and finally to the arms and legs. It lasts from four to seven days and may be accompanied by mild itching. There may be some light brown coloring to the skin lesions as the illness progresses.

How Measles Spreads

Measles is a highly contagious viral disease. It is spread by droplets from the mouth or throat and by direct contact with articles freshly soiled by nose and throat secretions. It may be spread during the period from three to six days before the appearance of the rash to several days after. Symptoms begin in a susceptible person approximately 8 to 12 days after exposure to the virus.

There are a number of complications of measles: sore throats, ear infections, and pneumonia are all common. Many of these complicating infections are due to bacteria and will require antibiotic treatment. The pneumonias can be life threatening. A very serious problem that can lead to permanent damage is measles encephalitis (infection of the brain); life-support measures and treatment of seizures may be necessary when this rare complication occurs.

Home Treatment

Treatment of symptoms is all that is needed for uncomplicated measles. Over-the-counter pain and fever medications (page 54) should be used to keep the fever down and to reduce discomfort. A vaporizer can be used for the cough. Avoid aspirin for children and teenagers because of the rare possibility of Reye's syndrome. Dim lighting in the room is often more comfortable because of the eyes' sensitivity to light.

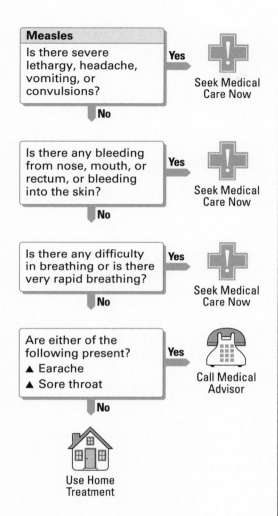

Measles

Is there severe lethargy, headache, vomiting, or convulsions? — **Yes** → Seek Medical Care Now

No ↓

Is there any bleeding from nose, mouth, or rectum, or bleeding into the skin? — **Yes** → Seek Medical Care Now

No ↓

Is there any difficulty in breathing or is there very rapid breathing? — **Yes** → Seek Medical Care Now

No ↓

Are either of the following present?
▲ Earache
▲ Sore throat
— **Yes** → Call Medical Advisor

No ↓

Use Home Treatment

Rash begins around hairline, on face and neck, behind ears

Rash spreads downward to chest and abdomen

Rash affects arms and legs last

Measles. Early signs include red, itchy eyes; "brassy" cough; and Koplik's spots inside mouth.

In general, the person feels "measley." The patient should be isolated until the end of the contagious period. All unimmunized people in contact with the patient should be immunized immediately. (People who have had the measles are considered immunized.)

What to Expect at the Doctor's Office

The history and physical examination will be directed at determining the diagnosis of measles and the nature of any complica-

tions. Bacterial complications, such as ear infections and pneumonia, can usually be treated with antibiotics. The person with symptoms suggestive of encephalitis (lethargy, stiff neck, convulsions) will be hospitalized, and a spinal tap will be performed. Very rarely, there may be a problem with blood clotting so that bleeding occurs. Usually this is first apparent as dark purple splotches in the skin. It is best, however, to avoid all of the problems through measles immunization (page 30).

Rubella

Rubella is also known as German measles and three-day measles. It is different from the disease called red measles, seven-day measles, or ten-day measles (page 216).

How to Recognize Rubella

Before the Rash. There may be a few days of mild fatigue. Lymph nodes at the back of the neck may be enlarged and tender.

The Rash. The rash first appears on the face as flat or slightly raised red spots. It quickly spreads to the trunk and the extremities, and the discrete spots tend to merge into large patches. A rubella rash is highly variable and is difficult for even the most experienced parents and doctors to recognize. Often there is no rash.

Fever. The fever rarely goes above 101°F (38°C) and usually lasts less than two days.

Pain. Joint pain occurs in about 10% to 15% of older children and adults with rubella. The pain usually begins on the third day of illness.

How Rubella Spreads

Rubella is a mild viral infection that isn't as contagious as measles or chicken pox. It is usually spread by droplets from the mouth or throat. It can be spread from seven days before the rash appears until five days afterward.

The incubation period is from 12 to 21 days, with an average of 16 days.

The specific questions on the decision chart are addressed to possible complications, which are extremely rare. The main concern with rubella is an infection in an unborn child. If three-day measles occurs during the first month of pregnancy, there is a 50% chance that the fetus will develop an abnormality such as cataracts, heart disease, deafness, or mental deficiency. By the third month of pregnancy, this risk decreases to less than 10%, and it continues to decrease throughout the pregnancy. Because of the problem of congenital defects, a vaccine for rubella has been developed.

Home Treatment

Usually no therapy is required. Occasionally, fever will require the use of over-the-counter fever medications (page 54). Isolation is usually not imposed. Children and teenagers should use only acetaminophen.

Women who could possibly be pregnant should avoid any exposure to the person with rubella. If a question of such exposure arises, the pregnant woman should discuss the risk with her doctor. Blood tests are available that will indicate whether a pregnant woman has had rubella in the past and is immune, or whether problems with the pregnancy might be encountered. In most states, these tests are required for a marriage license, and there are now few pregnant women who are at risk.

What to Expect at the Doctor's Office

Visits to the doctor's office are seldom required for uncomplicated rubella. Questions about possible infection of pregnant women are more easily and economically discussed over the telephone. Rubella vaccine, part of the

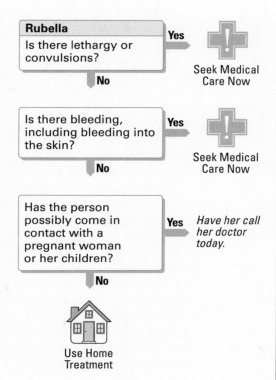

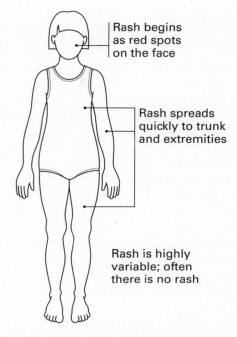

Rash begins as red spots on the face

Rash spreads quickly to trunk and extremities

Rash is highly variable; often there is no rash

Rubella. For a few days before the rash, the child may experience mild fatigue and have enlarged, tender lymph nodes at the back of the neck.

MMR shot, is usually given at about 15 months and 5 years of age. The question of immunization is complex. We discuss it in detail in our book with Dr. Robert Pantell, *Taking Care of Your Child.*

Roseola

Roseola is most common in children under the age of three but may occur at any age. Its main significance lies in the sudden high fever, which may cause a convulsion. Such a convulsion is due to the high temperature and doesn't indicate that the child has epilepsy. Prompt treatment of the fever is essential (page 284).

How to Recognize Roseola

Fever. There are usually several days of sustained high fever. Sometimes this fever can trigger a convulsion or seizure. Otherwise, the child appears well.

The Rash. The rash appears as the fever is decreasing or shortly after it is gone. It consists of pink, well-defined patches that turn white on pressure and first appear on the trunk. It may be slightly bumpy. It spreads to involve the arms, legs, and neck but is seldom prominent on the face or legs. The rash usually lasts less than 24 hours.

Other Symptoms. Occasionally, there is a slight runny nose, red throat, or swollen glands at the back of the head, behind the ears, or in the neck. Most often there are no other symptoms.

This disease is probably caused by a virus and is contagious. Contact with others should be avoided until the fever has passed. The incubation period is from 7 to 17 days.

Encephalitis (infection of the brain) is a very rare complication of roseola. Roseola is basically a mild disease.

Home Treatment

Home treatment is based on two principles. The first is effective treatment of the fever (page 284). Avoid aspirin in children and teenagers because of the rare possibility of Reye's syndrome. The second principle is careful watching and waiting. The patient with roseola should appear well and have no other significant symptoms once the fever is controlled. If symptoms of ear infection (a complaint of ear pain or tugging at the ear—page 130) or cough (page 138) occur, then the appropriate sections of this book should be consulted. Lethargy can be a warning sign of meningitis or encephalitis. If the problem is still not clear, a phone call to the doctor should help.

Remember that roseola shouldn't last more than four or five days. You should call your doctor if the symptoms persist.

What to Expect at the Doctor's Office

Patients are usually seen soon after the onset of the illness because of the high fever. As noted, at this stage, there is little else to be found in roseola. The ears, nose, throat, and chest should be examined. If the fever remains the only finding, then the doctor will recommend home treatment (control of the fever with careful waiting and watching to see if a roseola rash appears). There is no medical treatment for roseola other than that available at home.

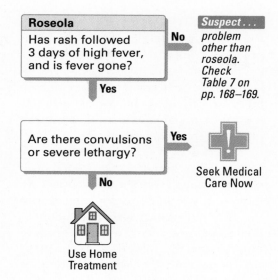

Roseola

Has rash followed 3 days of high fever, and is fever gone?

No → *Suspect . . .* problem other than roseola. Check Table 7 on pp. 168–169.

Yes

Are there convulsions or severe lethargy?

Yes → Seek Medical Care Now

No

Use Home Treatment

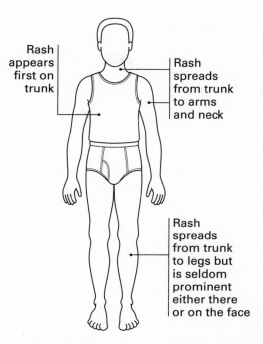

Rash appears first on trunk

Rash spreads from trunk to arms and neck

Rash spreads from trunk to legs but is seldom prominent either there or on the face

Roseola. Several days of sustained high fever may trigger a convulsion or seizure before the onset of the rash.

Scarlet Fever

Scarlet fever derived its name over 300 years ago from its characteristic red rash. The illness is caused by a streptococcal infection, usually of the throat. Strep throats are discussed in Sore Throat (page 128).

You can recognize the illness by its characteristic features.

▲ The rash appears 12 to 48 hours after the illness begins. It begins on the face, trunk, and arms and generally covers the entire body by the end of 24 hours. It is red, is very fine, and covers most of the skin surface. The area around the mouth is pale. The rash feels like fine sandpaper. Skin creases, such as in front of the elbow and the armpit, are more deeply red. Pressing on the rash will produce a white spot lasting several seconds.

▲ Fever and weakness are often accompanied by a headache, stomachache, and vomiting. A sore throat is usually but not always present.

▲ The intense redness of the rash lasts for about five days, although peeling of skin can go on for weeks. It isn't unusual for peeling, especially of the palms, to last for more than a month.

Examination often reveals a red throat, spots on the roof of the mouth (soft palate), and a fuzzy, white tongue that later becomes swollen and red. There may be swollen glands in the neck.

As with other streptococcal infections, the significance of scarlet fever is its connection with rheumatic fever (see Sore Throat, page 128).

Home Treatment

You can't treat scarlet fever yourself at home; you must see your doctor. Because scarlet fever is due to a streptococcal infection, a medical visit is required for antibiotic treatment. Streptococcal infections are quite contagious, and other members of the family should also be tested.

You can treat some of the disease's symptoms at home. To go along with the antibiotics, you should reduce the fever with over-the-counter medications (page 54), keep up with fluid requirements, and give plenty of cold liquids to help soothe the throat. (**Caution:** Aspirin never should be given to children or teenagers if the possibility of a viral infection exists.)

What to Expect at the Doctor's Office

Several rashes can be confused with scarlet fever, including those associated with measles and drug reactions. If the rash is sufficiently typical of scarlet fever, the doctor will probably begin antibiotics, usually penicillin (or erythromycin if the patient is allergic to penicillin), and take throat cultures from the rest of the family. If the doctor is uncertain of the cause of the rash, a throat culture may be taken before beginning treatment. Treatment that is delayed by a day or two while waiting for culture results will still prevent the complication that causes the greatest concern, rheumatic fever.

Scarlet Fever

Are both of the following present?

▲ Fever

▲ Fine, red rash on trunk and extremities that feels like sandpaper

No → *Suspect...* problem other than scarlet fever. Check Table 7 on pp. 168–169.

Yes ↓

Call Medical Advisor

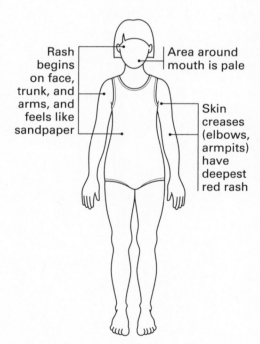

Rash begins on face, trunk, and arms, and feels like sandpaper

Area around mouth is pale

Skin creases (elbows, armpits) have deepest red rash

Scarlet fever. Fever and weakness are often accompanied by headache, stomachache, vomiting, and sore throat.

Ebola Virus

Ebola Hemorrhagic Fever was first identified in 1976 in Sub-Saharan Africa. The virus spreads by direct contact with body fluids, such as blood or semen, or through contact with an item recently contaminated by body fluids. It does not appear to be transmitted through the air.

The disease appears 2 to 21 days after exposure and kills about half of those infected. It can be carried in semen or breast milk for several months. Symptoms are high fever, sore throat, muscle pains, and decreased function of liver and kidneys, associated with low blood pressure and internal leaks of tissue fluids, followed by internal hemorrhaging, shock, and, too often, death. Usually, surviving patients improve within two or three weeks.

It is hoped that the West African outbreak of 2013–2016, with nearly 30,000 cases and more than 11,000 deaths, proves to be the largest outbreak that the world ever encounters. Management was almost entirely by isolation and containment, oral rehydration therapy, burial or cremation of those who died, strict isolation precautions for the sick, protective clothing, compulsive washing of hands and garments, and care for all potential contacts, including dialysis machines and other hospital equipment.

Experience gained with the containment measures should make contamination measures safer in the future, and improved fluid management should reduce complications. And an effective vaccine is on track for approval, most likely in 2017.

Fifth Disease

Consider the strange case of fifth disease, whose only claim to fame is that it might be mistaken for another disease. It is so named because it is always listed last (and least) among the five very common contagious rashes of childhood. Its medical name, *erythema infectiosum*, is easily forgotten.

It comes very close to not being a disease at all. It has no symptoms other than a rash, has no complications, and needs no treatment. It can be recognized because it causes a characteristic "slapped cheek" appearance in children. The rash often begins on the cheeks and is later found on the backs of the arms and legs. It often is very fine, lacy, and pink. It tends to come and go and may be present one moment and absent the next. It is prone to recur for days or even weeks, especially as a response to heat (such as a warm bath or shower) or irritation. In general, however, the rash around the face will fade within four days of its appearance, and the rash on the rest of the body will fade within three to seven days.

The only significance of fifth disease is that it could worry you or have you make an avoidable trip to the doctor's office.

Its recent resurgence makes this more likely. It is very contagious. Epidemics of fifth disease have resulted in unnecessary school closings. Fifth disease is caused by parvovirus B19; the incubation period is thought to be from 4 to 14 days. But parvovirus can cause serious problems in pregnant women, so contact the doctor if a pregnant woman has been exposed.

Home Treatment

There is no treatment. Just watch and wait to make sure you are dealing with fifth disease. Check that there is no fever. Fever is very unusual with fifth disease. No restrictions on activities are necessary.

What to Expect at the Doctor's Office

The doctor may be able to distinguish fifth disease from other rashes. If the rash fits the description given in this section, the doctor is going to make the same diagnosis that you might have made. Checking the child's temperature and looking at the rash can be expected. Because there are no tests currently available, laboratory tests are unlikely. Waiting and watching are the means of dealing with fifth disease.

Fifth Disease

Are all of the following present?
- ▲ No fever
- ▲ "Slapped cheek" rash is the first and only symptom
- ▲ Palms and soles are not involved

No → **Suspect...** problem other than fifth disease. Check Table 7 on pp. 168–169.

↓ **Yes**

Has a pregnant woman been exposed?

Yes → Have her call her doctor today.

↓ **No**

Use Home Treatment

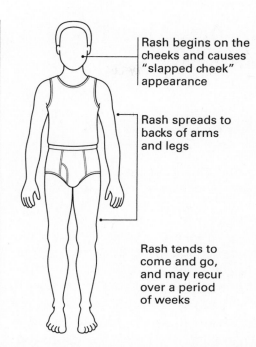

Rash begins on the cheeks and causes "slapped cheek" appearance

Rash spreads to backs of arms and legs

Rash tends to come and go, and may recur over a period of weeks

Fifth disease. Apart from the rash, there are no symptoms.

CHAPTER 8

Bones, Muscles, and Joints

Arthritis

"Arthritis" means joints that are painful to move. They may be red, warm, or swollen as well. Many people use the "arthritis" label for pain that is really in muscles, tendons, ligaments, or bones; we discuss this kind of musculoskeletal pain on page 228.

There are more than a hundred types of arthritis. The most common are listed below.

▲ Osteoarthritis can cause knobby swelling of finger joints. More seriously, it can affect knees, hips, neck, or spine. Some osteoarthritis happens to almost everyone in later life but is usually not too serious.

▲ Rheumatoid arthritis can cause you to feel sick and stiff all over, in addition to causing joint problems. It usually starts in midlife.

▲ Gout mostly affects men. It causes severe attacks of pain and swelling in one joint at a time, often the big toe, ankle, or knee.

▲ Ankylosing spondylitis affects the back. It causes chronic sore back and morning stiffness. A person with ankylosing spondylitis may be unable to touch the toes.

The complications of arthritis usually develop slowly. You can prevent these problems more easily than you can correct them, so you should manage the condition correctly and carefully.

When to See the Doctor

Few people with arthritis need to see a doctor right away. Urgent problems are:

▲ Infection
▲ Nerve damage
▲ Fractures near a joint
▲ Gout

The first three could result in serious joint damage. Gout can be so painful that the patient needs immediate help. Otherwise, if you can, use the "six-week rule." If it lasts beyond six weeks, check it out.

Home Treatment

You can reduce pain and swelling in the joints by taking an over-the-counter pain medication (page 54). Although acetaminophen can relieve pain, it doesn't reduce inflammation, so doctors seldom use it to treat arthritis other than osteoarthritis. Stomach irritation is the major concern. Bleeding from the stomach is a serious concern. Do not use these drugs for more than six weeks without talking with the doctor. Talk with the doctor if you are over 65 years of age.

Glucosamine and chondroitin sulphate are popular alternative treatments. They are safe and seem to help some people.

Resting an inflamed joint can speed healing. Heat can also help. Working a painful joint through its range of motion twice a day will help prevent stiffness.

If pain, swelling, or stiffness persists for six weeks without improvement, see a doctor.

What to Expect at the Doctor's Office

The doctor will examine the joints and may have blood tests and X-rays done.

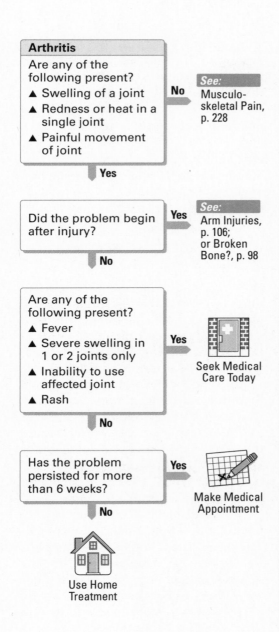

Arthritis

Are any of the following present?
- ▲ Swelling of a joint
- ▲ Redness or heat in a single joint
- ▲ Painful movement of joint

No → *See:* Musculo-skeletal Pain, p. 228

Yes ↓

Did the problem begin after injury?

Yes → *See:* Arm Injuries, p. 106; or Broken Bone?, p. 98

No ↓

Are any of the following present?
- ▲ Fever
- ▲ Severe swelling in 1 or 2 joints only
- ▲ Inability to use affected joint
- ▲ Rash

Yes → Seek Medical Care Today

No ↓

Has the problem persisted for more than 6 weeks?

Yes → Make Medical Appointment

No ↓

Use Home Treatment

He or she may use a needle to sample fluid from an affected joint.

A nonsteroidal anti-inflammatory drug (NSAID), such as Celebrex or Mobic, may be prescribed. Their effects are very similar to those of aspirin, ibuprofen, naproxen, or ketoprofen, but they may be less hazardous. Lower the risk of upset stomach by taking the tablets after meals or with an antacid.

Corticosteroid drugs such as prednisone can reduce inflammation but cause serious side effects after long-term use. Talk to your doctor if you take them for more than a few weeks. The doctor may inject a corticosteroid drug into a painful joint. This usually shouldn't be done more than three times.

Rheumatoid arthritis usually requires strong drugs such as methotrexate, gold salts, or hydroxychloroquine, or even stronger new drugs. Patients should be seen early by a specialist (rheumatologist) and should have periodic follow-ups.

Lyme Disease

Lyme disease is an infection spread by ticks, usually deer ticks. An oval "bull's-eye" skin rash is a distinctive sign of the infection. The rash appears 3 to 20 days after the bite of an infected tick. The person with Lyme disease may also have fever, headache, stiff neck, and backache. Some people with the illness then develop arthritis within 1 to 22 weeks. A few get heart or neurological problems. Call your doctor if you see the "bull's-eye" rash on your skin. (See Insect Bites or Stings, page 114.)

Musculoskeletal Pain

Pain in a muscle or joint with no swelling or redness can be caused by tension, viral infection, or unusual physical activity. Sometimes joint or muscle pain has no obvious cause. These pains aren't arthritis, and they rarely suggest a serious disease. Muscle or joint pain usually goes away by itself.

Muscle or joint pain may be caused by thyroid disease, cancer, polymyositis (inflammation of the muscles), or polymyalgia rheumatica (aching in the neck, shoulder, and hip muscles that can affect the elderly). Pain in the upper neck and at the base of the skull is usually minor.

Fibromyalgia is marked by muscle pain, fatigue, and difficulty getting restful sleep. The person with fibromyalgia may also have irritable bowel syndrome, morning stiffness, anxiety, memory loss, and other symptoms.

Make an appointment if you have fever, weight loss, or severe fatigue. Otherwise, try home treatment for several weeks.

Home Treatment

Rest and exercise and good sleep habits are important for musculoskeletal disorders. A program of slowly increasing exercise can help restore muscle tone. Walking, bicycling, and swimming are good activities. Take warm baths, have a massage, and do stretching exercises as often as possible.

Poor work habits are a common cause of muscle and joint pain. If you work on hard floors, try rubber-soled shoes. A better chair may help if you work at a desk. Many people feel better after a change in lifestyle, switching jobs, or moving. If your pain goes away when you're on vacation, stress may be part of the problem.

Over-the-counter pain medications may help relieve pain (page 54).

Hot or Cold?

You should apply cold or heat to painful areas at different times:

▲ Use cold for new injury and within 24 hours of the first inflammation.
▲ Use heat after the first stages of inflammation.

Cold right after an injury reduces the fluid and blood that escape into joints or muscles; this helps reduce the pain and swelling. Later, heat increases blood flow during healing, makes joints more flexible, and can relieve muscle spasm.

Exercise is the most important part of fibromyalgia treatment. Start and increase your exercise slowly. Stretch for flexibility. Increase your physical activity toward full aerobic cardiovascular conditioning (page 6). Walking, hiking, swimming, and bicycling are good activities. Avoid impact exercises such as jogging or tennis.

If you start an exercise program, the pain of fibromyalgia may get worse before it gets better. You have to persevere. Relief may be months away. Varying degrees of pain can persist for many years. But it will get better.

If you are not feeling better within three weeks, see your doctor.

What to Expect at the Doctor's Office

The doctor will do a physical exam and request blood tests. He or she will probably give advice similar to the home treatment described above.

Musculoskeletal Pain

Are any of the following present?

▲ Swelling of a joint

▲ Redness or heat in a joint

▲ Pain when a joint moves

Yes → *See:* Arthritis, p. 226

No ↓

Are any of the following present?

▲ Fever without flu-like symptoms

▲ Weight loss of 10 pounds (5 kg) or more

▲ Widespread pain lasting more than 3 weeks

Yes → Make Medical Appointment

No ↓

Use Home Treatment

If a specific joint in the body is causing the pain, a corticosteroid shot may help.

The doctor may manage fibromyalgia with drug regimens such as amitriptyline (Elavil) an hour or so before bedtime and an antidepressant (e.g., Prozac) in the morning. The goal of medication is to improve sleep without causing drowsiness during the day.

Neck Pain

Most neck pain, such as the common "stiff neck," is due to muscle strain or spasm. You can care for this kind of minor pain at home.

Neck pain can be part of a flu syndrome that includes fever, headache, and muscle aches. If the person with neck pain also has general muscle aches, a visit to the doctor probably won't help.

Causes of neck pain that require a doctor's attention are:

Meningitis. Neck pain accompanied by fever and headache (but without general muscle aches) can signal this serious inflammation of the brain covering. With a very stiff neck, the person with meningitis may be unable to touch the chin to the chest. If you aren't sure, you're better off seeing the doctor for an ordinary muscle spasm than ignoring this **emergency** sign.

Pinched Nerve. Arthritis or neck injury can result in a pinched nerve. You may feel pain running down one arm, or numbness or tingling in one arm or hand. The symptoms appear on only one side, and neck stiffness is not the main complaint.

Home Treatment

Morning neck pain may be due to poor sleeping habits. Sleep on a firm mattress. Stop using a pillow or use special pillows that keep the head from twisting and use a soft collar at night.

Warmth may help spasms and pain. You can use hot showers, hot compresses, or a heating pad. Be careful with heat—skin burns easily. Over-the-counter pain

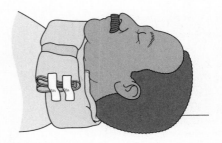

Bedtime neck pain relief. An ordinary bath towel can relieve neck pain. Before going to bed, fold a bath towel into a long strip four inches (10 cm) wide. Wrap it around the neck and secure it with tape or a safety pin. A soft neck collar from the drugstore works the same way. You usually will not need to wear the towel or collar during the day.

medications will help relieve pain and inflammation (page 54).

Neck pain is slow to improve and may take several weeks to resolve. Call the doctor if you aren't better in a week.

What to Expect at the Doctor's Office

If the doctor suspects meningitis, he or she will do a spinal tap and blood tests. You may have X-rays taken of the neck. The doctor may prescribe a neck collar. If he or she suspects nerve damage, the doctor may refer you to a neurologist or neurosurgeon.

The doctor may prescribe a muscle relaxer and perhaps a pain reliever. Prescription drugs aren't necessarily better than over-the-counter pain relievers. If you don't have infection or nerve damage, you're usually just as well off with home treatment.

Neck Pain

Is neck pain accompanied by fever and headache, or is person unable to touch chin to chest?

Yes →

Seek Medical Care Now

No ↓

Does pain travel down one arm, or is there tingling or numbness in the arm or hand?

Yes →

Seek Medical Care Today

No ↓

Use Home Treatment

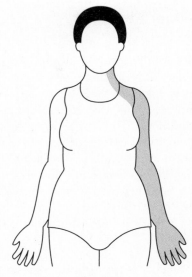

Sites of pinched nerve pain

Shoulder Pain

Pain located around the shoulder is common and almost never poses a serious threat to life. Nonetheless, it can persist for a long time and cause discomfort and disability. Most of the time, the pain comes from the soft tissues near the joint, not from the bones or the joint itself. These soft tissues include the ligaments (which connect one bone to another), tendons (which connect bone to muscle), and bursae (little fluid-filled sacs at the joints).

Bursitis. This is an inflammation of the bursae that starts with an uneasy feeling in the shoulder and may progress to considerable pain within 6 to 12 hours. There may be swelling at the tip of the shoulder. It is often seen in persons who have been cutting hedges, painting the house, or playing sports.

Rotator Cuff Tendinitis. This is an irritation of the tendons and muscles around the shoulder and is most likely to be seen in baseball pitchers and racket sports enthusiasts. Unlike bursitis, it is difficult to detect even a small amount of swelling, and the pain seems to occur in only a few positions.

Bicep Tendinitis. Much less common, this occurs in gymnasts and players of baseball and racket sports. The tenderness and pain are located in the front of the shoulder.

Because these three common problems of the shoulder are treated the same initially, you need not worry about which condition you have. However, there are problems that should be differentiated from these three conditions:

▲ **Injuries** require a slightly different approach (see Arm Injuries, page 106).
▲ **Infections** are quite unusual in the shoulder, but fever, swelling, and redness of the shoulder suggest the need for a doctor's help.
▲ **Complete inability to move the arm** suggests pain severe enough that consulting with a doctor is reasonable.

If none of these problems seems to fit your situation, give your doctor a call for advice. Often a visit will not be necessary.

Home Treatment
For bursitis, rotator cuff tendinitis, and bicep tendinitis, the key word is RIMS:

▲ Rest
▲ Ice
▲ Maintenance of mobility
▲ Strengthening

At the first sign of trouble, you should apply ice for 30 minutes, then let the shoulder rewarm for the next 15 minutes. Continue the cycle for the next one to two hours. Be careful not to freeze the skin.

Give the shoulder complete rest for the first 24 to 48 hours. You can use a sling if necessary (see Arm Injuries, page 106). After that time, gently put your arm through a full range of motion several times a day.

Complete immobilization of the arm may result in stiffness and loss of motion in the shoulder (frozen shoulder). Thus, maintenance of the shoulder's range of motion is an important part of the treatment. Wait three to six weeks before

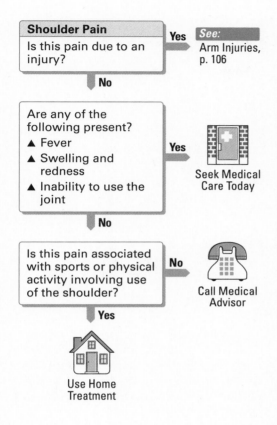

Shoulder Pain

Is this pain due to an injury? — **Yes** → *See:* Arm Injuries, p. 106

No ↓

Are any of the following present?
▲ Fever
▲ Swelling and redness
▲ Inability to use the joint — **Yes** → Seek Medical Care Today

No ↓

Is this pain associated with sports or physical activity involving use of the shoulder? — **No** → Call Medical Advisor

Yes ↓

Use Home Treatment

returning to the activity that caused the problem, depending on the problem's severity. Returning too soon will increase the probability of reinjury.

After the initial rest period, exercises should be started to gradually stretch and strengthen the muscles around the shoulder. This is especially important in rotator cuff tendinitis. At first, the exercise need consist only of putting the arm through a full range of motion. Next, a small amount of weight (1 to 1.5 pounds, or around half a kilogram) is held in the hand as the exercises are performed. Weight is gradually increased by a half pound (200 g) every 10 days. A similar

approach uses a towel held behind the back and moved around with tension to stretch and strengthen the backward motions of the shoulder. Ice is recommended after exercise.

Over-the-counter pain medications may help decrease pain and inflammation (page 54).

Call a doctor if the condition persists beyond six weeks.

What to Expect at the Doctor's Office

The doctor will examine the shoulder and prescribe a regimen similar to the one above, if one of the common causes of shoulder pain is diagnosed. If the problem is bursitis, a corticosteroid injection may be given. Such injections should be given only if home therapy doesn't work. There should be no more than two or three such injections. Nonsteroidal anti-inflammatory drugs (NSAIDs) may be given. These prescription drugs are similar to aspirin, ibuprofen, naproxen, and ketoprofen. They may decrease pain but don't speed the healing process. Expect instruction in rehabilitation exercises.

Surgery is the last resort and is a gamble. Satisfaction isn't guaranteed.

Sports-Related Problems

Some of the problems related specifically to racket sports, baseball pitching, or golf are due to poor technique. Coaching from a professional is well worth considering. It is less expensive than going to a doctor, and you will probably improve your game.

Elbow Pain

Aside from injuries, the main causes of elbow pain are bursitis and tennis elbow.

Bursitis

The elbow bursa is a fluid-filled sac located right at the tip of the elbow. When it is irritated, the amount of fluid increases, causing a swelling that looks very much like a small egg right at the end of the elbow. The swelling is the cause of discomfort. There should be no fever and only a little redness, if any.

Tennis Elbow

Of the cases of tennis elbow that reach the doctor's office, fewer than half are actually associated with playing tennis. The rest usually result from work that requires a twisting motion of the arm— such as using a screwdriver—or have no obvious cause. The doctor's help is needed only for prolonged cases that don't get better; perhaps 1 person in 1,000 needs such help.

The diagnosis of tennis elbow doesn't depend on tests or special examinations. Tennis elbow is simply defined as pain in the lateral (outer) portion of the elbow and upper forearm. The pain occurs after repeatedly rolling or twisting the

forearm, wrist, and hand. Tennis elbow is usually caused by the tremendous impact transmitted to the forearm when the tennis ball is hit with the backhand motion. The risk that this force will create tennis elbow is raised by:

▲ Hitting the ball with the elbow bent rather than locked in a position of strength
▲ Trying to put top spin on the ball by rolling the wrist on contact (this doesn't work)
▲ Holding the thumb behind the racket
▲ Using a racket that is head-heavy
▲ Switching to a faster court surface
▲ Using heavier balls, such as those of foreign make or the pressureless type
▲ Using a very stiff racket

According to the experts, the most important preventive measure for tennis players is to use a two-handed backhand stroke.

Home Treatment

Bursitis of the elbow is treated very much like bursitis of the shoulder (page 232).

At the first sign of tennis elbow, you should, of course, take preventive measures. But suppose that you already use a two-handed backhand, have switched to a light and supple metal racket, and so on. Or suppose your job or favorite hobby requires repeated use of screwdrivers or other tools that aggravate the problem. What now? Resting the arm will surely make it hurt less, but most likely taking two weeks off won't cure it forever. Interestingly, most authorities now think that you can "play with pain" and not cause permanent injury.

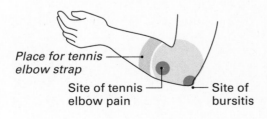

Place for tennis elbow strap

Site of tennis elbow pain

Site of bursitis

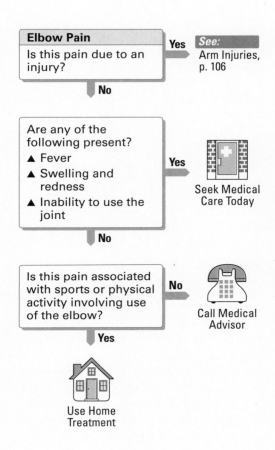

Elbow Pain
Is this pain due to an injury? — **Yes** → **See:** Arm Injuries, p. 106

No ↓

Are any of the following present?
▲ Fever
▲ Swelling and redness
▲ Inability to use the joint
— **Yes** → Seek Medical Care Today

No ↓

Is this pain associated with sports or physical activity involving use of the elbow? — **No** → Call Medical Advisor

Yes ↓

Use Home Treatment

Wrist flap. Move the wrist from full flexion to full extension. Do a session of 10 once daily.

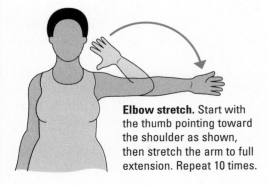

Elbow stretch. Start with the thumb pointing toward the shoulder as shown, then stretch the arm to full extension. Repeat 10 times.

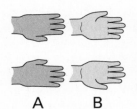

A   B

Arm twist. With your arms straight out in front of you, rotate the hands from palms down (A) to palms up (B). Repeat 10 times.

We advocate a commonsense approach to tennis elbow: cut down on your playing time. When you do play, warm up slowly and do some stretching exercises of the wrist and elbow before you begin to hit the ball. Using a tennis elbow strap may help. Get the strap at the drugstore and apply it about an inch *below* where it hurts. Applying ice after playing may also help a great deal.

What to Expect at the Doctor's Office

Bursitis of the elbow is treated by the doctor very much like bursitis of the shoulder. If you're the rare person with tennis elbow who has severe persistent pain, the next step is to inject a pain reliever and corticosteroid (cortisonelike drug) into the painful area. Three such injections are the limit. Surgery should be a last resort—an act of desperation. If you get to this point, perhaps it's time to take up another game.

Wrist Pain

The wrist is an unusual joint because stiffness or even complete loss of motion causes relatively little difficulty; however, if the joint is wobbly and unstable, this can pose real problems. The wrist provides the platform from which the fine motions of the fingers operate. It is essential that this platform be stable. The eight wrist bones form a rather crude joint that is very limited in motion compared with, for example, the shoulder. But this joint is strong and stable. The wrist platform works best when it is bent upward just a little. Almost no normal human activities require the wrist to be bent all the way back or all the way forward, and the fingers don't operate as well when the wrist is fully flexed or fully extended.

Causes of Pain

Fever and/or rapid swelling accompanying the onset of pain suggest the possibility of an infection. This requires prompt medical attention.

The wrist is very frequently involved in rheumatoid arthritis, and the side of the wrist by the thumb is very commonly involved in osteoarthritis (see Arthritis, page 226).

Carpal tunnel syndrome can cause pain at the wrist. In addition, this syndrome can cause pains to shoot down into the fingers or up into the forearm. Usually there is a numb feeling in the fingers as if they were asleep. In this syndrome, the median nerve is trapped and squeezed as it passes through the fibrous carpal tunnel in the front of the wrist. Generally the squeezing results from too

much inflamed tissue. Some causes of this inflammation are a blow to the front of the wrist, rheumatoid arthritis, playing tennis, paddling a canoe, or other activities that repeatedly flex and extend the wrist.

You can diagnose carpal tunnel syndrome pretty well yourself. The numbness in the fingers doesn't involve the little finger and often doesn't involve the half of the ring finger nearest the little finger. If you tap with a finger on the front of the wrist, you may get a sudden tingling in the fingers, similar to the feeling of hitting your funny bone. Tingling and pain in carpal tunnel syndrome may be worse at night or when the wrists are cocked down (flexed).

Home Treatment

The key to management of wrist pain is splinting. The strategy is to rest the joint in the position of best function. Wrist splints made of plastic or aluminum are available at hospital supply stores and many drugstores. Any that fit you are probably all right. The splint will cock your wrist back just a bit. You can put a cloth sleeve around the splint to make it more comfortable on your skin. Wrap the splint gently with an elastic bandage to keep it in place. That's all there is to it. Wear it all the time for a few days, then just at night for a few weeks. This simple treatment is all that is required for most wrist flare-ups.

No prescription pain medication should be necessary. Over-the-counter pain medications (page 54) are all right but probably won't help much. If you know what triggered the pain, work out a way to avoid that activity. Common sense means listening to the pain message.

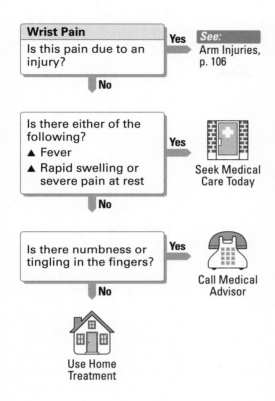

Wrist Pain

Is this pain due to an injury? — **Yes** → *See:* Arm Injuries, p. 106

No ↓

Is there either of the following?
▲ Fever
▲ Rapid swelling or severe pain at rest
— **Yes** → Seek Medical Care Today

No ↓

Is there numbness or tingling in the fingers? — **Yes** → Call Medical Advisor

No ↓

Use Home Treatment

If the problem persists after six weeks of home treatment, see the doctor.

What to Expect at the Doctor's Office

The wrist will be examined and advice similar to that above will be given. X-rays may be required, but only rarely. Anti-inflammatory drugs may be prescribed. Injection with a corticosteroid medication may be performed on occasion and is likely to help if carpal tunnel syndrome hasn't responded to splinting.

Several different kinds of surgery are available, and one or another procedure may be recommended in difficult cases. Carpal tunnel nerve compression may

Computer Posture

As everyone types on computers, there have been more worries about carpal tunnel syndrome. Research continues, but there seem to be two important factors: stress, especially from pressure to type quickly or without interruption, and poor hand positioning. Take brief rests, and consider using a different keyboard to help avoid pain.

For proper typing position, keep your elbows at a 90° angle, with your forearms parallel to the floor; keep your wrists in a neutral position, and use a wrist rest for support; and keep your feet flat on the floor.

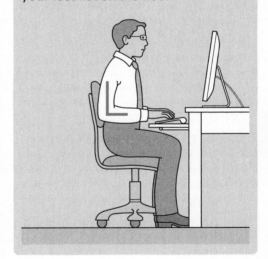

be released surgically. In rheumatoid arthritis, the synovial tissue that lines the tendon sheaths on the back of the hand may be removed to protect the tendons that run through the inflamed area (synovectomy). The wrist may be casted or the bones fused.

Finger Pain

Each hand has 14 finger joints, each like a small hinge. These joints are operated by muscles in the forearm that control them through an intricate system of tendons that runs through the wrist and hand. The small size and complex arrangement of these joints and tendons mean that any inflammation or damage to a joint is likely to result in some stiffness and lost motion. Even a small scar may limit motion.

You shouldn't expect that a problem with a small finger joint will resolve completely. Even after healing, some leftover stiffness and occasional twinges of discomfort are likely. Unrealistically high expectations lead to feelings that you did something wrong or that the doctor was no good. In fact, almost all of us have a few fingers that have been injured and remain a bit crooked or stiff.

Osteoarthritis frequently causes knobby swelling of the most distant joints of the fingers as well as swelling of the middle joints. It can also cause problems at the base of the thumb. If we live long enough, all of us get these knobby swellings. They cause most of the changed appearance that we associate with the aging hand. As a rule, they cause relatively

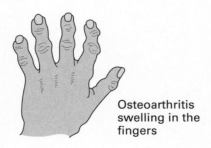

Osteoarthritis
swelling in the
fingers

little pain or stiffness and don't need specific treatment other than exercise.

Numbness or tingling may indicate a problem with nerves or circulation. A call to the doctor will help you make a decision about what to do.

Home Treatment

Listen to the pain message and avoid activities that aggravate pain *after* the exercise. Rest the finger joints so that they can heal, but use gentle stretching exercises to keep them limber and maintain motion. The key to managing finger problems is to use common sense. Exercise of all kinds (aerobic, strengthening, and stretching) is essential as long as it is relatively pain-free.

With a bit of ingenuity, you can find a less stressful way to do almost any activity that puts stress on the joints. Because everyone's activities are a bit different, you will have to invent some of these new methods yourself. Here are a few hints to get you going:

▲ A big handle can be gripped with less strain than a small handle. Wrap pens, knives, and other similar objects with tape.

▲ Lift smaller loads. Make more trips. Plan ahead rather than blundering through an activity.

▲ Find clothing that uses Velcro or large buttons instead of small buttons and snaps for fasteners.

▲ Use a gripper for opening tough jar lids or stop buying products that come in hard-to-open jars. When opening a tough lid, apply friction pressure on the top of the lid with your palm and twist with your whole hand, not with your grip.

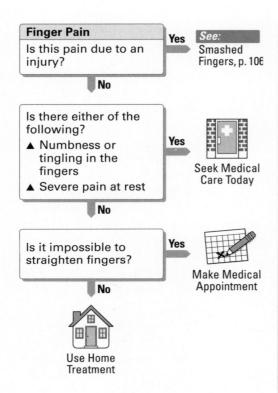

Finger Pain
Is this pain due to an injury?

Yes → *See:* Smashed Fingers, p. 106

No ↓

Is there either of the following?
▲ Numbness or tingling in the fingers
▲ Severe pain at rest

Yes → Seek Medical Care Today

No ↓

Is it impossible to straighten fingers?

Yes → Make Medical Appointment

No ↓

Use Home Treatment

Finger Exercises

Stretch your joints gently twice a day to maintain motion. Putting your hands in warm water before stretching may help you get more motion.

1. Straighten one hand out against the tabletop.

2. Make a fist and then cock the wrist to increase the stretch.

3. Use one hand to move each finger of the other hand through its full range of motion. Don't force, but stretch just to the edge of discomfort. If the motion of a joint is normal, one repetition is enough. If the motion is limited, do up to 10 repetitions.

▲ Don't put heavy objects too high or too low. Organize your kitchen, workshop, study, and bedroom.

Don't use strong medicines that mask your pain because these may lead you to overdo an activity. Over-the-counter pain medications (page 54) may help some. If the problem persists after six weeks of home treatment, see the doctor.

What to Expect at the Doctor's Office
The doctor will examine your hands and the finger motions. Sometimes an X-ray is taken, but usually not more often than every two years.

In rare cases, injecting corticosteroids into a particularly bad finger joint is helpful, but this is less effective with small joints such as fingers than with large ones. Surgery is also less effective with small joints and is often not appropriate. Operations such as replacement with plastic joints or removal of inflamed tissue usually succeed in making the hand look more normal and may decrease pain, but the hand often doesn't work much better than it did before the operation.

Low Back Pain

Low back pain is frustrating for doctors and patients alike. It's slow to heal and often comes back.

The cause of low back pain is usually an injury to the ligaments or other tissue, though it can be a herniated disk. The pain can be severe or moderate, or you can simply feel stiff. The pain is usually felt in the back, sometimes in the buttocks or upper leg as well.

Often the cause isn't clear. The pain may start immediately after a muscle strain or hours later. Severe pain usually lasts for 48 to 72 hours, followed by days or weeks of less severe pain.

Back pain that results from a severe blow or fall may require immediate attention.

Back pain may extend down the leg *below the knee* if a sciatic nerve is pinched. Doctors call this sciatica. This pain often responds to home treatment. You should see the doctor right away for sciatica, especially if there is:

▲ Loss of bladder or bowel control
▲ Weakness in the leg

Home Treatment

The low back pain syndrome is a vicious cycle: injury causes the pain of muscle spasm, and the spasm leads to more pain. To heal most rapidly, you must avoid reinjury and allow your back to recover.

▲ Avoid reinjury by limiting your physical activity. If necessary, rest flat on your back for the first 24 hours.
▲ After the first day, moderate activity—as much as the pain allows—is better than bed rest. Strenuous activity during the next six weeks can make the problem worse, however. After recovery, an exercise program will help prevent reinjury.
▲ If you suffer from low back pain, sleep without a pillow on a very firm mattress, a waterbed, or even the floor. A bed board under your mattress will make it firmer. You may find it more comfortable to sleep with a towel folded under the small of your back or a pillow beneath your knees.
▲ A heat pack applied to the back will help relieve pain.
▲ You can take over-the-counter pain medications (page 54).

If there is no nerve damage, you don't gain anything by going to the doctor for low back pain. Being careful and easing the symptoms will help your back recover. If severe back pain lasts more than a week, call the doctor.

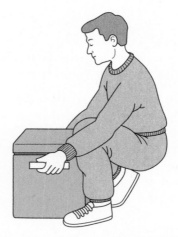

Lifting heavy objects. To avoid back strain, bend your knees but keep your back straight and erect.

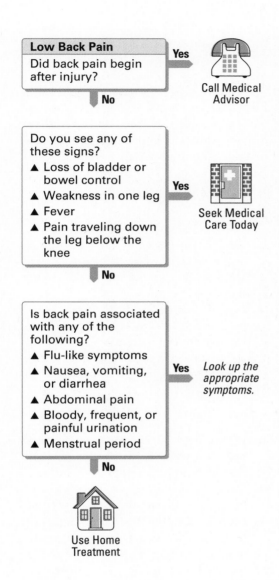

Low Back Pain

Did back pain begin after injury?

Yes → Call Medical Advisor

No ↓

Do you see any of these signs?

▲ Loss of bladder or bowel control

▲ Weakness in one leg

▲ Fever

▲ Pain traveling down the leg below the knee

Yes → Seek Medical Care Today

No ↓

Is back pain associated with any of the following?

▲ Flu-like symptoms

▲ Nausea, vomiting, or diarrhea

▲ Abdominal pain

▲ Bloody, frequent, or painful urination

▲ Menstrual period

Yes → *Look up the appropriate symptoms.*

No ↓

Use Home Treatment

What to Expect at the Doctor's Office

The doctor will ask questions and do a physical exam to look for causes of back pain. X-rays may be taken of the back, particularly if the pain is due to an injury. If the doctor suspects that nerves may have been hurt, special studies may be done, such as myelogram, computerized tomography (CT), or magnetic resonance imaging (MRI). In rare cases, when nerves are at risk, the doctor may hospitalize the person. Treatment may include traction or surgery.

Usually the doctor gives advice similar to the home treatment we describe above. He or she may prescribe a muscle relaxant or a pain reliever such as celecoxib or meloxicam. Back exercises, relaxation, and biofeedback may help chronic low back pain.

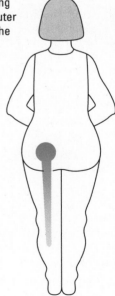

Sciatica. Pain extending down the leg on the outer part of the leg below the knee may be sciatica. See the doctor.

Hip Pain

Because the hip joint is so deep inside the body, identifying the source of hip pain can be difficult. An injury or disease of the hip may be felt in the groin, in the outer thigh, or down the leg to the knee. Pain felt in the hip may actually start in the lower back.

Although the hip is one of the body's strongest and best-protected joints, it is still subject to dislocation, fracture, and soft-tissue injury. The narrow neck of the thigh bone (femur) can break easily, particularly among elderly people who slip or fall. The artery to the end of that bone can get blocked, leading to the death of bone tissue and a form of arthritis called aseptic necrosis.

Other causes of hip pain are:

▲ Infection
▲ Bursitis—inflammation of the fluid-filled sacs over the joint
▲ Rheumatoid arthritis and osteo-arthritis (page 226)

A stiff hip may not be painful, but it can place extra strain on the lower back. The form of arthritis called ankylosing spondylitis can cause hip stiffness. Hip problems can lead to a flexion contracture, in which the hip joint becomes fixed in a slightly bent position, losing some range of motion.

Home Treatment

Pay attention to pain. Avoid activities that make your hip worse. Rest the joint after painful activities. Avoid pain medication as much as possible.

Use a cane or crutches if needed. Hold the cane in the hand *opposite* the painful hip. This allows the large muscles around the sore hip joint to relax. Move the cane forward along with the affected hip.

As the hip pain lessens, gradually introduce exercise. Use gentle motion exercises at first to free the hip and reduce stiffness. Repeat these exercises two or three times a day:

▲ Stand with your good hip by a table. Lean on the table with your hand. Swing the leg with the bad hip from side to side and front and back.
▲ Spread your legs as far as you can and bend from side to side.
▲ With your legs together, turn your feet outward like a duck.
▲ Lie on your back on the edge of your bed with your bad hip and leg hanging just off the mattress. Stretch your leg toward the floor while keeping your knees as straight as you can.

Introduce more activity to strengthen the hip muscles:

▲ Lie on your back and raise your legs one at a time. Keep the leg straight and lift until you reach a 45° angle.
▲ Swim. This stretches muscles and builds good tone.
▲ Bicycle or walk. When walking, start with short strides and gradually lengthen them as you loosen up. Gradually increase your effort and distance, but not by more than 10% each day.

A good, firm bed will help. The best sleeping position is on your back. Avoid pillows beneath the knees or under the lower back. Over-the-counter pain medications (page 54) may help.

If pain persists after six weeks of home treatment, see the doctor.

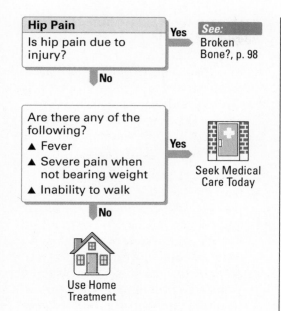

Hip Pain

Is hip pain due to injury?

Yes → *See:* Broken Bone?, p. 98

No ↓

Are there any of the following?
▲ Fever
▲ Severe pain when not bearing weight
▲ Inability to walk

Yes → Seek Medical Care Today

No ↓

Use Home Treatment

What to Expect at the Doctor's Office

The doctor will examine the hip and its range of motion. You may have X-rays taken. The doctor may prescribe anti-inflammatory medication. Rarely, the doctor may give you a shot.

The doctor may recommend surgery if your pain is intense and persistent, or if you are having problems walking. Total hip replacement is usually successful. An artificial hip lasts at least 10 to 15 years. You will be able to get up and around soon after surgery. Complications of surgery are rare.

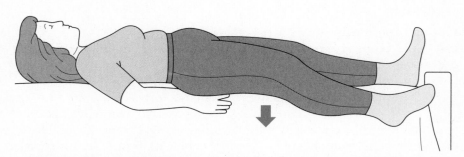

Hip exercise. With your shoulders, trunk, and one leg resting on the bed, allow the leg with the injured hip to dangle off the bed. Bend your knee as little as possible as you stretch the leg and hip backward, toward the floor.

Knee Pain

The knee is a large, strong joint, but it does not tolerate side stresses very well. The engineering of the knee makes it prone to both injury and degenerative disease. People are more likely to have these problems if they are overweight.

To work properly, the knee must bend and straighten while keeping stable support. The knee should not wobble from side to side. Make an appointment with the doctor if:

▲ Your knee is unstable or wobbles.
▲ You cannot completely straighten or bend the knee.

A knee that is red or feels hot may have an infection or gout. Pain or swelling in the calf below a sore knee suggests a blood clot or a cyst. See a doctor promptly if:

▲ You cannot walk.
▲ Your knee is very painful even when it's not bearing weight.
▲ You have pain or swelling in the calf or thigh.

Home Treatment

Pay attention to your pain. Avoid activities that make pain worse. Over-the-counter pain medications may ease pain (page 54), but don't use these medications to ignore what the pain is telling you.

If you have arthritis, make sure you take your medication as directed.

A cane may help reduce the stress on your knee. Most people use the cane on the *same* side as the painful knee.

Do not use a pillow under the knee while resting or sleeping. This can make your knee stiff.

Knee pain can result from foot problems; make sure your shoes fit properly and are in good shape.

Start exercising slowly. Increase your level of activity until you are exercising several times daily. Here is a gradual program:

▲ Start by bending and straightening the leg. Work at getting it straight and keeping it straight. You may find it more comfortable to sit or lie down while a friend moves the leg for you.
▲ Next, begin gentle exercises. Tighten your thigh muscles and hold for two seconds, then rest for two seconds. Do 10 repetitions three times a day.
▲ Introduce gentle activity. A bicycle in low gear is a good place to start. Stationary bicycles are fine. Be sure that the seat is high enough so your knee doesn't bend to more than a right angle as you pedal.
▲ Swimming and walking are very good activities for knees. Gradually increase your distance. Avoid exercise and activities that involve deep knee bends; these place too much stress on the knee.

See your doctor if your knee is painful after six weeks of home treatment.

What to Expect at the Doctor's Office

The doctor will examine your knee and other joints. You may have an X-ray done of your knee. The doctor may use a needle to draw fluid from the knee.

Several operations are helpful for knee problems, including surgery to trim or remove cartilage. Increasingly,

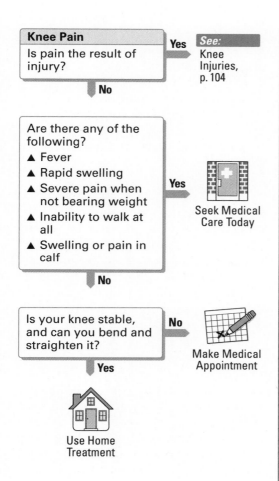

Knee Pain

Is pain the result of injury?

Yes → *See:* Knee Injuries, p. 104

No ↓

Are there any of the following?
▲ Fever
▲ Rapid swelling
▲ Severe pain when not bearing weight
▲ Inability to walk at all
▲ Swelling or pain in calf

Yes → Seek Medical Care Today

No ↓

Is your knee stable, and can you bend and straighten it?

No → Make Medical Appointment

Yes ↓

Use Home Treatment

Benefits of Exercise

Does exercise such as walking or running cause knee problems? No. If the knee isn't injured, exercise and weight bearing are good. They help nourish the cartilage, and they keep the side ligaments, the muscles, and the bones strong, which helps keep the knee stable. We have been studying 500 senior long-distance runners for the past 24 years. Only one has needed a knee replacement.

doctors are using an arthroscope to diagnose and treat knee problems. This is a minor procedure.

For severe and persistent problems, the doctor may suggest total knee replacement. This surgery is usually successful in giving total pain relief.

Leg Pain

Four types of problems account for most leg pain not associated with injuries:

▲ Inflammation and clots in veins—thrombophlebitis
▲ Infection of the calf—cellulitis
▲ Narrowing of arteries—intermittent claudication
▲ "Overuse" problems associated with vigorous exercise, collectively referred to as "shin splints" (page 248)

Thrombophlebitis is most likely to occur after a prolonged period of inactivity, such as a cramped, long car or plane ride. It is so common that it is called "economy class syndrome." If you have leg swelling before the flight or are over 50 years of age, your doctor may recommend aspirin (81 mg) *before* each flight to decrease the risk. The pain is aching and usually not localized, but sometimes a firm and tender vein can be felt in the middle of the calf. Swelling doesn't always occur or may be so slight that it's hard to detect.

Cellulitis is an infection of the leg tissues, usually limited to the calf and ankle regions. It can mimic thrombophlebitis. Treatment requires antibiotics.

A "Baker's cyst" behind the knee can, rarely, be the cause of leg pain and swelling. It may require injection of a corticosteroid medication or other measures.

In older people or heavy smokers, the arteries in the leg may become narrowed so that not enough blood reaches the muscles during even such mild exercise as walking. This pain is called intermittent claudication because the pain is brought on by exercise, but relief comes in a few minutes with rest.

Both thrombophlebitis and intermittent claudication require the help of the doctor, but thrombophlebitis is more urgent. A decision on treatment should be made as soon as possible.

Call the physician for leg pain that doesn't fit the description of intermittent claudication, thrombophlebitis, or shin splints.

What to Expect at the Doctor's Office

If thrombophlebitis is suspected, the crucial question is whether or not to prescribe anticoagulants (blood thinners). The purpose of anticoagulants is to minimize the risk of a clot going to the lungs—pulmonary embolism. However, the effectiveness of anticoagulants is far from complete, and the therapy itself carries substantial risks.

Compression ultrasonography and impedance plethysmography (IPG) are useful in detecting thrombophlebitis in the thigh. These are painless and require no surgery or injections. They are usually combined with a blood test called D-dimer to improve diagnostic accuracy. You and the doctor must come to an understanding about the risks and benefits of anticoagulant therapy before making a decision.

Intermittent claudication can usually be diagnosed from history and physical examination. However, an arteriogram (a special X-ray of the arteries of the legs) will be required to determine where the problem lies before treatment can be considered. Therapy, if required, is one of several surgical procedures, ranging from insertion of a special tube (balloon catheter) so that the artery is widened, to bypassing the obstructed segment with a synthetic graft.

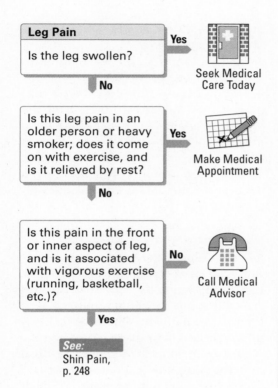

Leg Pain

Is the leg swollen?

Yes → Seek Medical Care Today

No

Is this leg pain in an older person or heavy smoker; does it come on with exercise, and is it relieved by rest?

Yes → Make Medical Appointment

No

Is this pain in the front or inner aspect of leg, and is it associated with vigorous exercise (running, basketball, etc.)?

No → Call Medical Advisor

Yes

See:
Shin Pain,
p. 248

Shin Pain

Shin pain is often called "shin splints," a catchall term that may indicate any one of four conditions associated with strenuous exercise, usually after a period of relative inactivity.

Posterior tibial shin splints are the "original" shin splints and account for about 75% of the problems affecting athletes in the front portion of their legs. Overstressing the posterior tibial muscle causes pain where the muscle attaches to the tibia, or shinbone, which is easily seen and felt in the front of your leg. Pain and tenderness are located in a three- to four-inch (8–10 cm) area on the inner edge of the tibia about midway between the knee and ankle. It is the muscle and the attachments to the bone that are painful; the front of the tibia itself, felt immediately beneath the skin, is not tender.

The front of the tibial bone is tender, however, in another form of shin splint, tibial periostitis. The pain and tenderness are similar to that in posterior tibial shin splints except that it is more toward the front of the leg and the bone itself is tender.

A third form of shin splint, anterior compartment syndrome, is located on the outer side of the front of the leg. You can readily feel the difference between the hard tibial bone and the muscles located in the anterior compartment. Pain arises when the muscles swell with blood during hard use. The compartment cannot increase in size so that the swelling squeezes the blood vessels and diminishes blood flow. The lack of adequate blood flow to the muscles causes the pain. After you rest for 10 to 15 minutes, the pain goes away.

Sharply localized pain and tenderness in the tibia one to two inches (3–5 cm) below the knee is typical of a stress fracture. Just as with stress fractures of the foot, these are likely to occur two to three weeks into an increased training program after the legs have taken a real pounding. As with stress fractures of the foot, stress fractures of the tibia aren't treated with casts, but with rest.

Home Treatment

Posterior Tibial Shin Splints. This condition will usually respond to a week of rest during which the area of tenderness is iced twice a day for 20 minutes. Over-the-counter pain medicines with every meal may also help (page 54). When the pain is gone, stretch the posterior tibial muscle using the exercises described for Achilles tendinitis (page 255). If you have flat feet, consider getting an arch support (orthotic) for your athletic shoe. Don't begin running again for another two to four weeks, and then only at half speed, with a gradual increase in speed and distance.

Tibial Periostitis. This is treated in the same way as posterior tibial shin splints, except that your gradual return to sports can begin after a week of rest; over-the-counter pain medicines; and ice therapy. Athletic shoes with good shock absorption, especially in the heel, are very important.

Anterior Compartment Syndrome. This condition will almost always go away as the muscles gradually become accustomed to vigorous exercise. You can help

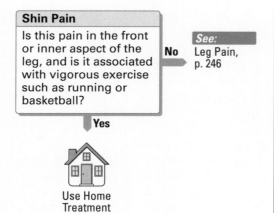

Shin Pain

Is this pain in the front or inner aspect of the leg, and is it associated with vigorous exercise such as running or basketball?

No → *See:* Leg Pain, p. 246

Yes ↓

Use Home Treatment

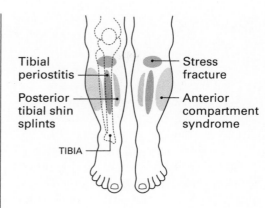

Tibial periostitis

Posterior tibial shin splints

TIBIA

Stress fracture

Anterior compartment syndrome

by resting for 10 minutes when pain occurs, and running slowly when you begin to run again. Cooling the leg with ice for 20 minutes after each workout may also help. Complete rest is not necessary. Shoes and pain relievers are unimportant in the treatment of anterior compartment syndrome. If you're the 1 person in 1,000 with anterior compartment syndrome for whom the problem doesn't go away with home treatment, surgery can be considered.

Stress Fractures. These require rest from running, usually for a month, before gradually starting to recondition your legs. Complete healing requires between four and six weeks. Crutches can be used but usually aren't necessary.

Note again that only anterior compartment syndrome has any treatment other than home treatment and that this treatment (surgery) is used only as a last resort. However, if you are unsure as to the nature of the problem or you have made no progress with home treatment after several weeks, consult the doctor.

What to Expect at the Doctor's Office

Home treatment will be prescribed for any of the four varieties of shin splints. In the very rare event that anterior compartment syndrome doesn't go away over time, the pressure can be relieved by splitting the tough, fibrous tissue (fascia) that surrounds the muscles. This is a relatively simple surgical procedure and can be accomplished without requiring a stay in the hospital.

Ankle Pain

The ankle is a large weight-bearing joint that is unavoidably stressed at each step. Several kinds of arthritis can involve the bones and cartilage of the ankle, but pain and instability are more frequently a result of problems in the ligaments.

With an ankle sprain, the ligament attaching the bump on the outer side of the ankle to the outer surface of the foot is injured at one or both ends; the ankle itself is all right.

With arthritis, injured ligaments may let the joint slip and wobble. This results in further stress on the ligaments, pain, and instability. Walking on an unstable joint increases the damage, but with a stable joint, walking is usually all right.

If you look at your leg when you are lying down and again when you are standing, you can tell if the joint is stable. If it is unstable, the line of your leg won't be straight down to the foot when you stand. Perhaps the foot will be slipped a half inch to an inch (1–3 cm) to the outside of where it should be. When you aren't bearing weight on it, it will move back in line toward a more normal position. The unstable joint may actually slip sideways if you try to move the foot with your hands. Instability is not just a swollen ankle (page 252); the ankle must be crooked to be unstable.

Home Treatment

Listen to the pain message. It is telling you to rest your ankle a bit more, to provide support for an unstable ankle, to back off your exercise program, or to use an aid to take weight off the ankle.

The unstable ankle should be supported for major weight-bearing activity.

Support is most simply obtained from high-lacing boots, but sometimes these will be too uncomfortable and you will need specially made boots or an ankle brace. Professional help is required for adequate fitting of such devices, and they can be quite expensive.

Crutches and even a cane can help you take the weight off the sore ankle.

For the stable ankle, an elastic bandage (page 73) and a shoe with a comfortable, thick heel pad will help. Jogging shoes are good. Light hiking boots, resembling running shoes that go above the ankle, are often excellent.

If you have arthritis, make particularly sure that you have been taking any prescribed medication exactly as ordered. Sometimes a patient gets a little bored and lax with the pill-taking routine and a few days later experiences pain or swelling.

As soon as the pain begins to decrease, you can gently begin to exercise the joint again. Swimming is good because you don't have to bear weight. Start easily and slowly with your exercises.

1. Sit on a chair, let the leg hang, and wiggle the foot up and down and in and out.

2. Later, walk carefully with an ankle bandage for support. Stretch the ankle by putting the forefoot on a

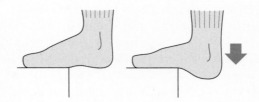

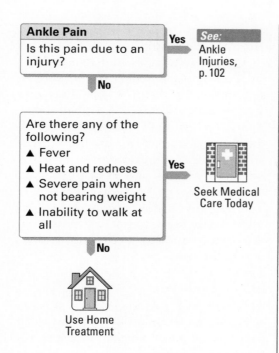

Ankle Pain
Is this pain due to an injury?

Yes → *See:* Ankle Injuries, p. 102

No ↓

Are there any of the following?
- ▲ Fever
- ▲ Heat and redness
- ▲ Severe pain when not bearing weight
- ▲ Inability to walk at all

Yes → Seek Medical Care Today

No ↓

Use Home Treatment

Using Crutches

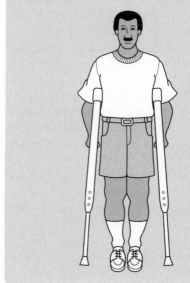

Crutches should be short enough so you don't injure the nerves in your armpits by leaning on the crutch. Take the weight on your hands or arms. When a person stands straight, crutches should reach from six inches to the side of the feet to two inches— or three to four fingers' width—below the armpits.

slightly raised surface, such as a step, and lowering the heel.

3. As the ankle gains strength, you can walk on tiptoe and walk on your heels to stretch and strengthen the joint.

Do the exercises several times a day. The ankle shouldn't be a lot worse after exercising if you aren't overdoing it. Keep at it, take your time, and be patient.

What to Expect at the Doctor's Office
The ankle and the area around it will be examined. X-rays may be necessary. The doctor may prescribe anti-inflammatory medications or increase the dosage if you are already taking them. Special shoes or braces may be prescribed.

Surgery is occasionally necessary. Fusing some of the ankle bones together is generally the most useful procedure. A fixed, pain-free ankle is far preferable to an unstable and painful one. The artificial ankle joint isn't yet satisfactory for most people, but engineers are making rapid progress in this area.

Ankle and Leg Swelling

Painless swelling of the ankles is a common problem, and the swelling usually affects both legs and may extend up the calves or even the thighs.

Usually the problem is fluid accumulation (edema). This is most pronounced in the lower legs because of the effects of gravity. If there is excess fluid and you press firmly with your thumb on the area that is swollen, it will squeeze the fluid out of that area and leave a deep impression. The depression will stay for a few moments.

Fortunately, most swelling is due to local causes. Often, breakdowns in the veins over time have made it difficult for blood to be returned to the heart fast enough. This increases pressure in the smallest blood vessels (capillaries) and causes fluid to leak out into the tissues, which causes the leg swelling. This is what happens in "varicose veins," but the problem can happen with larger, deeper veins as well as with capillaries.

Serious Problems

If just one leg becomes swollen rapidly, thrombophlebitis (a blood clot in the vein) may be present, and a doctor is needed (page 246). Thrombophlebitis usually causes pain and redness also, but this isn't always true.

Accumulation of fluid in the body as a result of heart failure can also result in swollen ankles. With serious lung disease, such as emphysema, blood may "back up" through the heart, increase pressure in the veins, and thus cause ankle swelling. More rarely, a problem with the kidneys can result in swelling of the ankles. With serious liver disease, retention of fluid is very common. This fluid tends to accumulate primarily in the abdomen but is also frequently present in the legs.

Home Treatment

If there is an associated medical problem, the most important treatment will come from your doctor. However, all kinds of ankle swelling can be helped by things you can do yourself. First, you need to exercise your legs. As you work the muscles, the fluid tends to work back into the veins and lymphatic channels, and the swelling tends to go down.

Ankle swelling is almost always a signal that your body has too much salt. A low-salt diet helps decrease the fluid retention and the ankle swelling.

Elevating your legs can help the fluid drain back into more proper parts of your circulatory system. Lie down and

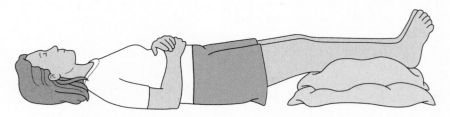

Reducing swelling. Rest with your legs higher than your heart.

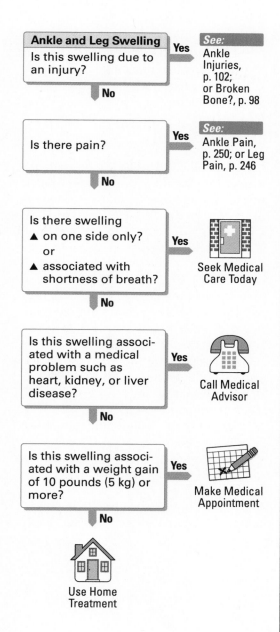

Ankle and Leg Swelling

Is this swelling due to an injury? — **Yes** → *See:* Ankle Injuries, p. 102; or Broken Bone?, p. 98

No ↓

Is there pain? — **Yes** → *See:* Ankle Pain, p. 250; or Leg Pain, p. 246

No ↓

Is there swelling
▲ on one side only? or
▲ associated with shortness of breath? — **Yes** → Seek Medical Care Today

No ↓

Is this swelling associated with a medical problem such as heart, kidney, or liver disease? — **Yes** → Call Medical Advisor

No ↓

Is this swelling associated with a weight gain of 10 pounds (5 kg) or more? — **Yes** → Make Medical Appointment

No ↓

Use Home Treatment

prop your legs up so they are higher than your heart as you rest. One or two pillows under the calves will help. Be sure not to place anything directly under the knees and don't wear any constricting clothing or garters on the upper legs.

Avoid sitting or standing without moving for long periods of time. If you must be in these positions, work the muscles in your calves by wiggling your feet and toes frequently. Support stockings, by applying constant external pressure, help reduce ankle swelling.

What to Expect at the Doctor's Office

The doctor will conduct a thorough examination including heart and lungs as well as the legs. Blood tests may be taken to check the function of your kidneys, heart, and liver and to measure the proteins in your blood. The specific treatment will be directed at whatever underlying cause is found. Diuretics (pills that decrease fluids in the body by increasing urination) may be prescribed. These are effective, but, of course, they have some side effects, such as causing loss of potassium from the body. If home treatment is successful, it is generally better than using drugs.

Heel Pain

The most frequent causes of heel pain are sometimes referred to as injuries, but they aren't due to a single event such as a fall or twist. Each of the following problems usually brings tenderness and some swelling.

Plantar fasciitis is a sprain of the tendon that is attached to the front of the heel bone and runs forward along the bottom of the foot. There are four main causes of plantar fasciitis:

▲ Feet that flatten and roll inwardly (pronate) excessively when walking or running
▲ Shoes with inadequate arch support
▲ Sudden turns that put great stress on the ligaments
▲ Running on hard surfaces or up hills

The retrocalcaneal bursa is a fluid-filled sac that surrounds the back of the heel. This may become inflamed (bursitis) due to pressure from shoes. For this reason, it is sometimes called a "pump bump." The inferior calcaneal bursa is located underneath the heel. Inflammation here is usually caused by landing hard or awkwardly on the heel.

The Achilles tendon is the large tendon that connects the calf muscles to the back of the heel. Achilles tendinitis occurs when the calf muscles repeatedly contract hard or suddenly. There are four factors that contribute to Achilles tendinitis:

▲ Shortening of and lack of flexibility in the calf muscle—Achilles tendon unit (the main cause)
▲ Shoes that don't provide good stability and shock absorption for the heel

▲ Sudden inward or outward turning of the heel when striking the ground (this is due to the shape of the foot, an inherited trait)
▲ Running on hard surfaces such as concrete or asphalt, or running on hills

Home Treatment

Plantar Fasciitis. Give your feet as much rest as possible for a week or so. Pain relievers can be used for comfort (page 54). Use that time to get proper-fitting shoes—that is, shoes with adequate arch supports and flexible soles. A one-quarter-inch (6 mm) heel pad is a good idea. Some people need to wear only well-padded shoes, such as running shoes. Lace the top two eyelets very firmly to take some tension off your ligaments. Get a plantar fasciitis strap at the drugstore and place it about an inch forward of the tender spot; this is often the best treatment. Try an orthotic device (obtained through a podiatrist or orthopedic surgeon), especially if there is excessive pronation of the foot. Be very patient. This problem can take a long time to go away.

Bursitis. Resting for 7 to 10 days and taking an over-the-counter pain medi-

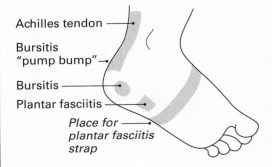

Achilles tendon

Bursitis "pump bump"

Bursitis

Plantar fasciitis

Place for plantar fasciitis strap

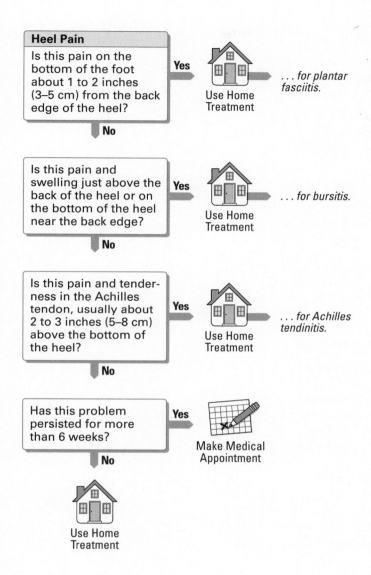

cation with each meal will help relieve the initial problem (page 54). For retrocalcaneal bursitis, getting a new shoe or stretching the old shoe so that there is no rubbing against the heel is recommended. Moleskin may be used to relieve pressure from the "pump bump."

Achilles Tendinitis. Stop exercising, apply ice twice daily to the tendon, and take an over-the-counter pain medication with each meal for a week (page 54). After that, stretching is the most important treatment. Remember to stretch and hold the stretched position. Do not bounce.

One method of stretching the Achilles tendon is wall push-ups:

1. Stand two feet (0.7 m) from a wall, hands outstretched and placed on the wall.

2. Bend elbows so that body moves closer to the wall. Keep heels on the ground.

3. Hold for a count of 10 and push away from wall.

4. Repeat 10 times per session, three sessions a day.

Slow improvement is the rule in most cases. If things are getting worse despite home treatment or if there is little progress after a month, see your doctor.

What to Expect at the Doctor's Office

Plantar Fasciitis and Bursitis. Cortisone injections, no more than three, may be tried if adjustments to the shoe and the use of orthotics and plantar fasciitis strap haven't been successful. They usually don't work. Surgery is a last resort and is seldom necessary.

Achilles Tendinitis. A stronger oral anti-inflammatory medicine may be prescribed, but cortisone injections aren't done because they may weaken the tendon and lead to rupture. In particularly resistant cases, a walking cast may be tried. Surgery is almost never recommended.

Foot Pain

There are some common problems that often lead to unnecessary pain or an unnecessary visit to the doctor's office.

The nerves that supply sensation to the front portion of your foot and your toes run between the long bones of the foot, the metatarsals. (There is a metatarsal just behind each toe.) Tight-fitting shoes can squeeze the nerves between the bones, and this may cause swelling in a nerve, a Morton's neuroma. The swelling is very sensitive, and pressure can cause intense pain. If pressure is constant, some numbness between the toes may also occur. Morton's neuroma occurs most commonly between the third and fourth metatarsals (between the middle toe and the next toe toward the outside of the foot).

If your big toe points toward the other four toes on that foot, the end of the metatarsal behind the big toe may rub against the shoe. The skin thickens over the end of the metatarsal, and the metatarsal itself may develop a bony spur at that point. This is a bunion, and if it becomes inflamed and sore, it can make life miserable.

Corns and calluses are the results of friction, and friction is usually caused by ill-fitting shoes. Corns appear as lumps of thickened skin that may be hard with a clear core or soft and moist. They are usually found on the tops of toes. Calluses also appear as thickened skin but are less lumpy and are most often found across the ball of the foot.

Plantar warts are caused by a virus and are often found on the ball of the foot. They may be distinguished from calluses by small black dots within the wart, the interruption of normal skin lines, and the inward growth of the wart.

Unaccustomed heavy use of the feet, such as in the beginning of training for running or basketball, may produce enough stress to produce a crack—stress fracture—in the metatarsals. The fourth metatarsal is most vulnerable to this. A stress fracture usually occurs several weeks into an increased training session or other activity involving strenuous use of the feet. Pain usually comes on gradually.

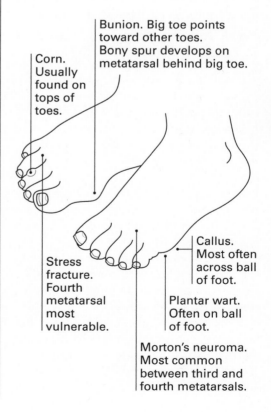

Corn. Usually found on tops of toes.

Bunion. Big toe points toward other toes. Bony spur develops on metatarsal behind big toe.

Stress fracture. Fourth metatarsal most vulnerable.

Callus. Most often across ball of foot.

Plantar wart. Often on ball of foot.

Morton's neuroma. Most common between third and fourth metatarsals.

Home Treatment

Morton's Neuroma. Shoes with adequate room around the balls of the feet are necessary. Over-the-counter pain relievers for two to three weeks may also help (page 54).

Bunion. Place a small sponge or pad between the big and second toes so that the big toe becomes aligned with the other four toes. Moleskin or padding around the bunion may help relieve pressure. Shoes that are wide enough in the balls of the feet so that pressure isn't applied will help. Acetaminophen or other over-the-counter pain medication may be used as above (page 54).

Corns and Calluses. The first step is to make sure your shoes fit properly. Sandals, if practical, and cushioning socks can be helpful. The "corn plasters" containing 40% salicylic acid, available without a prescription, are effective. Be sure to follow the directions: cut the plaster so that it is smaller than the corn or callus, and be careful in removing the dead skin that the plaster produces. A doctor's visit is rarely needed.

Plantar Warts. Good shoes and corn plasters can be effective for plantar warts also, but the removal of dead skin may be more difficult and time-consuming. For this reason, people with plantar warts end up in the doctor's office more often than people with corns and calluses. See the doctor if you are making no progress in decreasing the size of the problem. Meanwhile, wear slippers or bath shoes to decrease the likelihood of passing the virus on to someone else.

Metatarsal Stress Fracture. You are going to have to give your foot a rest. Using crutches for a week or so may be helpful in getting pressure off the foot if it is particularly painful. Remember that it may take from six weeks to three months for the fracture to heal completely so that you can return to full activity. A cast doesn't reduce the healing time and may create other problems, so most doctors avoid any kind of cast if at all possible.

What to Expect at the Doctor's Office

Morton's Neuroma. Cortisone injections, no more than three, may be tried if relief hasn't been obtained with oral medication and switching shoes. If these fail, the neuroma can be removed surgically. The operation usually leaves a region of skin on the foot permanently numb.

Bunion. If the bunion is particularly inflamed, a cortisone injection can provide temporary relief. If the big toe is so crooked that adjusting the shoes and using moleskin don't help, then surgery to realign the big toe may be needed.

Plantar Warts. The doctor may use cold (liquid nitrogen), heat (electrocoagulation), or surgery to remove a plantar wart. Unfortunately, plantar warts often recur.

Metatarsal Stress Fracture. The doctor has little to offer to relieve metatarsal stress fractures. You can get crutches at the drugstore. Casts are to be avoided if at all possible, and surgery is virtually never done. A walking cast for an incredibly painful foot is about the only thing the doctor can do that you can't.

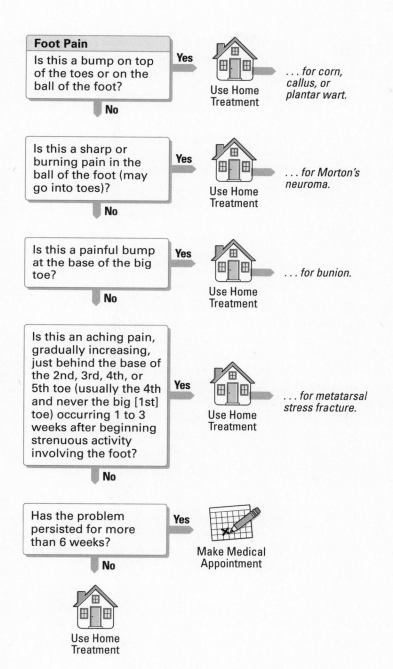

Foot Pain

Is this a bump on top of the toes or on the ball of the foot?

Yes → Use Home Treatment → *. . . for corn, callus, or plantar wart.*

No

Is this a sharp or burning pain in the ball of the foot (may go into toes)?

Yes → Use Home Treatment → *. . . for Morton's neuroma.*

No

Is this a painful bump at the base of the big toe?

Yes → Use Home Treatment → *. . . for bunion.*

No

Is this an aching pain, gradually increasing, just behind the base of the 2nd, 3rd, 4th, or 5th toe (usually the 4th and never the big [1st] toe) occurring 1 to 3 weeks after beginning strenuous activity involving the foot?

Yes → Use Home Treatment → *. . . for metatarsal stress fracture.*

No

Has the problem persisted for more than 6 weeks?

Yes → Make Medical Appointment

No → Use Home Treatment

CHAPTER 9

Chest, Abdominal, and Urinary Problems

Chest Pain

Chest pain is a serious symptom meaning "heart attack" to most people. However, many things in the chest can cause pain. Often it's hard even for a doctor to figure out the cause.

There's no easy rule to decide which pains you may treat at home. If you have any doubts about chest pain or if you have other symptoms such as shortness of breath, call 911 immediately.

The heart almost never causes pain for healthy men under 30 years of age or women under 40. Heart pain remains rare among men in their 40s and women in their 50s. Until middle age, chest pain is usually caused by something other than the heart:

▲ A brief, shooting pain is common in healthy young people and means nothing. So is a "catch" at the end of a deep breath.

▲ Hyperventilation is a common cause of chest pain, particularly in young people (page 298).

▲ If you press at the spot of discomfort and cause or worsen the pain, it is probably coming from the chest wall, not the heart. You can treat this pain at home.

▲ Angina is heart pain, but not a heart attack (see box on facing page).

▲ The pain of pleurisy (an inflammation of the chest cavity) gets worse with a deep breath or cough. Call your doctor.

▲ If the pain throbs with each heartbeat, the covering of the heart may be inflamed (pericarditis). Call your doctor.

▲ Pain from an ulcer is worse on an empty stomach and gets better with food. Call your doctor.

▲ Pain from the gallbladder is often more intense after a meal. Call your doctor.

Home Treatment

Treat pain in the chest wall with over-the-counter pain medicines (page 54) or topical treatments (e.g., Bengay, Vicks VapoRub). Rest and heat will also help. See the doctor if chest pain lasts for more than five days.

What to Expect at the Doctor's Office

The doctor will take the history and do a physical examination. Most likely, the doctor will run an electrocardiogram (ECG) and blood tests. The doctor may do additional tests if the cause of chest pain remains unknown. The person with chest pain may need to stay in the hospital. The doctor may prescribe pain medication.

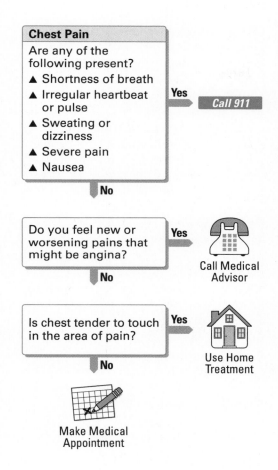

Chest Pain

Are any of the following present?

▲ Shortness of breath
▲ Irregular heartbeat or pulse
▲ Sweating or dizziness
▲ Severe pain
▲ Nausea

Yes ➤ *Call 911*

No

Do you feel new or worsening pains that might be angina?

Yes ➤ Call Medical Advisor

No

Is chest tender to touch in the area of pain?

Yes ➤ Use Home Treatment

No

Make Medical Appointment

Heart Attack and Angina

The chest pain of a heart attack is usually intense, though it can be mild. Sometimes the sensation is more like pressure or squeezing on the chest. Usually the pain or discomfort is centered beneath the breastbone. The pain may radiate to the jaw or down the inner part of either arm.

A person having a heart attack may experience nausea, sweating, dizziness, or shortness of breath. Call 911 immediately if you suspect a heart attack.

Heart pain that occurs with exertion and goes away with rest isn't an actual heart attack. Doctors call this angina pectoris, or angina. The risk of a heart attack is highest when you feel worse or new angina pain. Call your doctor immediately if you have new angina pains.

Shortness of Breath

This symptom is normal under circumstances of strenuous activity. The medical use of "shortness of breath" doesn't include shortness of breath after heavy exertion, being "breathless" with excitement, or having clogged nasal passages. These instances aren't cause for alarm.

Rather, shortness of breath is a problem if you:

▲ Get "winded" after slight exertion or at rest

▲ Wake up in the night out of breath

▲ Have to sleep propped up on several pillows to avoid becoming short of breath

This is a serious symptom that should be promptly evaluated by your doctor.

If wheezing is present, the problem is probably not as serious, but attention is needed just as promptly. In this instance, you may have asthma or early emphysema. See Wheezing (page 142).

A sudden onset of a new symptom of shortness of breath can, rarely, be a symptom of a blood clot in the lungs called a pulmonary embolus. There may have been leg swelling or pain before. This is a medical **emergency,** even if the shortness of breath is not too severe.

Hyperventilation syndrome (page 298) is a common cause of shortness of breath in previously healthy young people and is almost always the problem if the fingers are tingling. In this syndrome, the patient is actually overbreathing due to anxiety but has the sensation of shortness of breath.

Another emotional problem that may include the complaint of difficult breathing is mental depression (page 302). Deep, sighing respirations are a frequent symptom in depressed individuals.

Home Treatment

Rest, relax, and use the treatment described for hyperventilation syndrome (page 298) if indicated. If the problem persists, see a doctor. There isn't much you can do for shortness of breath at home.

What to Expect at the Doctor's Office

The doctor will thoroughly examine the lungs, heart, and upper airway passages. Electrocardiograms (ECGs), chest X-rays, and blood tests will sometimes be necessary. Depending on the cause and severity of the problem, the doctor may prescribe hospitalization, fluid pills, heart pills, or asthma medicine. Oxygen is less frequently helpful than commonly imagined and can be hazardous for patients with emphysema.

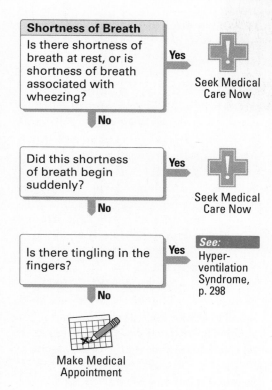

Shortness of Breath

Is there shortness of breath at rest, or is shortness of breath associated with wheezing?

Yes → Seek Medical Care Now

No ↓

Did this shortness of breath begin suddenly?

Yes → Seek Medical Care Now

No ↓

Is there tingling in the fingers?

Yes → *See:* Hyper-ventilation Syndrome, p. 298

No ↓

Make Medical Appointment

Palpitations

Everyone experiences palpitations. A pounding heart seems serious but is usually trivial. It can be brought on by strenuous exercise or intense emotion or can just happen. It is seldom associated with serious disease. Most people who complain of palpitations don't have heart disease but are overly concerned about the possibility of such disease and thus overly sensitive to normal heart actions. Often this anxiety stems from heart disease in parents, other relatives, or friends.

Understanding the Pulse

The pulse can be felt on the inside of the wrist, in the neck, or over the heart itself. During your next checkup, ask the nurse or doctor to check your method of taking pulses. Take your own pulse and those of your family, noting the variation with respiration. There is a normal variation in the pulse with respiration (faster when breathing in, slower when breathing out). Even though the pulse may speed up or slow down, the normal pulse has a regular rhythm.

Occasional extra heartbeats, felt as "flip-flops" or thumps in the chest, occur in nearly everyone. The most common time to notice these extra beats is just before going to sleep. They are of no consequence unless they're frequent (more than five per minute) or if they occur in runs of three or more.

Rapid pulses may also mimic palpitations. In adults, a heart rate greater than 120 beats per minute (without exercise) is cause to check with your doctor. Young children may have normal heart rates in that range, but they rarely complain of the heart pounding. If one does, check the situation with your doctor.

Causes

Keep in mind that the most frequent causes of rapid heartbeat (other than exercise) are anxiety (page 296) and fever (page 284). The presence of shortness of breath (page 262) or chest pain (page 260) increases the chances of a significant problem. Hyperventilation may also cause pounding and chest discomfort, but the heart rate remains less than 120 beats per minute (page 298).

Home Treatment

If a person seems stressed or anxious, focus on this rather than on the possibilities of heart disease. If anxiety doesn't seem a likely cause and the person has none of the other symptoms on the decision chart, discuss the problem with the doctor by phone. If it persists, see the doctor.

What to Expect at the Doctor's Office

Tell the doctor the exact rate of the pulse and whether or not the rhythm was regular. Usually the symptoms will disappear by the time you see the doctor, so the accuracy of your story becomes crucial. The doctor will examine your heart and lungs. An electrocardiogram (ECG) is unlikely to help if the problem is not present when the test is being done. A chest X-ray is seldom needed.

Don't expect reassurance from a doctor that your heart will be sound for the next month, year, or decade. Your doctor has no crystal ball, nor can he or she perform an annual tune-up or oil change. You, not the doctor, are in charge of the preventive maintenance of your heart (see Chapter 1).

Palpitations

Is there shortness of breath, or is there chest pain?

Yes → 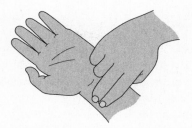 Seek Medical Care Now

No ↓

Are extra beats more than 4 per minute or coming in runs of 3 or more?

Yes → Seek Medical Care Today

No ↓

Is the pulse more than 120 beats per minute?

Yes → Seek Medical Care Today

No ↓

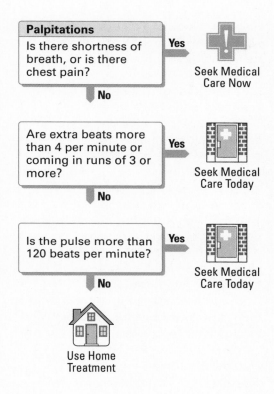 Use Home Treatment

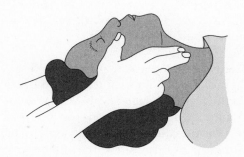

Wrist pulse. This drawing shows the technique for taking a pulse from the inside of the wrist. (Caution: Do not use your thumb, which has its own pulse.)

Neck pulse. This drawing shows the technique for taking a pulse from either side of the neck. (Caution: Do not take pulse from both sides of the neck at the same time.)

Nausea and Vomiting

Medications are the most common cause of nausea and vomiting in the elderly, whereas viral infections are the most common cause in children and young adults. When viruses are to blame, diarrhea is usually present as well.

Food poisoning is often blamed for stomach problems but is actually one of the less frequent causes of nausea and vomiting. In any event, nausea and vomiting caused by food poisoning are treated the same way as any other kind.

Dangers of Vomiting

Dehydration is the real threat with most vomiting. The speed with which dehydration develops depends on the size of the individual, the frequency of the vomiting, and the presence of diarrhea. Thus, infants with frequent vomiting and diarrhea are at the greatest risk. Signs of dehydration are:

▲ Marked thirst
▲ Infrequent urination or dark yellow urine
▲ Dry mouth or eyes that appear sunken
▲ Skin that has lost its normal elasticity. To determine this, gently pinch the skin on the stomach using all five fingers. When you release it, it should spring back immediately; compare with another person's skin if necessary. When the skin remains tented up and doesn't spring back normally, the person may be dehydrated.

Bleeding (bloody or black vomit) or severe abdominal pain also requires a doctor's attention immediately. Some abdominal discomfort accompanies almost every case of vomiting, but severe pain is unusual.

Head injuries may be associated with vomiting (page 108).

When pregnancy, diabetes, or medications cause nausea and vomiting, getting the doctor's advice by phone is usually sufficient to determine the approach you should take.

Headache and stiff neck along with vomiting are sometimes seen in meningitis, so an early visit to the doctor's office for further advice is wise. Lethargy or marked irritability in a young child has a similar implication.

Persistent nausea without vomiting is often due to medication, and occasionally to ulcers or cancer.

Home Treatment

The objective of home treatment is to take in as much fluid as possible without upsetting the stomach any further. Sip clear fluids such as water or ginger ale. Suck on ice chips if nothing else will stay down.

Don't drink much at any one time, and avoid solid foods. As your condition improves, try soups, bouillon, Jell-O, and applesauce. Milk products may help but sometimes aggravate the situation. Work up to a normal diet slowly. Popsicles or iced fruit bars often work well with children.

Unfortunately, drugs for vomiting (anti-emetics) don't work very well, if at all.

If vomiting persists for more than 72 hours, or if the person isn't hydrated enough after that time, check with your doctor.

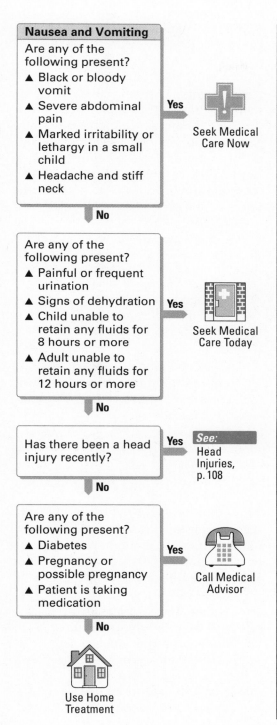

Nausea and Vomiting

Are any of the following present?

▲ Black or bloody vomit

▲ Severe abdominal pain

▲ Marked irritability or lethargy in a small child

▲ Headache and stiff neck

Yes → Seek Medical Care Now

No ↓

Are any of the following present?

▲ Painful or frequent urination

▲ Signs of dehydration

▲ Child unable to retain any fluids for 8 hours or more

▲ Adult unable to retain any fluids for 12 hours or more

Yes → Seek Medical Care Today

No ↓

Has there been a head injury recently?

Yes → *See:* Head Injuries, p. 108

No ↓

Are any of the following present?

▲ Diabetes

▲ Pregnancy or possible pregnancy

▲ Patient is taking medication

Yes → Call Medical Advisor

No ↓

Use Home Treatment

If a medication might be responsible, call the doctor to see if you should keep taking it. If it might be from an over-the-counter medicine you have taken yourself, stop taking it. The most common medications that can cause nausea and vomiting are nonsteroidal anti-inflammatory drugs (NSAIDs), including aspirin, naproxen, Aleve, Motrin, and many others.

If nausea persists for four weeks, call the doctor.

What to Expect at the Doctor's Office

The history and physical examination will focus on determining the degree of dehydration, as well as the possible causes. Blood tests and a urinalysis may be ordered but aren't always necessary. Ordinary X-rays of the abdomen are usually not very helpful, but special X-ray procedures may be necessary in some cases. If dehydration is severe, intravenous fluids may be given. This may require hospitalization, although it can often be done in the doctor's office. The use of antivomiting drugs is controversial, and they should be used only in severe cases.

Diarrhea

Many of the considerations with respect to diarrhea are the same as those in Nausea and Vomiting (page 266). Viruses are the most common cause, and dehydration is the greatest risk. Diarrhea is often accompanied by nausea and vomiting. Vomiting and fever both increase the risk of dehydration. Bacteria or bacterial toxins (food poisoning) may also produce diarrhea, but antibiotics are rarely helpful and may make things worse. As with viral infections, the major danger in bacterial problems is dehydration, and the treatment is essentially the same.

Dangers of Diarrhea

Black or bloody diarrhea may signal significant bleeding from the stomach or intestines. However, medicines containing bismuth subsalicylate (Pepto-Bismol, etc.) or iron may also turn the stool black. Cramping and intermittent gaslike pains are usual with diarrhea, but severe, steady abdominal pain isn't. Bleeding or severe abdominal pain requires the immediate attention of a doctor.

Many medications may cause diarrhea. Frequent culprits include the following:

▲ A nonsteroidal anti-inflammatory drug (NSAID), especially meclofenamate (Meclomen)—these are often prescribed for arthritis
▲ Antibiotics
▲ Blood pressure drugs
▲ Acid-blocking drugs
▲ Antacids containing magnesium
▲ Digitalis
▲ Anticancer drugs

If you are taking such medications, call the doctor who prescribed them.

Home Treatment

As with vomiting, the objective in treating diarrhea is to get as much fluid in as possible without upsetting the intestinal tract any further. Sip clear fluids; plain old tap water is best. If nothing will stay down, sucking on ice chips is usually tolerated and provides some fluid. Avoid juices or sodas for children. Pedialyte is essential for infants.

Once the patient tolerates clear fluids, it is time to eat the foods that spell BRAT:

▲ Bananas
▲ Rice
▲ Applesauce
▲ Toast

Avoid milk and fats for several days.

Nonprescription preparations such as Pepto-Bismol or Kaopectate (bismuth subsalicylate) may reduce stool amount and frequency (page 68). Adults may try loperamide, but this should be avoided in children. If symptoms persist for more than 96 hours, call your doctor.

What to Expect at the Doctor's Office

A thorough history and physical examination with special attention to assessing dehydration will be completed. The abdomen will be examined. Frequently the stools will be examined under the microscope, and occasionally a culture will be taken. A urine specimen may be examined to assist in assessing dehydration. An antibiotic may be prescribed. A narcotic-like preparation (such as Lomotil) may also be prescribed for adults to decrease the frequency of stools.

Chronic diarrhea may require more extensive evaluation of the stools, blood tests, and often X-ray examinations of the intestinal tract. As with vomiting, severe dehydration will require intravenous fluids. This may be taken care of in the doctor's office or may require hospitalization.

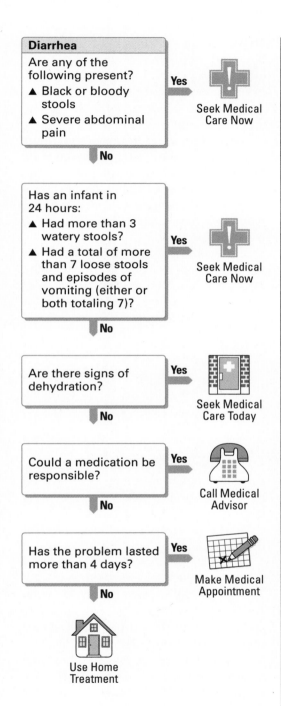

Diarrhea

Are any of the following present?
▲ Black or bloody stools
▲ Severe abdominal pain

Yes → Seek Medical Care Now

No

Has an infant in 24 hours:
▲ Had more than 3 watery stools?
▲ Had a total of more than 7 loose stools and episodes of vomiting (either or both totaling 7)?

Yes → Seek Medical Care Now

No

Are there signs of dehydration?

Yes → Seek Medical Care Today

No

Could a medication be responsible?

Yes → Call Medical Advisor

No

Has the problem lasted more than 4 days?

Yes → Make Medical Appointment

No

Use Home Treatment

Dehydration

Severe and prolonged diarrhea can lead to dehydration. Fever and vomiting increase fluid loss and raise the risk of dehydration. People with the lowest tolerance for dehydration are infants, the elderly, and those with health problems. Signs of dehydration are:

▲ Marked thirst
▲ Scanty urination or dark yellow urine
▲ Dry mouth
▲ Eyes that appear sunken
▲ Skin that has lost its normal elasticity. Normally skin springs back if you pinch it; when a person is dehydrated, the skin may remain tented up after pinching.

Heartburn

Heartburn is irritation of the stomach or the esophagus, the tube that leads from the mouth to the stomach. The stomach lining is usually protected from the effects of its own acid. Certain factors, however, such as smoking, caffeine, aspirin, and stress, cause this protection to be impaired. The esophagus is not protected against acid, and a backflow of acid from the stomach into the esophagus causes irritation. There may be a sour taste in the mouth.

Ulcers of the stomach or the upper bowel (duodenum) may also cause pain. Treatment for ulcers is the same as for uncomplicated heartburn, provided that pain isn't severe and there's no evidence of bleeding. Long-lasting stomach ulcers may demand antibiotic treatment (see Abdominal Pain, page 272).

Vomiting black, "coffee ground" material or bright red blood means you should give the doctor a call. Black stools, rather like tar, have the same significance; however, iron supplements and bismuth subsalicylate (Pepto-Bismol) will also cause black stools.

Heartburn pain ordinarily doesn't go through to the back. Such pain may signal involvement of the pancreas or a severe ulcer.

Rarely, "indigestion" or heartburn can signal a heart attack. If you are over 40 years of age and the heartburn is a new problem, check out the chest pain discussion (page 260).

Home Treatment

Avoid substances that aggravate the problem. The most common irritants are coffee, tea, alcohol, aspirin, ibuprofen, and naproxen. The contributing effect of smoking or stress must be considered in every sufferer.

Relief is often obtained by using nonabsorbable antacids (Maalox, Mylanta, Gelusil, etc.) every one to two hours (page 59). Baking soda may provide quick relief but isn't suitable for repeated use. Nonfat milk may be substituted for antacid but adds calories. If the pain continues, you can try acid neutralizers (page 59).

If the pain is worse when lying down, the esophagus is probably the problem. Measures that help prevent backflow of acid from the stomach into the esophagus should be employed:

▲ Avoid lying down or reclining after eating.
▲ Elevate the head of the bed with blocks four to six inches (10–15 cm).
▲ Don't wear tight-fitting clothes (girdles, tight jeans).
▲ Avoid eating or drinking for two hours before going to bed.

If the problem could have been caused by a medication, call the prescribing doctor.

If the problem lasts for more than three days, call your doctor.

What to Expect at the Doctor's Office

The doctor will determine if the problem is due to stomach acid, a peptic acid syndrome. If so, treatment will be similar to that outlined above. Medications to reduce secretion of acid may be prescribed. X-rays of the esophagus and stomach (upper GI) may be done, after the patient has swallowed barium, to determine the presence of ulcers and

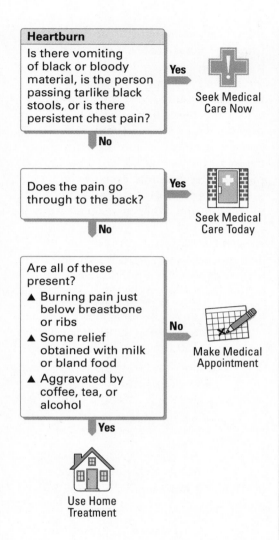

Heartburn

Is there vomiting of black or bloody material, is the person passing tarlike black stools, or is there persistent chest pain?

Yes → Seek Medical Care Now

No ↓

Does the pain go through to the back?

Yes → Seek Medical Care Today

No ↓

Are all of these present?

▲ Burning pain just below breastbone or ribs
▲ Some relief obtained with milk or bland food
▲ Aggravated by coffee, tea, or alcohol

No → Make Medical Appointment

Yes ↓

Use Home Treatment

to note if backflow of acid from the stomach into the esophagus, or hiatal hernia, is present. If the doctor says you have "GERD" (gastroesophageal reflux disease), remember this is just heartburn. Because the treatment for any acid syndrome is essentially the same, an X-ray is usually not done on the first visit. Any indication of bleeding will require a more vigorous approach to therapy.

Abdominal Pain

Abdominal pain can be a sign of a serious condition. Fortunately, minor causes are much more frequent. Location of the pain can help in suggesting the cause.

▲ **Appendix pain** usually occurs in the right lower quarter of the abdomen
▲ **Diverticulitis** usually hurts in the left lower quarter of the abdomen
▲ **Kidney pain,** the back
▲ **Gallbladder,** the right upper quarter
▲ **Stomach,** the upper abdomen
▲ **Bladder** or **female organs,** the lower areas

Exceptions to these rules do occur.

Pain from hollow organs—such as the bowel or gallbladder—tends to be intermittent and resembles gas pains or colic. Pain from solid organs—kidneys, spleen, liver—tends to be more constant. Stomach ulcers tend to create burning pain in the upper abdomen, which usually gets better after a meal or a dose of antacid. There are exceptions to these rules as well.

When to See a Doctor

If the pain is very severe or if bleeding from the bowel occurs, see a doctor. Similarly, if there has been a significant recent abdominal injury, see the doctor—a ruptured spleen or other major problem is possible.

Pain during pregnancy is potentially serious and must be evaluated. An "ectopic pregnancy"—in the fallopian tube rather than in the uterus—can occur before a woman is even aware she is pregnant. Pain in only one area suggests a more serious problem than generalized pain; again,

there are exceptions. Pain that recurs with the menstrual cycle, especially premenstrually, is typical of endometriosis; see Difficult Periods (page 318).

Stomach ulcers are made worse by excess acid and better by antacids. It's now known that a bacterium called helicobacter pylori is responsible for many, if not most, stomach ulcers. So if your pain isn't completely eased by antacids and acid reducers in a week, see the doctor to consider other forms of therapy.

Appendicitis

The most constant signal of appendicitis is the *order* in which symptoms occur:

1. Pain—usually first around the belly button or just below the breastbone; only later in the right lower quarter of the abdomen

2. Nausea or vomiting or, at the very least, loss of appetite

3. Local tenderness in the right lower quarter of the abdomen

4. Fever ranging from 100° to 102°F (38° to 39°C)

The following signs make appendicitis unlikely:

▲ Fever precedes or is present at the time of initial pain
▲ There's *no fever* or a *high fever,* greater than 102°F (39°C), in the first 24 hours
▲ Vomiting accompanies or precedes the first bout of pain

Home Treatment

To treat abdominal pain, sip water or other clear fluids, but avoid solid foods. A bowel movement, passage of gas through

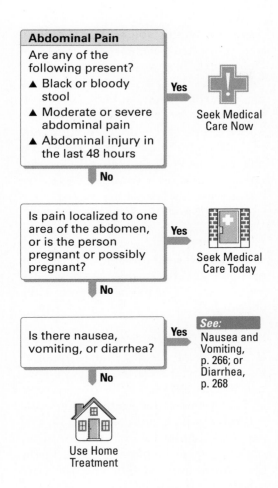

Abdominal Pain

Are any of the following present?
- ▲ Black or bloody stool
- ▲ Moderate or severe abdominal pain
- ▲ Abdominal injury in the last 48 hours

Yes → Seek Medical Care Now

No

Is pain localized to one area of the abdomen, or is the person pregnant or possibly pregnant?

Yes → Seek Medical Care Today

No

Is there nausea, vomiting, or diarrhea?

Yes → *See:* Nausea and Vomiting, p. 266; or Diarrhea, p. 268

No

Use Home Treatment

the rectum, or a good belch may give relief—don't hold back. A warm bath helps some patients.

Antacid treatment for heartburn, indigestion, or suspected stomach ulcer should usually begin with an antacid every four hours (page 59). You may also use liquid antacids and periodic drinks of nonfat milk. If antacids fail, try one of the nonprescription medications that help stop stomach acid secretion (page 60). And if these don't work either, a visit to the doctor is in order.

The key to home treatment is periodic reevaluation; any persistent pain should be treated at the emergency room or the doctor's office. Home treatment should be reserved for mild pains that resolve within 24 hours or are clearly identifiable as stomach flu, heartburn, or other minor problems.

What to Expect at the Doctor's Office

The doctor will give a thorough examination, particularly of the abdomen. Usually a white blood cell count and urinalysis, and often other laboratory tests, will be recommended. X-rays are generally not important for pain of short duration, but they are sometimes needed. Observation in the hospital may be required. If the initial evaluation is negative but pain persists, reevaluation is necessary.

Doctors have achieved impressive results treating stomach ulcers with antibacterial agents to kill the helicobacter pylori. If your doctor diagnoses a stomach ulcer, ask about such treatment.

Constipation

Many people are overly preoccupied with constipation. Concern about the shape of the stool, its consistency, its color, and the frequency of bowel movements is often reported to doctors. Such complaints are medically trivial. Only rarely (and then usually in older patients) does a change in bowel habits signal a serious problem.

Weight loss and thin, pencil-like stools suggest a tumor of the lower bowel.

Abdominal pain and a swollen abdomen suggest the possibility of a bowel obstruction.

Home Treatment

We like to encourage a healthy diet for the bowel, followed by a healthy lack of interest in the details of the stool-elimination process. The diet should contain fresh fruits and vegetables for their natural laxative action and adequate fiber residue. Fiber is present in brans, celery, and whole-grain breads and is absent from foods that have been overly processed. Fiber draws water into the stool and adds bulk; thus, it decreases the transit time from mouth to bowel movement and softens the stool.

Bowel movements may occur three times daily or once every three days and still be normal. The stools may change in color, texture, consistency, or bulk without need for concern. They may be regular or irregular. Don't worry about them unless there is a major deviation.

If you need to use laxatives, we prefer a bulk laxative such as Metamucil (page 67). Milk of magnesia is satisfactory, but it and stronger traditional laxatives should not be used over a long period. A suppository (such as Dulcolax) can give quick relief, often within the hour. Remember that (just like everything else) exercise can help.

Increasingly, bulk laxatives such as Miralax, which act to draw water into the stool osmotically, are gaining favor for effectiveness and gentleness. Glycerin rectal suppositories work the same way but are usually less expensive and may cause less violent bowel movements.

For an acute problem, an enema may help. Fleet's enemas are handy and disposable. If such remedies are needed more than occasionally, ask your doctor about the problem on your next routine visit.

What to Expect at the Doctor's Office

If you have had a major change in bowel habits, expect a rectal examination and, usually, inspection of the lower bowel and sometimes the entire colon with a flexible tube called a sigmoidoscope. An X-ray of the lower bowel (using a barium enema) is often needed. These procedures are generally safe and only mildly uncomfortable. If you have only a minor problem, you may receive advice similar to that under Home Treatment, without examination or procedures.

Constipation

Is constipation associated with the following?

▲ Very thin, pencil-like stools

▲ Abdominal pain and bloating

▲ Weight loss

Yes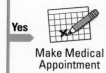

Make Medical Appointment

No

Use Home Treatment

Rectal Problems

Seldom is a rectal problem major, but the discomfort it can cause may make life miserable. Unlike most other medical problems, rectal pain doesn't yield the dividend of a good topic for social conversation.

Hemorrhoids, or "piles," are the most common rectal problem. There is a network of veins around the anus, and they tend to enlarge with age, particularly in individuals who sit a great deal during the day. Straining to have a bowel movement and passing hard, compacted stools tend to irritate these veins, and they may become inflamed, tender, or clogged. They may bleed or bulge outside the anus. The veins themselves are the "hemorrhoids." They may be outside the anal opening and visible (external), or they may be inside and invisible (internal). Pain and inflammation usually disappear within a few days or a few weeks, but this interval can be extremely uncomfortable. After healing, a small flap, or "tag," of vein and scar tissue often remains.

Bleeding from the digestive tract should be taken seriously, especially blood from higher in the digestive tract. This blood will be burgundy or black. Iron supplements or bismuth subsalicylate (Pepto-Bismol) may also turn the stool black. Blood from hemorrhoids may be on the outside of the stool, but usually is not mixed into the stool substance and frequently will be seen only on the toilet paper after wiping. Such bleeding from hemorrhoids isn't medically significant unless it is heavy or persists for several weeks.

Sometimes a child will suddenly awake soon after going to bed and complain of rectal pain. This almost always means pinworms. Though these small worms are seldom seen, they're quite common. They live in the rectum, and the female emerges at night and secretes a sticky and irritating substance around the anus into which she lays her eggs. Occasionally the worms move into the vagina, causing pain and itching in that area.

If rectal pain persists more than a week, consult the doctor. In such cases, a crack in the wall of the rectum may have developed, or an infection or other problem may be present.

Home Treatment

Soften the stool by including more fresh fruits and fiber (bran, celery, whole-grain bread) in the diet, or by using fiber bulk laxatives (page 67). Keep the area clean. Use the shower or sitz bath as an alternative to rubbing with toilet paper.

For external hemorrhoids, after gently drying the painful area, apply zinc oxide paste or powder (page 70). This will protect against further irritation. The various proprietary hemorrhoid preparations are less satisfactory. We prefer not to use compounds with a local anesthetic agent because these compounds may sensitize and irritate the area and may prolong healing. Such compounds have "-caine" in the brand name or in the list of ingredients.

Internal hemorrhoids sometimes may be helped by using a soothing suppository in addition to stool-softening measures. If relief isn't complete within a week, see the doctor. Even if the problem resolves quickly, mention it to your doctor on your next visit.

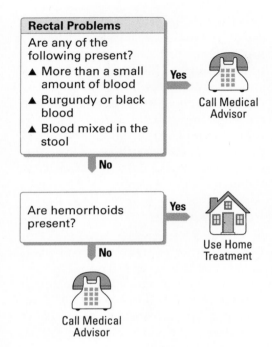

Rectal Problems

Are any of the following present?

▲ More than a small amount of blood

▲ Burgundy or black blood

▲ Blood mixed in the stool

Yes → Call Medical Advisor

No ↓

Are hemorrhoids present?

Yes → Use Home Treatment

No ↓

Call Medical Advisor

Pinworms are effectively treated with pyrantel (Pin-X, etc.). Follow directions on the label.

What to Expect at the Doctor's Office

The doctor will examine the anus and rectum. If a clot has formed in a hemorrhoid, the vein may be lanced and the clot removed. Major hemorrhoid surgery is seldom required and should be reserved for the most persistent problems. Usually, advice such as that given in Home Treatment will be given.

There are prescription drugs for pinworms that may be more convenient to take (and more expensive), but not a lot more effective than pyrantel.

Incontinence

Incontinence is the inability to hold feces or urine. We're all born incontinent, and as we grow older, there's a tendency for this problem to return. Incontinence is a complicated issue because there are many causes and many treatments. It isn't a hopeless condition. The vast majority of people can be greatly helped.

Effects of Aging

In women, the uterus and pelvic floor sag with aging. This changes the angle of the urethra (the tube leading from the bladder) and disposes it to leak urine.

In men, harmless enlargement of the prostate gland tends to block passage of urine until finally the bladder must overflow.

With age, there are sometimes sudden contractions of the bladder muscles. This results in increased pressure at unexpected times. There can be decreased sensitivity to the presence of a full bladder, and once the condition is realized, it can be difficult to get to the toilet in time.

Causes of Incontinence

Drugs such as diuretics ("water pills") can cause major surges in urine flow. Other drugs, such as tranquilizers, sedatives, anticholinergics, pain pills, and antidepressants, can block the normal voiding mechanisms; this results in retention of urine and then incontinence.

Infections of the urinary tract can cause an urgency for which there is no time to react.

Fecal Incontinence

Fecal incontinence is usually due to the presence of hard or impacted stool in the rectum. This results in diarrhea and incontinence around the impacted stool. Problems with fecal incontinence should be reported to your doctor. This isn't a complaint to be shy about. If you let it persist, it will begin to affect every part of your life, including your self-image.

Home Treatment

For fecal incontinence, it's important that your diet contain adequate fiber, water, and bulk. A soft stool passed twice a week is normal, but you should consider a hard, impacted stool (even if passed in small amounts twice daily) a problem. Fiber—as in whole grains, bran, celery, fresh fruits, and vegetables—is helpful. Preparations (Metamucil, Fiberall, etc.) can be used to add bulk (page 67). Because the presence of impacted feces in the rectum can make you feel bad all over, it is important to get this taken care of immediately. The doctor will help.

Performance of the bladder can often be improved by exercising the muscles that control the urinary outlet. Practice stopping urination in midstream and then starting again. This exercise is often difficult, especially for women, but it will build stronger sphincter muscles. Deliberately contracting the muscles around your anus and urinary tract for a second or two, then relaxing, then repeating, will build strength in these muscles and help tighten the pelvic floor. Many doctors recommend that these exercises be done up to 100 times daily.

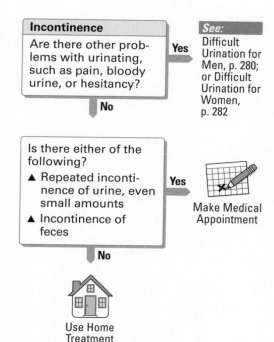

Incontinence

Are there other problems with urinating, such as pain, bloody urine, or hesitancy?

Yes →

See:
Difficult Urination for Men, p. 280; or Difficult Urination for Women, p. 282

No ↓

Is there either of the following?

▲ Repeated incontinence of urine, even small amounts

▲ Incontinence of feces

Yes →

Make Medical Appointment

No ↓

Use Home Treatment

Double voiding techniques can be helpful. Here, you empty the bladder as much as you can, wait a minute or so and then empty it again. It is surprising how much additional urine will sometimes be present. "Bladder drill" consists of urinating at fixed intervals, perhaps every four hours, during the day, whether the sensation of urgency is present or not; this can help. If you have trouble getting to the toilet on time, consider keeping a urine receptacle close at hand. Absorbent underwear (Depends, etc.) can help avoid embarrassment.

Always suspect that drugs that you're taking might be aggravating the problem; be sure to bring this possibility to the attention of your doctor.

What to Expect at the Doctor's Office

The doctor will perform a complete examination, with emphasis on the abdomen, rectum, and urinary opening. Urinalysis will usually be performed. If there are abnormalities, cystoscopy (inspection of the inside of the bladder) may be performed.

The gynecologist and the urologist are the specialists most familiar with these problems. If simple treatments don't work, a variety of specialized tests may pinpoint the problem.

For women, the doctor will sometimes prescribe a local estrogen cream, which can be surprisingly effective. Uterine or pelvic suspension operations are sometimes needed.

Men may choose prostatectomy, drugs, or simple "watchful waiting." Internal or external tubes (catheters) are sometimes used.

Difficult Urination for Men

Infections of the bladder may be signaled by:

▲ Pain or burning upon urination
▲ Frequent, urgent urination
▲ Blood in the urine

These symptoms aren't always caused by infection due to bacteria. They can be due to a viral infection or excessive consumption of caffeine-containing beverages (coffee, tea, and some soft drinks), or they may have no known cause and be blamed on "nerves."

Prostatitis—inflammation of the prostate gland—may cause symptoms similar to those of a bladder infection. Difficulty in starting urination, dribbling, or decreased force of the urinary stream—symptoms of *prostatism*—may also be present. However, prostatism is much more likely to be due to benign prostatic hypertrophy (BPH) than prostatitis. Some degree of BPH is universal in elderly men. Prostatic cancer may also cause prostatism.

Vomiting, back pain, or teeth-chattering, body-shaking chills aren't typical of bladder or prostate infections. They suggest kidney infection. This requires a more vigorous treatment and follow-up. A history of kidney disease (infections, inflammations, and kidney stones) also alters the treatment.

Most, if not all, bacterial bladder infections will respond to home treatment. Nevertheless, using antibiotics has become standard medical practice. Given this and the difficulty of distinguishing between bladder infection and prostatitis, see a doctor unless the symptoms respond quickly and completely to home treatment. Prostatitis and prostatism require the doctor's help.

Home Treatment

For symptoms of a bladder infection:

▲ Drink a lot of fluids. Increase fluid intake to the maximum (up to several gallons of fluid in the first 24 hours). Bacteria are literally washed from the body during the resulting copious urination.
▲ Drink fruit juices. Putting more acid into the urine, while less important than the quantity of fluids, may help bring relief. Cranberry juice may be the most effective because it contains a natural antibiotic, mandelic acid. This medicinal acid is marketed as mandelamine.

Begin home treatment as soon as symptoms are noted. If symptoms persist for 24 hours or recur, see the doctor.

What to Expect at the Doctor's Office

A urinalysis and culture should be performed. The back and abdomen are usually examined. With symptoms of prostatitis or prostatism, a rectal examination (so that the prostate can be felt) should be expected. With preexisting kidney disease or symptoms of kidney infection, a more detailed history and physical as well as extra laboratory studies may be needed.

If bacterial infection is determined, the doctor will prescribe an antibiotic. A surgical procedure—there are several—may be chosen to relieve prostatism, but drugs or simple "watchful waiting" may be best for you.

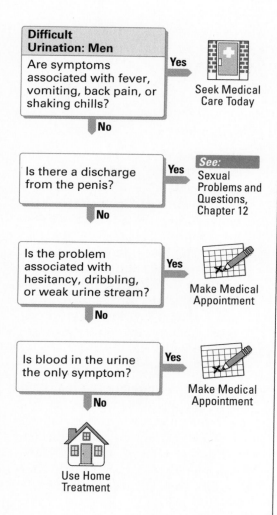

Difficult Urination: Men

Are symptoms associated with fever, vomiting, back pain, or shaking chills?

Yes → Seek Medical Care Today

No

Is there a discharge from the penis?

Yes → *See:* Sexual Problems and Questions, Chapter 12

No

Is the problem associated with hesitancy, dribbling, or weak urine stream?

Yes → Make Medical Appointment

No

Is blood in the urine the only symptom?

Yes → Make Medical Appointment

No

Use Home Treatment

Difficult Urination for Women

The best-known symptoms of bladder infections are:

- ▲ Pain or burning on urination
- ▲ Frequent, urgent urination
- ▲ Blood in the urine

These symptoms aren't always caused by infection due to bacteria. They can be due to a viral infection, excessive use of caffeine-containing beverages (coffee, tea, and cola drinks), or bladder spasm, or they can have no known cause (i.e., "nerves").

Bladder infections are far more common in women than in men. The female urethra, the tube leading from the bladder to the outside of the body, is only about one-half inch (1 cm) long—a short distance for bacteria to travel to reach the bladder. Sometimes bladder infections are related to sexual activity; hence, "honeymoon cystitis" has become a well-known medical syndrome.

Bladder infections are common during pregnancy. Treatment may be more difficult and must take the pregnancy into account.

Vomiting, back pain, or teeth-chattering, body-shaking chills aren't typical of bladder infections. They suggest kidney infection. This requires more vigorous treatment and follow-up. A history of kidney disease (infections, inflammations, and kidney stones) also alters the treatment.

Most, if not all, bacterial bladder infections will respond to home treatment alone. Nevertheless, using antibiotics has become standard medical practice, and it is possible that they

shorten the illness. Antibiotics may be more important in recurrent bladder infections.

Home Treatment

Begin home treatment as soon as you note symptoms.

- ▲ Drink a lot of fluids. Increase fluid intake to the maximum (up to several gallons of fluid in the first 24 hours). Bacteria are literally washed from the body during the resulting copious urination.
- ▲ Drink fruit juices. Putting more acid into the urine, although less important than the quantity of fluids, may help bring relief. Cranberry juice may be the most effective, as it contains a natural antibiotic, mandelic acid. This medicinal acid is marketed as mandelamine.

If relief isn't substantial in 24 hours and complete in 48, call the doctor.

For women with recurrent problems, an important preventive measure is to wipe from front to back after urination. Most bacteria that cause bladder infections come from the rectum.

What to Expect at the Doctor's Office

A urinalysis and culture will be performed. The back and abdomen are usually examined. In women with a vaginal discharge, an examination of both vagina and discharge is often necessary. With preexisting kidney disease or symptoms of kidney infection, a more detailed history and physical are needed, and extra laboratory studies may be necessary. If tests prove there is a urinary tract infection, the doctor will prescribe an antibiotic.

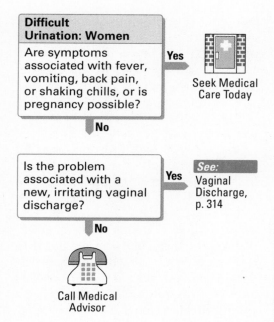

Difficult Urination: Women

Are symptoms associated with fever, vomiting, back pain, or shaking chills, or is pregnancy possible?

Yes → Seek Medical Care Today

No

Is the problem associated with a new, irritating vaginal discharge?

Yes → *See:* Vaginal Discharge, p. 314

No

Call Medical Advisor

CHAPTER 10

Generalized Problems

Fever

A high temperature is not always a sign of illness. Normal body temperature varies from person to person and is usually lower in the morning. Physical activity, excitement, anxiety, food, and heavy clothing can all raise body temperature. Hormones can cause a monthly change in body temperature in fertile women. Children usually have a higher temperature than adults, and their temperatures go up and down more during the day.

The point at which an elevated temperature becomes a fever is not well defined. To make it easy, we say that a fever is a temperature over 100°F (38°C) taken with an oral thermometer. A temperature that remains around 99° to 100°F (38°C) for a week or more also deserves attention.

Causes

The most common causes of fever are viral and bacterial infections, such as colds, sore throats, earaches, diarrhea, urinary infections, roseola, chicken pox, mumps, and measles. Pneumonia, appendicitis, and meningitis are also occasional causes.

A fever can cause the brain's temperature center to register cold, triggering the body's systems to produce more heat, such as by shivering. The person with a fever may look pale, as blood is shunted away from the skin. He or she may have goose bumps. Children will sometimes curl up in a ball to conserve heat. Don't bundle up the person with chills in blankets. This will only cause the fever to go higher.

Home Treatment

You can reduce the body temperature of a person with a high fever by sponging the skin with lukewarm water. (Cool water may be uncomfortable. Do not use alcohol because the fumes can be dangerous.) You can also cool the person in a tub of water about 70°F (21°C). Wetting the hair will feel good and help carry away heat. After drying, have the person rest in a cool room wearing little or no clothing. You can cover a child with a light sheet.

Medication

You don't need to do anything for a mild fever. If the fever is high enough to interfere with a person's sleep, work, or other activities, you can treat it with an over-the-counter remedy.

Starve a Fever?

You may have heard the old saying that begins, "Starve a fever." Unfortunately, it's not a helpful old saying. There are many reasons why people should eat during a fever. A person whose body temperature is high burns calories faster and therefore needs to consume more.

Even more important than food for someone with a fever are fluids. Never withhold liquids from a feverish person (unless he or she is in the middle of a seizure). Even if the fever makes the person so uncomfortable that he or she won't eat, it is still essential that the person drink fluids.

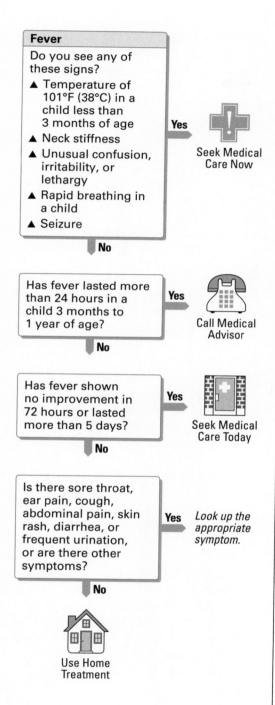

Fever

Do you see any of these signs?

▲ Temperature of 101°F (38°C) in a child less than 3 months of age

▲ Neck stiffness

▲ Unusual confusion, irritability, or lethargy

▲ Rapid breathing in a child

▲ Seizure

Yes → Seek Medical Care Now

No ↓

Has fever lasted more than 24 hours in a child 3 months to 1 year of age?

Yes → Call Medical Advisor

No ↓

Has fever shown no improvement in 72 hours or lasted more than 5 days?

Yes → Seek Medical Care Today

No ↓

Is there sore throat, ear pain, cough, abdominal pain, skin rash, diarrhea, or frequent urination, or are there other symptoms?

Yes → *Look up the appropriate symptom.*

No ↓

Use Home Treatment

Call the doctor if a fever lasts for more than 48 hours or if it stays above 103°F (39.5°C) after an hour of home treatment.

What to Expect at the Doctor's Office

The medical professional will take a history and do a physical examination to assess fever and other symptoms. If a person appears very sick, a doctor may run blood and urine tests. In rare cases, a doctor may order a chest X-ray. If the person has had a seizure for the first time, a doctor may order a spinal tap to check for meningitis. If the person has a bacterial infection, a doctor or physician assistant may prescribe an antibiotic.

Often the medical professional will suggest sponging or over-the-counter medication, as we describe above. If you have no infection or other symptoms, the doctor may advise "watchful waiting."

Headache

Headache is the single most common complaint of modern times. Usually tension and muscle spasms in the neck, scalp, and jaw cause headaches. They are annoying but invariably get better with time.

If your headaches are worse in the morning, consider having your blood pressure measured. High blood pressure can cause headaches.

Migraines are a type of severe headache causing pain on one side of the head only. A migraine often causes nausea or vomiting and may be preceded by flashes of light or seeing "stars."

Some people prone to headaches worry that they have a brain tumor. Unless you have some other dramatic signs, such as paralysis or a personality change, the chance that an occasional headache is a brain tumor is exceedingly remote.

When accompanied by other symptoms, a headache might be the sign of an **emergency:**

▲ After a head injury (page 108), a headache accompanied by vomiting or difficulty seeing suggests a dangerous increase in pressure inside the skull.

▲ A headache, a fever, and the inability to touch the chin to the chest suggest that the covering of the brain and spinal cord might be inflamed (meningitis, page 230).

▲ Headaches that are accompanied by difficulty in using the arms or legs, or by slurring of speech, require immediate medical attention.

Home Treatment

Over-the-counter pain medicines are usually quite effective in relieving headache (page 54). You can take these medications with food to prevent stomach irritation. Do not give aspirin to children or teenagers. For migraine headaches, medications that include caffeine (Excedrin) are often best.

You may relieve headache by resting with the eyes closed and the head supported. You may find a massage or heat applied to the back of the neck soothing. Relaxation techniques such as meditation may also work.

Talk to your doctor about persistent headaches that don't respond to home treatment. Call the doctor if headaches quickly become more frequent or severe.

What to Expect at the Doctor's Office

The health professional will ask for a medical history and do a physical examination. He or she will pay special attention to the head and neck and to neurological function. Doctors rarely do imaging studies such as CT or MRI unless a headache doesn't respond to therapy.

Doctors treat most tension headaches with the basic home treatment approach we describe above. Your doctor may prescribe medication for headaches not due to tension, such as migraine.

If there is tenderness to pressure in the back of the neck where the muscles meet the skull, then a cervical collar (see Neck Pain, page 230), worn at night, can sometimes help.

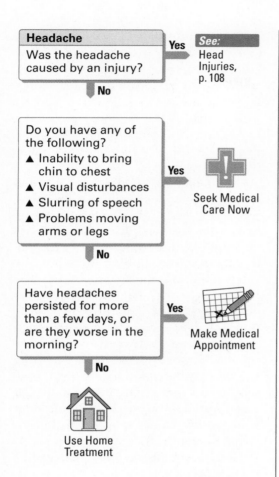

Headache

Was the headache caused by an injury? — **Yes** → *See:* Head Injuries, p. 108

No ↓

Do you have any of the following?
- ▲ Inability to bring chin to chest
- ▲ Visual disturbances
- ▲ Slurring of speech
- ▲ Problems moving arms or legs

Yes → Seek Medical Care Now

No ↓

Have headaches persisted for more than a few days, or are they worse in the morning? — **Yes** → Make Medical Appointment

No ↓

Use Home Treatment

Sleep Disorders

Almost everybody suffers from sleep problems now and then. Millions of people snore each night. Many people have occasional insomnia. And for 15 million to 20 million Americans, sleeplessness is an ongoing problem.

Medical problems can affect the quality of your sleep. Conditions that cause pain or shortness of breath may make sleep difficult. Depression and stress can also affect sleep. In these cases, treating the underlying cause is the best way to sleep soundly again.

For many people, snoring is just a noisy annoyance. However, a few snorers actually stop breathing (apnea) for 30 or more seconds several times during the night. This condition, called obstructive sleep apnea, has these associated signs:

▲ Loud, repeated snoring
▲ Feeling tired during the day and taking naps

By contrast, a person with central sleep apnea produces no loud, repeated snoring, but still stops breathing briefly during sleep. The associated signs of this condition are:

▲ Waking up many times during the night, often feeling short of breath
▲ Seldom taking naps, though one may feel tired

Most central sleep apnea occurs in men.

Doctors have linked sleep apnea with heart disease, high blood pressure, and impotence in men. Fortunately, doctors offer a range of effective treatments for it.

Home Treatment

Often a sleeping partner is the first to know of a serious snoring problem. If you've heard complaints, avoid sleeping on your back, which allows the tongue to rest against the back of the throat. Losing weight is one of the least expensive and most effective treatments for snoring.

Many people turn to alcohol or drugs to help them sleep. These substances interfere with normal sleep and can make your problems worse.

While alcohol has a sedating effect, it can also act as a stimulant and may keep you awake. Nonprescription sleep remedies seem to depend on the placebo effect: they work because you expect them to. Some contain antihistamines that may cause you to feel drowsy during the day. Stronger prescription sedatives can knock you out but do not give a normal, restful sleep. Often sleeping pills make insomnia worse. You should deal with possible causes of insomnia before trying sleeping pills.

Here are some tips for a good, restful night's sleep:

▲ Stop smoking. Smokers have more sleep trouble than nonsmokers.
▲ Exercise regularly.
▲ Avoid drinking alcohol in the evening.
▲ Avoid caffeine for at least two hours before bedtime—coffee, tea, soda, and chocolate.
▲ A bedtime snack seems to help many people, as does the traditional glass of warm milk. But don't eat a big meal within three hours of going to bed.
▲ Develop a sleeping routine with a regular bedtime, but don't go to bed if you feel wide awake.

Sleep Disorders

Do you still have insomnia after 3 weeks of home treatment, or do you still snore despite losing 10% of excess weight?

Yes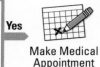

Make Medical Appointment

No

Use Home Treatment

▲ Break your chain of thought before going to bed; read, watch television, take a bath, or listen to music to relax your mind.

▲ Once in bed, use creative imagery and relaxation techniques to keep your mind free of distracting thoughts.

▲ If all else fails (or even if it doesn't), sex is one of the most effective natural sleep inducers.

It may take you several weeks to establish a normal sleep routine. Talk to your doctor if you still have sleep problems after trying these methods.

What to Expect at the Doctor's Office

The doctor will ask about your sleeping schedule, sources of stress and anxiety, and other sleep factors. In some cases, you may have brain activity monitored (electroencephalogram, or EEG) as you sleep. Rarely, the doctor may have more sophisticated tests done during a sleep study at the hospital (polysomnography).

In rare cases where weight loss and home treatment don't stop snoring, the doctor may discuss surgery of the nose and throat.

Weakness and Fatigue

Weakness and fatigue are often considered to be similar, but in medicine, they have distinct and separate meanings.

Weakness refers to lack of *strength*. Weakness is usually the more serious condition and is particularly important when it is confined to one area of the body. Such weakness in one area is often due to a problem in the muscular or nervous system, such as a stroke.

Fatigue is lack of *energy*. It is tiredness or lethargy. Fatigue is typically associated with a viral infection or with feelings of anxiety, depression, or tension. It's caused by a large variety of illnesses.

Hypoglycemia means "low blood sugar." Many patients fear that this problem is the cause of their tiredness. A few individuals do, in fact, feel shaky several hours after a meal because their blood sugar level drops at that point. However, they do *not* feel fatigued. Low blood sugar throughout the day can cause fatigue, but this is a rare condition.

Chronic fatigue is common; about one in every four adults seen in doctors' offices say it is one of their problems. But chronic fatigue syndrome (CFS) is unusual; perhaps only one in a thousand of the adults who complain of chronic fatigue meet the criteria for this diagnosis.

CFS created a stir in the 1980s because some doctors believed it to be a new disease, probably due to an acute infection (perhaps Epstein-Barr virus, or even yeast). However, a link to infection has never been demonstrated, and there is little evidence that treating for infection is useful. As a result, other doctors believe that CFS is actually a collection of diseases that have been with us for a long time under such names as neurasthenia and even "the vapors." To try to resolve this issue, groups of experts have created a standard list of criteria for diagnosing chronic fatigue immune-deficiency syndrome (CFIDS, pronounced "see-fids"). This list excludes almost all people with chronic fatigue. But the problem still may be one such as fibromyalgia (page 228) or depression (page 302).

Home Treatment

There is time and need for careful reflection on the causes of fatigue. Many young and middle-aged women come to the doctor's office complaining of fatigue and requesting tests for anemia or thyroid problems. Many adult women are mildly iron-deficient, and thyroid problems may cause fatigue, but it is very unusual for one of these conditions to be the cause of fatigue. In most cases, fatigue is more closely related to lack of physical activity and/or mental challenge, boredom, unhappiness, some disappointment, or just plain hard work. The patient should consider these possibilities before consulting the doctor.

Vitamins are rarely helpful, but in moderation, they don't hurt.

If fatigue lasts for more than two weeks, see your doctor.

What to Expect at the Doctor's Office

If the problem is weakness of only part of the body, the doctor will concentrate the examination on the nerve and muscle functions. A typical stroke will be identified by such an examination, whereas more uncommon ailments may require further testing and special procedures.

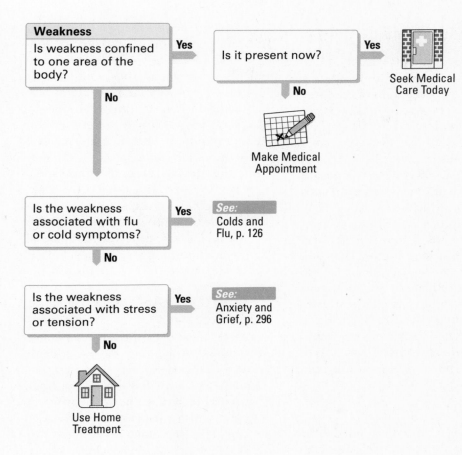

Weakness

Is weakness confined to one area of the body?

Yes → Is it present now? **Yes** → Seek Medical Care Today

No → Make Medical Appointment

No

Is the weakness associated with flu or cold symptoms? **Yes** → *See:* Colds and Flu, p. 126

No

Is the weakness associated with stress or tension? **Yes** → *See:* Anxiety and Grief, p. 296

No

Use Home Treatment

If the problem is fatigue, the medical history is the most important part of the encounter. Physical examination of the heart, lungs, and thyroid gland can be expected. The doctor may test for anemia and thyroid dysfunction, as well as other problems. Inquiry into the patient's lifestyle and feelings is important.

There are no direct cures for the most common fatigue syndromes. Pep pills don't work, and the downswing when the pills wear off usually makes the problem worse. Tranquilizers generally intensify fatigue. Vacations, job changes, undertaking new activities, and making marital adjustments are far more helpful.

Up to 80% of people with CFS have depression or anxiety as a part of the problem, and many doctors feel that treating those problems is the best way to deal with CFS.

Dizziness and Fainting

Three different problems are frequently introduced by the complaint of dizziness or fainting: loss of consciousness, vertigo, and lightheadedness.

Unconsciousness

True unconsciousness includes a period in which the victim has no control over the body and of which there is no recollection. Therefore, if consciousness is lost while standing, the victim will fall and may sustain injury in doing so. The common symptom of "blackout," in which the person finds it difficult to see and needs to sit or lie down but can still hear, isn't true loss of consciousness. Such blackouts may be related to changes in posture or to emotional experiences. True loss of consciousness needs to be investigated promptly by a doctor.

Vertigo

Vertigo is caused by a problem in the balance mechanism of the inner ear. Because this balance mechanism also helps control eye movements, there is loss of balance and the room seems to be spinning around. Walls and floors may seem to lurch in crazy motions. Most vertigo has no definite cause and is thought to be due to a viral infection of the inner ear. A doctor should be seen.

Feeling Lightheaded

"Lightheadedness" is by far the most common of these problems. It is that woozy feeling that is such a common part of flu or cold syndromes. If such a feeling is associated with other flu or cold symptoms, see page 126.

Lightheadedness that isn't associated with other symptoms is usually not serious either. Many people with this condition are tense or anxious. Others have low blood pressure and regularly feel lightheaded when standing up suddenly. This is called "postural hypotension" and doesn't require treatment. Many medications, especially antihypertensives, may cause lightheadedness. If lightheadedness is associated with the use of drugs, the doctor should be contacted to determine if the drug should be discontinued.

Alcohol is also a frequent cause of lightheadedness. If you suspect excess drinking may be the real cause of the problem, see page 304.

Home Treatment

A person most often feels a momentary blackout after he or she moves suddenly from reclining or sitting to standing upright. Blood stops flowing to the brain for an instant, and the person may notice a fleeting loss of vision or a lightheaded feeling. This phenomenon is called postural hypotension. Most people will experience it at one time or another, but it becomes more frequent as we grow older. The therapy is to avoid sudden changes in posture. Unless postural hypotension suddenly becomes worse, you don't need to visit the doctor. You may report the feeling on your next routine visit.

A persistent lightheaded feeling without any other symptoms doesn't indicate a brain tumor or other hidden disease. This type of lightheadedness often disappears when the person resolves anxiety. Not infrequently, it's a problem the person must learn to live with.

If the problem persists for more than three weeks, call the doctor.

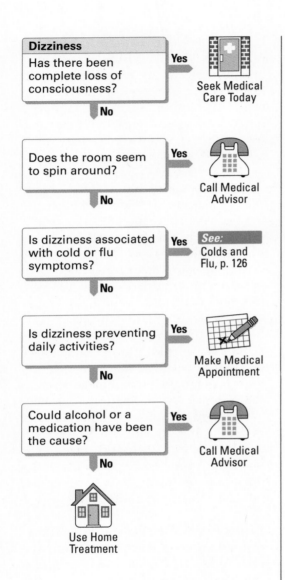

Dizziness

Has there been complete loss of consciousness? — **Yes** → Seek Medical Care Today

No ↓

Does the room seem to spin around? — **Yes** → Call Medical Advisor

No ↓

Is dizziness associated with cold or flu symptoms? — **Yes** → *See:* Colds and Flu, p. 126

No ↓

Is dizziness preventing daily activities? — **Yes** → Make Medical Appointment

No ↓

Could alcohol or a medication have been the cause? — **Yes** → Call Medical Advisor

No ↓

Use Home Treatment

What to Expect at the Doctor's Office

The doctor will obtain a history with emphasis on making the distinctions outlined above. If loss of consciousness is the problem, the heart and lungs will be examined and nerve function will be tested. Special testing for irregular heartbeat or sudden drop in blood pressure may be necessary. If vertigo is the problem, the head, ears, eyes, and throat will be examined, along with neurological testing. Sometimes, further tests of hearing or balance may be required. A search for predisposing factors, such as anxiety, will be made. Often a period of "watchful waiting" will be advised.

High Blood Pressure

High blood pressure (hypertension) is one of the most common and most treatable chronic health problems. It affects 30 million to 40 million Americans—more than 1 in 10. High blood pressure is a silent disease, often causing no symptoms until it is too late. A catastrophic heart attack, a stroke, or kidney disease is often the first sign of disease.

Two numbers make up the blood pressure reading. The upper number, or systolic, represents the maximum pressure in the arteries when the heart pumps. The lower number, or diastolic, is the pressure while the heart is at rest.

A typical blood pressure may be 120/80, but what is "normal" varies over a wide range. In general, the lower the blood pressure, the better. Blood pressure has been considered high if the upper (systolic) pressure is above 140, or if the lower (diastolic) number is above 90. More recently, "normal" has been defined as less than 135/85 or even less than 120/80. Lower readings are usually seen in children and adults in excellent physical condition.

Don't panic over one blood pressure result. Several readings over several weeks are needed to be meaningful. At least a third of those whose first reading is high have a normal reading when blood pressure is later rechecked.

Monitoring Your Blood Pressure

Have your blood pressure checked at least once a year. Blood pressure measurement is painless, quick, and reliable. The doctor's office may not be the best place to have your pressure checked, however, because being nervous can raise your blood pressure. Free blood pressure checks are often available at health fairs, businesses, and health agencies. Many stores, such as drugstores, have blood pressure machines available for public use, and these are reasonably accurate.

Is it worth buying a home blood pressure cuff or measuring machine? Many reliable, affordable models are on the market. If you have high blood pressure, you'll want to check yourself frequently so you can report any changes or difficulties to your doctor; a home blood pressure monitor is essential for you. Get one that goes around the upper arm, not the wrist or the finger.

If You Have High Blood Pressure

It is important to understand that you must manage high blood pressure yourself. You are responsible for controlling your weight, maintaining a proper level of activity, not smoking, limiting the salt and fats in your diet, and taking your medicine properly. Expect only a few doctor appointments for this condition, but make the most of these visits.

Keep in Shape. Make exercise, weight control, and a good diet part of your routine. Although a person in good shape can have high blood pressure, your risk is much greater if you're overweight and out of shape. Reducing your weight is a reliable way of lowering your blood pressure. Exercise conditions your cardiovascular system.

Diet. Decreasing the salt, fat, and cholesterol in your diet and increasing the potassium and calcium help lower blood

My Home Blood Pressure Chart

	Mon	Tue	Wed	Thu	Fri	Sat	Sun
Date	11/4						
Drug #1, a.m. Atenolol	7:30						
#1, p.m. —	—						
Drug #2, a.m. Cozaar	7:30						
#2, p.m. Cozaar	9:00						
Drug #3, a.m. HCTZ	7:30						
#3, p.m. —	—						
BP, a.m.	135/80						
BP, p.m.	130/78						

Your home blood pressure chart (example). "Monday" has been filled in as an illustration. Take your blood pressure before you take your medication.

pressure and decrease the risk of heart disease. Potassium-based salt substitutes are good, particularly if you are taking a diuretic blood pressure medication such as hydrochlorothiazide.

Managing Drugs. If the doctor prescribes medication to control your blood pressure, understand how to manage the drugs. Ask the doctor about side effects and warning signs. Set a target blood pressure with your doctor. (Frequently, this might be 135/85.) Take your blood pressure at least once or twice a week. The best time is in the evening, before any evening medication. You want to be at (or below) the target blood pressure *all* of the time unless you get dizzy or have other problems. We have learned that it is not enough to just be on blood pressure medicine. You must be on enough, but not too much, of the right medicines. You need to keep a careful chart record, especially for the seven days just before your doctor visits. Record your blood pressure medicines and when you took them, and your blood pressure in the morning and evening. Take

the chart with you to the doctor and be sure that you discuss it. With this record, you and your doctor can make the important decisions about managing your high blood pressure wisely. Drug therapy is effective but is expensive and has risks and side effects. Through good self-care and risk reduction, some people can control their blood pressure without the need for medication. Others can reduce the drug dosage required to control the blood pressure, saving money as well as lowering risks and side effects. Aim to reduce your drug intake—but don't change your therapy unless your doctor says so after going over your chart.

Stick with It. Managing high blood pressure is a lifelong job. Don't stop your program because you feel good. Don't miss any doses of your medicines unless your doctor agrees. Don't wait for signs and symptoms before you take preventive measures. If you take good care of high blood pressure, it will probably never cause you a major problem. If you ignore it, you are needlessly endangering your life and well-being.

Anxiety and Grief

Stress isn't a disease; it's a fact of life. Our reactions can vary tremendously, sometimes in ways that are not good.

Anxiety is a common reaction to powerful stress, such as money troubles. People who react to daily stress with anxiety probably need counseling, though they may not realize that. They may instead focus on the common symptoms of anxiety:

▲ Insomnia
▲ Nervousness
▲ Rapid heart rate
▲ Inability to concentrate
▲ "Lump in the throat," or even difficulty swallowing (page 300)
▲ Hyperventilation (like "lump in the throat," most common in young adults, especially women—see page 298)

Grief is a normal reaction to loss, such as the death of a loved one or the end of a job. Working through grief is an important part of dealing with loss. While family and community resources can provide some support, the only therapy for grief is time.

A grieving person may turn to alcohol, tranquilizers, or other prescription medication. While drugs may give short-term relief, they don't solve problems. Alcohol and drugs are crutches that interfere with normal recovery. You must address the underlying issues.

Home Treatment

Recognizing the signs of anxiety is the first step to finding and treating its cause. You may find it helpful to talk with friends, family, or a member of the clergy. Agencies in your community provide services and referrals. Occasionally, the person may require long-term therapy with a counselor. No single type of therapy is better for all people. Your choice should depend on what works for you.

Too much caffeine can cause chronic anxiety. Cutting down on caffeine may help you relax. Caffeine is found in coffee, soft drinks, tea, chocolate, non-prescription stimulants (e.g., NoDoz, Vivarin), and a variety of cold and headache remedies.

Relaxation techniques (page 300) and a program of regular physical exercise can help reduce anxiety.

What to Expect at the Doctor's Office

The doctor will get the medical history and do a physical exam. Health providers may take an electrocardiogram (ECG) and chest X-rays. The doctor will evaluate anxiety and determine whether you need a medication or a referral to a mental health professional.

For hyperventilation syndrome, the doctor may have the person breathe into a paper bag to restore normal breathing. The doctor may also ask the person to lie down and voluntarily hyperventilate (50 deep breaths) to understand how the symptoms arise. He or she may prescribe a tranquilizer.

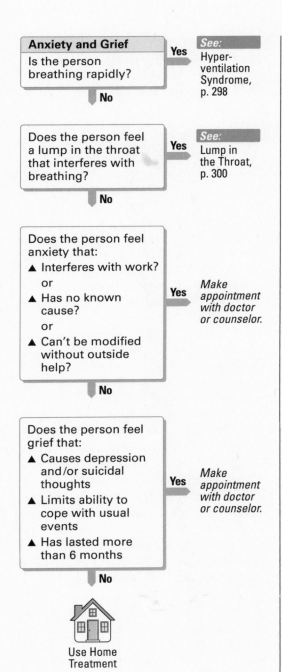

Anxiety and Grief

Is the person breathing rapidly?

Yes → *See:* Hyper-ventilation Syndrome, p. 298

No

Does the person feel a lump in the throat that interferes with breathing?

Yes → *See:* Lump in the Throat, p. 300

No

Does the person feel anxiety that:
▲ Interferes with work?
or
▲ Has no known cause?
or
▲ Can't be modified without outside help?

Yes → *Make appointment with doctor or counselor.*

No

Does the person feel grief that:
▲ Causes depression and/or suicidal thoughts
▲ Limits ability to cope with usual events
▲ Has lasted more than 6 months

Yes → *Make appointment with doctor or counselor.*

No

Use Home Treatment

Hyperventilation Syndrome

Anxiety, especially unrecognized anxiety, can lead to physical symptoms. The hyperventilation syndrome is such a problem. In this syndrome, a nervous or anxious person becomes concerned about his or her breathing and feels unable to get enough air into the lungs. This is often associated with chest pain or tightness.

The sensation of being out of breath leads to overbreathing and a lowering of the carbon dioxide level in the blood. The lower level of carbon dioxide brings on symptoms of numbness and tingling of the hands, and dizziness. The numbness and tingling may extend to the feet and may also be noted around the mouth. Occasionally, muscle spasms may occur in the hands.

This syndrome is almost always a condition of young adults. While it is more common in women, it is also frequently seen in men. Usually this syndrome afflicts people who recognize themselves as being nervous and tense. It often happens when such people have additional stress, use alcohol, or are in situations where it is advantageous to have a sudden, dramatic illness. A classic example is the occurrence of the hyperventilation syndrome during separation or divorce proceedings, so that the event becomes a call for help to the estranged spouse.

However, hyperventilation is also a natural response to severe pain. When in doubt, take a person who is hyperventilating to the doctor's office rather than discount a potentially serious problem.

Home Treatment

The symptoms of hyperventilation syndrome are due to carbon dioxide loss from overbreathing. If the person breathes into a paper bag, so that the carbon dioxide is taken back into the lungs rather than being lost into the atmosphere, the symptoms will be alleviated. This usually requires 5 to 15 minutes with a small paper bag held loosely over both the nose and the mouth. This isn't always as easy as it sounds because a major feature of the hyperventilation syndrome is panic and a feeling of impending suffocation. Approaching such a person with a paper bag for the mouth and nose may prove difficult, so be sure to reassure the person first.

Repeated attacks may occur. Once the person has honestly recognized that the problem is anxiety rather than a disease, the attacks will stop because the panic component won't come into play; convincing the person is the main obstacle. Having the person voluntarily hyperventilate (50 deep breaths while lying on a couch) to demonstrate that this reproduces the symptoms of the previous episode is frequently helpful. People are usually afraid that they are having a heart attack or are on the verge of a nervous breakdown. Neither is true, and when the fear has dissipated, hyperventilation usually ceases.

What to Expect at the Doctor's Office

The doctor will obtain a history and will direct attention primarily to the examination of the heart and lungs. In the young person with a typical syndrome, with a normal physical examination and no abdominal pain, the diagnosis of hyperventilation is easily made.

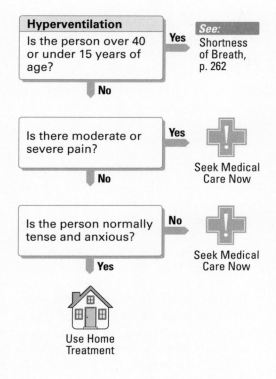

Hyperventilation

Is the person over 40 or under 15 years of age?

Yes → *See:* Shortness of Breath, p. 262

No ↓

Is there moderate or severe pain?

Yes → Seek Medical Care Now

No ↓

Is the person normally tense and anxious?

No → Seek Medical Care Now

Yes ↓

Use Home Treatment

Electrocardiograms (ECGs) and chest X-rays are seldom needed. These procedures may occasionally be necessary in less clear-cut cases.

If hyperventilation syndrome is diagnosed, the doctor will usually provide a paper bag and the instructions given above. A tranquilizer may be administered; we prefer merely to reassure the patient. It is seldom possible to deal effectively with the cause of the anxiety during the hyperventilation episode because the anxiety often takes some time to dissipate, and for the thinking to become more coherent. The patient shouldn't assume that the underlying problem is solved simply because the hyperventilation has been controlled.

Lump in the Throat

The feeling of a "lump in the throat" is a classic anxiety symptom. There may even be some difficulty swallowing, although eating is possible if an effort is made. The sensation is intermittent and is made worse by tension.

The difficulty in swallowing is worst when the person concentrates on swallowing and on the sensations within the throat. As an experiment, try to swallow rapidly several times without any food or liquid, and concentrate on the resulting sensation. You will then understand this symptom.

Several serious diseases can cause difficulty swallowing. In these cases, the symptom begins slowly, is noticed first with solid foods and then with liquids, results in loss of weight, and is more likely to be found in those over age 40. "Lump in the throat," like the hyperventilation syndrome, is likely to be found in young adults, most frequently women.

Home Treatment

The central problem isn't the symptom but, rather, the underlying cause of the anxiety state (see Anxiety and Grief, page 296). Recognition that the symptom is minor is crucial to its disappearance.

Relaxation techniques may be helpful. One such technique is called progressive relaxation:

1. Imagine that your toes weigh a thousand pounds and you couldn't move them if you wanted to. Let them go completely limp.

2. Do the same with each part of your body, relaxing the muscles and working your way up to the top of your head.

3. Don't neglect the facial muscles. Tension often centers in the forehead or jaw and keeps you from relaxing.

An alternative is to imagine that your breath is coming in through the toes of your right foot, all the way up to your lungs, and back out through the same foot. Do this three times. Repeat the procedure for the left foot and then for each of your arms.

What to Expect at the Doctor's Office

After taking a medical history and examining the throat and chest, a doctor may sometimes believe that X-rays of the esophagus are necessary. If an abnormality of the esophagus is found, further studies may be performed. Reassurance will probably be the treatment given.

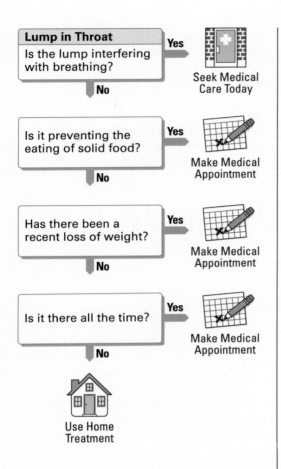

Lump in Throat

Is the lump interfering with breathing?

Yes → Seek Medical Care Today

No ↓

Is it preventing the eating of solid food?

Yes → Make Medical Appointment

No ↓

Has there been a recent loss of weight?

Yes → Make Medical Appointment

No ↓

Is it there all the time?

Yes → Make Medical Appointment

No ↓

Use Home Treatment

Depression

Everybody gets the blues sometimes. Depression can range from a lack of energy to an overwhelming sense of hopelessness. It can seem like a general fatigue or a vague sense of ill health. You may feel poorly and not know why. The future holds no promise. You have a sense of loss.

Most depression is a normal response to an unhappy event. It is natural to be depressed by the death of a loved one or after a big disappointment at work. However, if depression continues and starts to interfere with your work or family life, make an appointment to see your doctor.

Ask yourself these questions:

▲ Are you sad or blue for most of the day, for more days than not?
▲ Do you often cry even though you aren't sure why?
▲ Do you think that unhappiness is the rule in your life?
▲ Do you no longer get pleasure from things you used to like?
▲ Do you often have feelings of hopelessness?

If you answered yes to any of these questions, you are likely to be depressed.

Consider how your emotional condition is affecting your life:

▲ Do you have a poor appetite, or do you overeat?
▲ Do you not sleep enough, or do you sleep too much?
▲ Do you have low energy or fatigue?
▲ Do you feel bad about yourself in general?
▲ Do you have trouble concentrating or making decisions?

If you answered yes to any of these questions, you may have serious depression. Seek help from your doctor or a mental health counselor.

Home Treatment

Activity is the natural antidote for depression. Regular exercise can be as effective for mild depression as the drugs prescribed by doctors.

Stay involved with other people and let them support you. Tell someone about your problems. Don't push everyone away, and don't let your depression drive them away.

Drugs can cause depression, including tranquilizers, high blood pressure medicines, corticosteroids (e.g., prednisone), codeine, and indomethacin. If you are concerned about prescription medication, talk with your doctor. Reduce your alcohol and other drug use.

What to Expect at the Doctor's Office

The doctor will ask about issues and events related to depression. The doctor may offer suggestions for activities and exercise. He or she may adjust the dosage of medication that may be causing depression.

The doctor may prescribe antidepressant medication. You may be hospitalized if there is a risk of suicide.

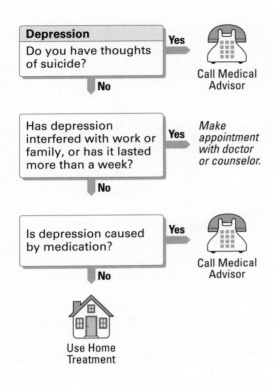

Depression

Do you have thoughts of suicide?

Yes → Call Medical Advisor

No ↓

Has depression interfered with work or family, or has it lasted more than a week?

Yes → *Make appointment with doctor or counselor.*

No ↓

Is depression caused by medication?

Yes → Call Medical Advisor

No ↓

Use Home Treatment

Suicidal Feelings

If the depression is so severe that you are thinking of suicide, call the doctor immediately. Many communities have telephone hotlines for crisis counseling. If there is no hotline in your community, go to the nearest emergency room.

Alcoholism

Alcohol, in moderation (2 drinks or less in a day), is neutral or even beneficial to health. But millions of persons abuse alcohol, and for them, this is a serious health problem. This section can help you identify the person with problems, even if it is you. A person with a drinking problem seldom changes this harmful behavior alone. Although recovery must come from within, the decisive nudge often comes from a relative, friend, or coworker. If, like most people, you know someone who drinks too much, you can provide that help.

We used to worry mostly about alcoholic liver disease, which affects only the drinker. Now, we are even more concerned about alcohol and automobile crashes, small airplane crashes, spousal abuse, homicide, and suicide.

If in reading this section you recognize yourself, be your own best friend and get help now.

Warning Signs of Problem Drinking:

▲ Drinking to get drunk
▲ Trying to solve or avoid problems by drinking
▲ Becoming loud, angry, or violent after drinking
▲ Drinking at inappropriate times, such as in the morning, before driving, or before going to work
▲ Drinking that causes problems, harm, or concern to others
▲ Developing an ulcer or gastritis
▲ Binge drinking, six or more drinks over a few hours
▲ "Passing out" after drinking

Warning Signs of Alcoholism:

▲ Spending time thinking about drinking, or planning where and when to get the next drink
▲ Receiving citations for driving while intoxicated, or having an automobile accident after any alcohol intake
▲ Starting to drink without planning to, and losing track of the amount of alcohol consumed, or denying the amount of alcohol consumed
▲ Needing a drink before stressful situations
▲ Having no memory of what occurred while drinking, although the alcoholic may have appeared normal to others at the time
▲ Incurring malnutrition and neglect
▲ Suffering from withdrawal symptoms, including delirium tremens (DTs)

A pregnant woman who drinks heavily is at risk of harming the fetus in her womb, a condition called fetal alcohol syndrome.

What to Say to the One You Care For
Pick a good time: not when the person is drunk but not long after a crisis. Tell the person what you have observed and how it causes problems. Describe your feelings and ask how the person feels about the situation. Suggest a way out. Try not to sound as if you are charging the person with a crime. Don't try to punish, bribe, or emotionally blackmail the person. Remain calm, detached, and factual. Make sure you leave the responsibility for the negative behavior and for changing it with the drinker.

Most will deny having a problem. Stating your concern and pointing out examples of trouble may be all you can

Alcoholism

Has the person displayed 2 or more of these signs?

▲ Mentioned a need to cut down on drinking

▲ Acted annoyed when someone criticized his or her drinking

▲ Expressed guilt feelings about drinking

▲ Taken an "eye-opener" first thing in the morning

Yes → *The odds are overwhelming that the person is an alcoholic. Seek counseling.*

No ↓

Has the person displayed any of the warning signs on p. 304?

Yes → *The person may have a drinking problem. Discuss how it has affected your relationship.*

No ↓

Suspect . . .
other problems if the person does not exhibit any of the warning signs on p. 304.

do the first time. When the problem recurs, you may talk again.

Most experts believe that most alcoholics will not seek help if only one person talks with them. A group approach—family, friends, employers, counselors, and neighbors together confronting the alcoholic and making it clear that the only option is to seek help—can be a powerful intervention. See page 306 for more information.

Home Treatment

Alcoholism isn't a problem that is easily solved at home, but a doctor can't cure it either. The focus of any treatment must be on the drinker changing his or her behavior. There are many worthwhile methods, some involving physicians or professional counselors and some not. Some techniques insist on abstinence, and others aim to reduce drinking to within acceptable limits.

The route to recovery pioneered by Alcoholics Anonymous (AA) has been as successful as any and more so than most. AA uses a self-help format to encourage the problem drinker to face up to his or her alcoholism and come to grips with the consequences. Almost all clinic- and hospital-based alcohol treatment programs refer their patients to AA once they have gotten off to a good start.

Allied with AA are Al-Anon (for people affected by a family member's alcoholism) and Alateen (for teens with family members or friends who are alcoholics). The most important ingredient in every program is commitment on the part of the drinker.

What to Expect at the Doctor's Office

Tell your doctor if you are recovering from alcoholism or suspect you have a drinking problem. A history of drinking can affect many aspects of your medical care.

If you ask your doctor for help for an alcoholic friend, the doctor will probably suggest counseling for your friend. Since the cost of outpatient treatment is less than one-tenth the cost of inpatient care, hospitals best serve patients who require acute detoxification; patients who may go into severe withdrawal, requiring medical care; or patients who suffer from profound psychological problems beyond alcoholism.

Where to Find Help

Start by looking in your phone book or doing a web search under "alcohol abuse"; there are many information hotlines that operate around the clock. For more information:

▲ Alcoholics Anonymous (AA)
   General Service Office
   P.O. Box 459
   Grand Central Station
   New York, NY 10163
   (212) 870-3400
   www.aa.org

▲ Al-Anon and Alateen Family Group
   Headquarters
   1600 Corporate Landing Parkway
   Virginia Beach, VA 23454-5617
   (757) 563-1600
   (888) 4AL-ANON, (888) 425-2666
   (Toll-free)
   www.al-anon.org

▲ National Council on Alcoholism
   and Drug Dependence
   20 Exchange Place, Suite 2902
   New York, NY 10005
   (212) 269-7797 "HOPE LINE"
   (800) 622-2255 (Toll-free)
   www.ncadd.org

▲ National Clearinghouse for Alcohol
   and Drug Information
   Substance Abuse and Mental Health
   Services Administration
   5600 Fishers Lane
   Rockville, MD 20857
   (877) SAMHSA-7
   (877) 726-4727 (Toll-free)
   www.additiona.com

Drug Abuse

From 5% to 13% of adults in the United States abuse or depend on some kind of psychoactive substance other than alcohol. This problem extends beyond illegal drugs, such as cocaine and some narcotics, to abuse of prescription drugs. People addicted to drugs need someone to push them into getting help. You, as a loved one or colleague, can start that process and improve both your lives.

Overdoses and withdrawal symptoms are just two of the dangers of drug dependency. Abusers need the substance so much that they will harm themselves or others in order to have it, causing many more medical and nonmedical problems. The craving for a drug may lead people to steal, share needles, engage in risky sex, neglect their health, and take other risks. Addictions also make abusers more emotionally volatile and, thus, more prone to violence. At least one-half of all spouse abuse cases and one-third of all child abuse and suicide cases are related to substance abuse.

There are, of course, degrees of difference among persons who use illegal drugs. Intravenous drug use over a long time is more problematic by far than light social use of marijuana. We are hard on illegal drug users here because (1) drugs are illegal (the medical and recreational marijuana laws have changed or are changing in many states, and (2) there remains concern that light drug use may lead to heavy drug use and lighter drugs to heavier. So, help the person find a nonjudg-mental health professional who can guide and advise on complex and individual issues.

Home Treatment

It isn't your role to treat a drug problem. Let the professionals do that. Your first task is to recognize the situation. The decision chart lists some of the signs of substance abuse. Unfortunately, they aren't all as easy to spot as the chronic runny nose of a cocaine abuser.

Legal drugs, most prominent prescription pain relievers, are the most problematic in the United States, now causing 28,000 deaths each year, more than hard narcotics or gun violence. This is an epidemic, and we are just beginning to solve it.

Flush leftover pain pills down the toilet or take them to a facility where you can turn in leftover drugs (visit fda.gov for procedures and "take back" locations) resist the doctor's suggestion of prescription pain relievers. Change doctors if you are concerned about the prescription.

If you suspect that a person is abusing drugs, talk to counselors, self-help groups, and your doctor. Phone hotlines are available locally and nationwide. Groups like Nar-Anon can provide support for you during this troubled period.

You may then be able to confront the drug abuser with your worry: "I'm concerned about your behavior. You seem troubled. Why not speak to someone about it?" See Alcoholism (page 304) for more advice on bringing up the subject. If the person agrees to seek help, share your knowledge about counseling services.

Many substance abusers resist such advice, however. Regardless, don't assist the drug abuser in continuing to abuse by:

▲ Covering up his or her behavior from others
▲ Taking over the abuser's responsibilities in the home or at work
▲ Cooperating in buying, selling, or using the drug

What to Expect at the Doctor's Office

For the drug abuser who refuses your entreaty to get help, a doctor or other professional advisor might recommend a method called group intervention. After meeting several times with an advisor, family members and friends confront the user. Led by the advisor, they express their concerns, citing specific examples. If the abuser agrees to get help, he or she immediately enters a treatment program. If the abuser still refuses help, it is critical that family and friends receive counseling so that they don't inadvertently enable the abuser to continue his or her behavior.

After diagnosing substance abuse, most doctors will refer the patient to a treatment program run by specialists. There is no cure for substance dependence; the craving can persist for life. But it can be controlled. Treatment programs are geared to the long haul. Successful rehabilitation or recovery can be expected for 50% to 70% of all substance abusers.

Sometimes, a short stay in a hospital is necessary to prevent a patient from dying of an overdose or withdrawal, to hold a dangerously unstable person, or to treat complications of drug abuse, such as infection. The average stay for drug abuse problems is 12 days. The hospital should guide the patient to continuing treatment after discharge.

Steroid Use

Anabolic steroids are drugs that target the muscles instead of the brain, encouraging muscle cell growth. They have positive medical uses, but taking them without a prescription can lead to dependency. Anabolic steroids have become very popular among young men and teenage boys, both those involved in athletics and those who want larger muscles to improve their appearance. Ironically, steroid abusers risk acne, stunted growth, impaired fertility, and psychological problems.

Drug Abuse

Does the person exhibit any of these signs?

▲ Unhealthy lifestyle— neglect of appearance
▲ Secretive behavior
▲ Frequently being absent or late
▲ Mood swings
▲ Weight loss
▲ Money problems
▲ Anxiety and nervousness
▲ Impulsive behavior
▲ Troubled relationships
▲ Denial that problem exists
▲ Frequent attempts to obtain prescriptions for pain relievers, often from different physicians.

Yes *Make appointment with doctor or counselor.*

No

Consider *other problems.*

Where to Find Help

Narcotics Anonymous (NA) and Cocaine Anonymous (CA) are self-help groups organized on the principles of Alcoholics Anonymous. Nar-Anon serves people affected by a family member's drug abuse. These organizations are listed in most phone directories. You can contact these central offices:

▲ Narcotics Anonymous (NA)
World Service Office
P.O. Box 9999
Van Nuys, CA 91409
(818) 773-9999
www.na.org

▲ Cocaine Anonymous (CA)
World Service Office
21720 S. Wilmington Avenue
Suite 304
Long Beach, CA 90810-1641
(310) 559-5833
www.ca.org

▲ Nar-Anon Family Group
Headquarters
22527 Crenshaw Boulevard, #200B
Torrance, CA 90505
(800) 477-6291 (Toll-free)
www.nar-anon.org

For immediate help, look in your phone book's white pages or do a web search under "drug abuse." Here are two national numbers:

▲ National Institute on Drug Abuse Hotline
(800) 662-HELP, (800) 662-4357 (Toll-free)

▲ Cocaine Hotline
24-hour information and referral
(800) NODRUGS, (800) 663-7847 (Toll-free)

CHAPTER 11

Women's Health

Breast Self-Examination

One in eight women will have a breast cancer. Most are curable if caught early. Most lumps in the breast are not cancerous. Most women will have a lump in a breast at some time during their lives. Many women's breasts are naturally lumpy (so-called benign fibrocystic disease). Obviously, every lump or possible lump cannot and should not be subjected to surgery.

Regular breast self-examination improves your chances of avoiding serious consequences. Self-examination should be done monthly, just after the menstrual period.

The technique is as follows:

1. Examine your breasts in the mirror, first with your arms at your sides (A1) and then with both arms over your head (A2). The breasts should look closely similar. Watch for any change in shape or size or for dimpling of the skin. Occasionally, a lump that is difficult to feel will be quite obvious just by looking.

2. Next, while lying flat, examine the left breast using the inner fingertips of the right hand and pressing the breast tissue against the chest wall. Don't pinch the tissue between the fingers; all breast tissue feels a bit lumpy when you do this. The left hand should be behind your head while you examine the inner half of the left breast (B1) and down at your side when you examine the outer half (B2). Don't neglect the part of the breast underneath the nipple or that which extends outward from the breast toward the underarm (B3). A small pillow under the left shoulder may help.

3. Repeat this process on the opposite side.

Any lump detected should be brought to the attention of your doctor. Regular self-examination will tell you how long it has been present and whether it has changed in size. This information is very helpful in deciding what to do about the lump; even the doctor often has difficulty with this decision. Self-examination is an absolute necessity for a woman with naturally lumpy breasts. She is the only one who can really know whether a lump is new or old, or has changed size. For all women, regular self-examination offers a better hope that surgery will be performed when, and only when, it is necessary. Many doctors recommend repeating a self-examination in the shower, where smooth, slightly soapy skin can make lumps easier to detect.

Professional Prevention

Breast self-examination is a supplement to other screening tests for breast cancer, not an alternative. Mammography can detect smaller lumps, particularly in women with large or lumpy breasts. Hence, we strongly recommend mammography yearly after age 50 and after age 40 for women with a strong history of breast cancer in their family. The physi-

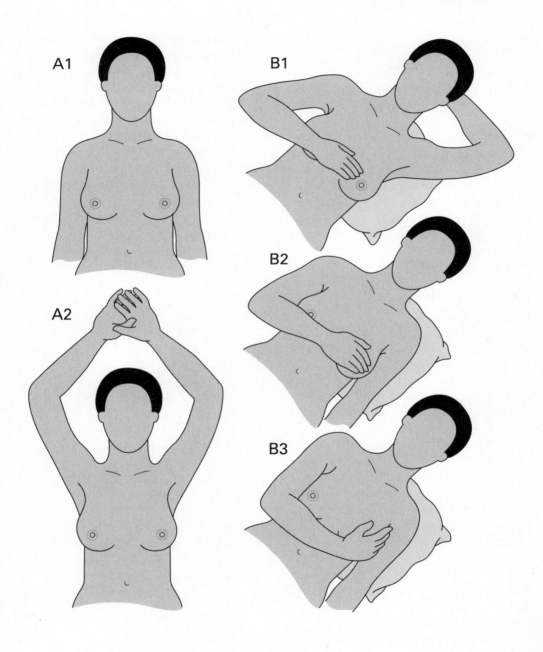

cian or other health worker examination also can be of benefit. The reason for careful monthly self-examination is that a cancer may not be present at mammography one year and be at an incurable stage at mammography a year later.

Gynecological Examination

Examination of the female reproductive organs, usually called a "pelvic examination," may be expected for complaints related to these organs, along with the annual Pap smear. This examination yields a great deal of information and is often absolutely essential for diagnosis. By understanding the phases of the examination and your role in them, you can make it possible for an adequate examination to be done quickly and with a minimum of discomfort.

Positioning. Lying on your back, put your heels in the stirrups (the nurse may assist in this step). With your knees bent, move down to the very end of the examination table. Get as close to the edge as you can. Now let your knees fall out to the sides as far as they will go. Don't try to hold the knees closed with the inner muscles of the thigh. This will tire you and make the examination more difficult.

The key word during the examination is "relax"; you may hear it several times. The vagina is a muscular organ, and if the muscles are tense, a difficult and uncomfortable examination is inevitable. You may be asked to take several deep breaths in an effort to promote relaxation.

External Examination. Inspection of the labia, clitoris, and vaginal opening is the first step in the examination. The most common findings are cysts in the labia, rashes, and so-called venereal warts. These problems have effective treatments or may need no treatment at all.

Speculum Examination. The speculum is the "duck-billed" instrument used to spread the walls of the vagina so that the inside may be seen. It is not a clamp. It may be constructed of metal or plastic. The plastic ones will click open and closed; don't be alarmed.

If a Pap smear or other test is to be made, the speculum examination usually will come before the finger (manual) examination. The speculum will be lubricated with water only; otherwise the results of the Pap smear may be spoiled. If these tests aren't needed, the manual examination may come first.

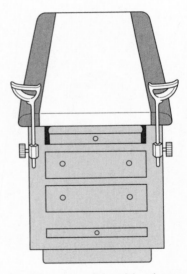

Examination table with stirrups

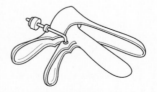

Speculum

The speculum also opens the vagina so that insertion of an intrauterine device (IUD) or other procedures can be accomplished.

Manual Examination. By inserting two lubricated, gloved fingers into the vagina and pressing on the lower abdomen with the other hand, the doctor can feel the shape of the ovaries and uterus as well as any lumps in the area. The accuracy of this examination depends on both the degree of relaxation of the patient and the skill of the doctor. Obese women can't be examined as easily; this is another reason not to be overweight.

Usually the best pelvic examinations are done by those who do them most often. You don't need a gynecologist, but be sure that your internist or family practitioner does "pelvics" on a regular basis before you request a yearly gynecological exam. A nurse-practitioner who does pelvic examinations regularly is usually an expert also. Doing the Pap smear alone doesn't require a great deal of experience.

Many doctors will also perform a rectal or recto-vaginal (one finger in rectum and one in vagina) examination. These examinations can provide additional information. Usually during the examination there is a drape over your knees and the doctor sits on a stool out of your line of sight. Ask the doctor to explain what is going on.

The Pap Smear

You should be familiar with the basics of this test, in which a scraping of the cervix and a sample of the vaginal secretions are obtained with the aid of a speculum. This provides cells for study under the microscope. A trained technician (a cytologist) can then classify the cells according to their microscopic characteristics.

Your doctor will explain the approach to confirming the diagnosis and starting treatment.

A single Pap smear detects up to 90% of the most common cancers of the womb and 70% to 80% of the second most common. Both of these common types of cancer grow slowly. Current evidence indicates that it may take 10 years or more for a single focus of cancer of the cervix to spread. Thus, there is an excellent chance that regular Pap smears will detect the cancer before it spreads.

Cancer of the cervix is more frequent with moderate to heavy sexual activity, especially, and perhaps only, if you have multiple partners. It can follow from sexually transmitted diseases. Regular Pap testing probably should begin when regular sexual activity begins or at age 21, whichever is earlier. Testing is done annually for the first three years. If these first Pap smears are normal, then tests are done every three years. Some experts suggest that the tests can be discontinued at age 65 if all previous tests have been normal. While this recommendation probably carries little risk, we think that a Pap smear every three years is a small burden and prefer to continue the tests.

Vaginal Discharge

Normal vaginal secretions are thin, clear, and painless. Abnormal vaginal discharge is common, however, and can have many causes.

Hormonal changes can cause vaginal dryness and irritation in older women. You may need a prescription cream if the symptoms bother you. Forgotten tampons and other foreign bodies can cause vaginal irritation and discharge. Abdominal pain and bleeding between periods (page 316) suggest the possibility of a serious problem.

Bacteria, viruses, and other microbes can cause vaginal discharge:

▲ A mixture of bacteria may be responsible (nonspecific vaginitis)
▲ A yeast infection (monilia) can cause a white, cheesy discharge
▲ Trichomonas, a common microbe, can cause intense itch and a white, frothy discharge

These infections aren't serious, but they are bothersome. Often the infection will go away by itself. Make an appointment with the doctor if the discharge lasts more than a few days.

See the doctor if it's possible you have been exposed to a sexually transmitted disease (STD). Don't feel ashamed. Doctors treat STDs all the time. You'll be asked to name your sexual contacts. Be frank about naming people with whom you had contact—for their benefit. Information is kept strictly confidential and may prevent spreading the disease.

Other signs to seek medical care:

▲ The discharge is more than slight.

▲ The discharge is yellow-green, gray, cheesy, smelly, or bloody.
▲ The affected area hurts or itches.
▲ The discharge lasts more than a few days.
▲ A girl with vaginal discharge has not reached puberty.

Home Treatment

Patience and good hygiene are the home treatment for vaginal discharge.

Wear cotton underwear, use condoms, and take a daily shower.

Nonprescription anti-yeast creams may help you if your discharge is similar to a previously diagnosed yeast infection.

Call your doctor if you are taking an antibiotic for some other condition. Your doctor may change the medication.

See the doctor if symptoms get worse or persist after a few days of home treatment. Do not douche for 24 hours before your doctor's appointment.

What to Expect at the Doctor's Office

The doctor will do a pelvic examination. He or she may obtain a culture from the vagina for laboratory analysis.

Suppositories or creams are the usual treatment of vaginal discharge. The doctor may prescribe oral medication for severe cases of fungal or trichomonas infection. If a sexually transmitted disease is possible, the doctor will prescribe an antibiotic. Your sexual partner(s) may require treatment too.

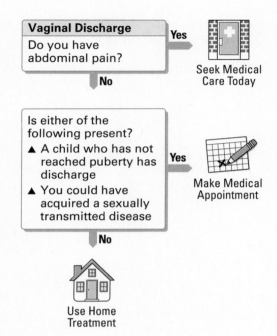

Vaginal Discharge

Do you have abdominal pain?

Yes → Seek Medical Care Today

No ↓

Is either of the following present?

▲ A child who has not reached puberty has discharge

▲ You could have acquired a sexually transmitted disease

Yes → Make Medical Appointment

No ↓

Use Home Treatment

Bleeding Between Periods or After Menopause

Most often the interval between two menstrual periods is free of bleeding or spotting. Many women experience such bleeding, however, even though no serious condition is present. Women with an intrauterine birth control device (IUD) are particularly likely to have occasional spotting. If the bleeding is slight and occasional, it may be ignored.

Serious conditions such as cancer and abnormal pregnancy may be first suggested by bleeding between periods. However, many less serious problems, such as fibroids (benign tumors in the uterus), may have the same sign. If bleeding is severe or occurs three months in a row, a doctor must be seen. Often a serious problem can be detected best when the bleeding isn't active. The gynecologist or the family doctor is a better resource than the emergency room.

Any bleeding after menopause should be evaluated by a doctor.

Home Treatment

Relax and use pads or tampons. Avoid taking aspirin, ibuprofen, naproxen, ketoprofen, or other NSAIDs (page 54) if possible; it may prolong the bleeding. If in doubt about the effect of any medication, call your doctor.

The relationship between tampons and toxic shock syndrome is a subject of medical controversy, but many doctors believe that leaving tampons in place too long increases the risk of this problem. Change tampons regularly, at least twice daily. Be sure that tampons are removed: it is surprisingly easy to forget about them. We don't think tampons should be avoided but believe they should be used with care.

What to Expect at the Doctor's Office

Some personal questions, a pelvic examination, and a Pap smear should be expected (see Gynecological Examination, page 312). If bleeding is active, the pelvic examination and Pap smear may be postponed but should be performed within a few weeks.

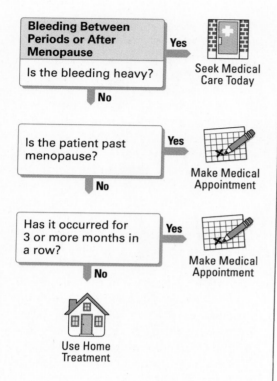

Bleeding Between Periods or After Menopause

Is the bleeding heavy?

Yes → Seek Medical Care Today

No

Is the patient past menopause?

Yes → Make Medical Appointment

No

Has it occurred for 3 or more months in a row?

Yes → Make Medical Appointment

No

Use Home Treatment

Difficult Periods

Adverse mood changes and fluid retention are very common in the days just prior to a menstrual period. Such problems are vexing and can be difficult to treat but are a result of normal hormonal variations during the menstrual cycle.

The menstrual cycle varies from woman to woman. Periods may be regular, irregular, light, heavy, painful, pain-free, long, or short, and yet still be normal. The rhythm of a menstrual cycle is medically less significant than bleeding, pain, or discharge between periods. Only when problems are severe or recur for several months is medical attention required. The doctor can find problems such as endometriosis—the presence of the sort of tissue that lines the uterus in other parts of the body, where it can cause problems. Emergency treatment is seldom needed.

Home Treatment

Diuretics (pills that help the body get rid of fluids through increased urination) and hormones are rarely needed. As we have said in other sections of this book, we prefer the simple and natural to the complex and artificial. We have all too frequently seen hormone treatment lead to mood changes that are worse than premenstrual tension, and diuretics lead to potassium loss, gouty arthritis, and psychological drug dependency.

Salt tends to hold fluid in the tissues. The most natural way to start fluids moving is to cut down on salt intake. In the United States, the typical diet has 10 times the required amount of salt. Many authorities feel that this is one cause of high blood pressure and arteriosclerosis. If you can eliminate some salt, you may have less swelling and fluid retention. If food tastes flat without salt, try using lemon juice as a substitute. Commercial salt substitutes are also satisfactory. Products with the word "sodium" or the chemical symbol "Na" anywhere in the list of ingredients contain salt.

For menstrual cramps, use ibuprofen or other NSAIDs (page 54). Products claimed to be designed for menstrual cramps often have ibuprofen as the main ingredient. Many patients swear by such compounds, and they are fine if you want to pay the premium. We don't understand why, on a scientific basis, they should be any better than plain ibuprofen. Ibuprofen or naproxen is usually most effective, but occasionally aspirin or acetaminophen may be preferred.

What to Expect at the Doctor's Office

The doctor will give you some advice. Frequently, a prescription for diuretics or hormones will be given. For menstrual cramps, ibuprofen (Motrin, etc.) or another prostaglandin-inhibiting drug is often prescribed. Note that ibuprofen is also available in lower doses (Advil, Nuprin, Midol, etc.) without a prescription (page 54).

Pelvic examination is often unrewarding and sometimes may not be performed. However, if endometriosis is suspected, the pelvic exam should be done during the premenstrual phase of the menstrual cycle.

In cases of heavy bleeding, dilatation and curettage, or "D and C," may be required.

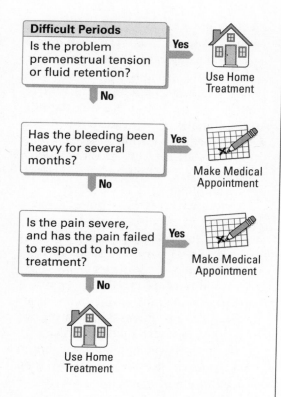

Difficult Periods

Is the problem premenstrual tension or fluid retention? — **Yes** → Use Home Treatment

No ↓

Has the bleeding been heavy for several months? — **Yes** → Make Medical Appointment

No ↓

Is the pain severe, and has the pain failed to respond to home treatment? — **Yes** → Make Medical Appointment

No ↓

Use Home Treatment

The removal of the uterus (hysterectomy) shouldn't be performed for this complaint alone. If a tumor is found, surgery will sometimes be required, but the common fibroid tumor will often stop growing by itself, and surgery may not be needed. Such tumors often grow slowly and often stop growing at menopause, so an operation can be avoided by waiting. If the Pap smear is positive, however, surgery is usually required.

Missed Periods

Although pregnancy is often the first thought when a period is missed, there are many reasons for being late. Obesity, excessive dieting, strenuous exercise, and stress may cause missed or irregular periods. Diseases such as hyperthyroidism that upset the hormonal balance of the body may also be the cause of missed periods, but this is only infrequently the case. It is normal for periods to be irregular before they stop completely with menopause.

Pregnancy Tests

Testing for pregnancy has become faster, easier, and more sensitive in the last decade. Home test kits that provide a reasonable degree of accuracy are now available and may show a positive result as early as two weeks after the missed period. The most sophisticated laboratory test available through your doctor's office may turn positive within a few days after the period should have started. In both instances, a negative result is less reliable when the test is used soon after the period is missed. Thus, it is common to repeat the test after a negative result if periods don't resume.

Because a positive result is less likely to be misleading than a negative one, the rule is to believe a positive test, but not to trust a negative test until it has been repeated at least once.

Other Causes

Two opposites, obesity and starvation, often lead to irregular periods. If either of these conditions is severe and persistent, it can cause the complete cessation of periods. At the other end of the health spectrum, women who are undergoing rigorous athletic training often have irregular periods. The missed periods themselves do not harm the athlete, but there is some concern that the hormonal imbalance that causes the missed periods may also lead to loss of calcium from bones. Currently, it isn't possible to determine if this poses any real risk to women athletes.

Emotional as well as physical stress may result in irregular periods. Indeed, anxiety over possible pregnancy may cause a missed period, thereby increasing the anxiety even further.

Missed periods, rarely, can be a first clue to a metabolic problem or other disease. If the problem persists over two or more cycles, seek medical advice.

If you've reached the age when menopause is possible or likely, then this inevitable event must move to the top of your list of possible causes for the missed period. You may have already experienced some of the other symptoms of menopause. Your periods may also be irregular for a considerable time before they cease altogether. (See Menopause, page 322, for more information.)

Home Treatment

In this instance, home treatment consists of giving yourself some time to consider the various causes of missed periods. You can do something about obesity (see Chapter 1). If you are dieting to the point of starvation, you may have a condition known as anorexia nervosa, and you should consult a doctor or a psychotherapist. If you are following a course of strenuous physical exercise, be alert for further infor-

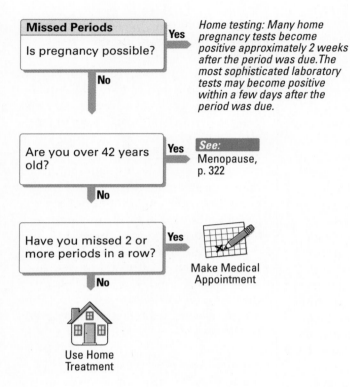

Missed Periods

Is pregnancy possible? — **Yes** → *Home testing: Many home pregnancy tests become positive approximately 2 weeks after the period was due. The most sophisticated laboratory tests may become positive within a few days after the period was due.*

↓ **No**

Are you over 42 years old? — **Yes** → *See:* Menopause, p. 322

↓ **No**

Have you missed 2 or more periods in a row? — **Yes** → Make Medical Appointment

↓ **No**

Use Home Treatment

mation concerning the possible harmful effects of hormonal imbalance associated with missed periods. Finally, knowing that emotional stress may lead to missed periods will help you focus on the cause of the stress rather than on a potential symptom.

If you feel that there is no satisfactory explanation for the missed period or you are unable to develop a plan for dealing with the cause on your own, a phone call to your doctor should provide the advice you need.

What to Expect at the Doctor's Office

Because diseases are relatively infrequent causes of missed periods, most doctors won't rush into a series of tests in an effort to detect these diseases. The doctor will consider the common causes of missed periods discussed above; this is best done with a careful history and physical examination. If pregnancy is the only real possibility, the doctor may refer you by phone to the laboratory for a pregnancy test so that you can avoid an unnecessary office visit.

Menopause

Many women expect that menopause will be a time of difficulty and unhappiness. Understanding the changes that take place during menopause—and what you can do about them—is the best way to approach this time of your life. You may even find that, on balance, menopause is a positive experience.

During menopause, the ovaries reduce their production of female hormones (estrogen and progesterone). Menstrual periods usually become lighter and irregular, and then stop altogether. The halt of menstrual periods means the end of fertility. After menopause, a woman no longer needs contraception to prevent pregnancy. This is one aspect of menopause that many women consider positive.

Hot flashes—sudden feelings of intense heat lasting two or three minutes—are an annoying sign of menopause. They can happen anytime during the day but are most common in the evening. Caffeine and alcohol may make hot flashes worse. Exercise may reduce their effects. For most women, hot flashes gradually decrease over about two years and eventually disappear altogether.

Many women also have mood swings during menopause. It isn't clear whether menopausal hormonal changes cause the mood swings. The moods many women report aren't necessarily unpleasant, just unexpected. For example, one may feel alert in the middle of the night, but not uncomfortable.

Menopausal changes may also prompt a woman to worry, which is why it's good to know what changes are common.

A woman in menopause may be depressed, but menopause does not cause depression.

Female hormones are responsible for the production of natural lubricants in the vagina. Loss of estrogen can cause vaginal dryness. This may lead to irritation, itching, and soreness during and after intercourse.

Osteoporosis, a condition that makes bones more fragile, begins with menopause but causes no symptoms for years. Usually, the first sign of osteoporosis is a broken bone, often a hip, later in life. Such fractures are especially serious because they may lead to prolonged physical inactivity. Also, once bones become thin enough to fracture easily, it is difficult to reverse the process and strengthen the bones.

Home Treatment

Staying cool is the key to treating hot flashes. Keep the home or office cool, dress lightly, and drink plenty of water. Reduce your consumption of alcohol and caffeine, and maintain a regular exercise program. There's no need for medicines such as acetaminophen or aspirin.

You can get relief from vaginal dryness with lubricants such as water-based gels (e.g., Lubifax, K-Y) or other over-the-counter products (e.g., Lubrin). Many women also find that the soreness of intercourse decreases with regular sexual activity.

Regular exercise and adequate dietary calcium are important to prevent osteoporosis. An aerobic exercise program—30 minutes a day, four days a week—is good, but any physical activity will help keep bones strong (page 7). Calcium is essential to maintain strong bones. Post-

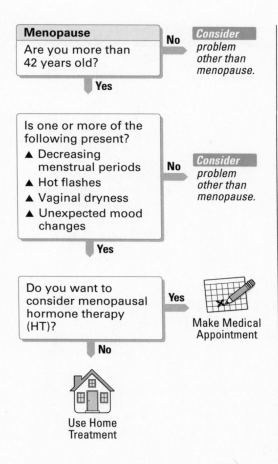

Menopause
Are you more than 42 years old?

No → *Consider* problem other than menopause.

Yes ↓

Is one or more of the following present?
▲ Decreasing menstrual periods
▲ Hot flashes
▲ Vaginal dryness
▲ Unexpected mood changes

No → *Consider* problem other than menopause.

Yes ↓

Do you want to consider menopausal hormone therapy (HT)?

Yes → Make Medical Appointment

No ↓

Use Home Treatment

menopausal women should have 1,200 to 1,500 mg of calcium per day, about as much as in a quart (1 L) of skim milk. You can use a calcium supplement if you can't get enough from dairy products.

What to Expect at the Doctor's Office

The doctor will take the history and do a physical examination to confirm menopause.

The major issue you should discuss with the doctor is menopausal hormone therapy (HT). HT can reduce many symptoms of menopause. It can help prevent osteoporosis and colon cancer.

But it appears to increase the risk for heart disease, stroke, blood clots, breast cancer (more than 4 years of use), and gallstones. Clearly, the use of HT cannot be recommended for all women. But, some will decide to use it after a complete discussion of risks and benefits with their doctor.

Your doctor might prescribe estrogen combined with progestin, a hormone similar to progesterone, but this is no longer generally recommended. This combination is not a good one and may increase the risk of high blood pressure, heart disease, and stroke.

Estrogen treatment alone is seldom suggested unless you have had a hysterectomy because there may be an increased risk of uterine cancer.

Many doctors now prescribe estrogen skin patches, which have a low dose and few side effects. However, some estrogen patches are not strong enough to strengthen the bones.

For vaginal dryness the doctor may prescribe estrogen-containing creams or vaginal suppositories (e.g., Vagifem). These work well and cause few side effects.

Talk over the risks and benefits of estrogen replacement therapy with your doctor.

CHAPTER 12

Sexual Problems and Questions

Sexually Transmitted Diseases

There are many types of sexually transmitted diseases (STDs). Their symptoms range from annoying to deadly. Fortunately, there are now treatments for all of them. Furthermore, it is important for you to know if you have an STD and may thus infect your sexual partner. For these reasons, you must not let embarrassment block you from seeking medical care.

The table opposite lists the symptoms of six STDs. If you think you might have any of these, you need the help of a doctor. On page 326, you'll find information about genital herpes, the only type of STD you might be able to treat at home.

Table 8: Sexually Transmitted Diseases	
Disease	**Symptoms**
Gonorrhea	MEN: discharge from penis; burning feeling while urinating WOMEN: usually none; sometimes vaginal discharge and abdominal discomfort
Syphilis	FIRST SIGN: chancre sore in genital, anal, or mouth area LATER: rash, slight fever, swollen joints
Chlamydia	Similar to gonorrhea, if any
Genital warts	Small, fleshy "condyloma" growths in genital or anal area: soft and reddish inside the body, darker growths outside
Pubic lice	▲ Itching worse at night ▲ Lice visible in pubic hair ▲ Eggs ("nits") attached to pubic hair
AIDS (acquired immuno-deficiency syndrome)	▲ Unusual susceptibility to illness ▲ Persistent fatigue and fever ▲ Night sweats ▲ Unexplained weight loss ▲ Swollen glands ▲ Persistent diarrhea ▲ Dry cough

Diagnosis	Treatment	Special Concerns
▲ Culture of a suspected infection ▲ Examination of vaginal discharge by microscope	Antibiotics	Untreated can lead to: ▲ Severe pelvic inflammation in women ▲ Infertility ▲ Arthritis ▲ Other problems
▲ Examination of fluid from chancre ▲ Blood test	Penicillin or other antibiotics	Untreated can lead to: ▲ Blindness ▲ Brain damage ▲ Heart disease ▲ Birth defects
▲ Culture of a suspected infection ▲ Examination of vaginal discharge by microscope	Antibiotics	Untreated can lead to: ▲ Pelvic inflammation ▲ Infertility in women ▲ Pregnancy complications
▲ Physical examination	Large growths may be removed surgically or burned off	Can return after treatment
▲ Physical examination	Medication to kill the lice	None
▲ Blood test for antibodies to the human immunodeficiency virus (HIV)	Treatment can now help fight the virus and slow the disease, but there is still no cure.	Symptoms may not appear until years after infection. See page 328 for more information.

Genital Herpes

Millions of Americans are infected with one of the two types of herpes virus.

▲ Herpes type 1 is usually spread by kissing. It causes the common fever blisters and cold sores of the lips and mouth, but it can also affect the genitalia.

▲ Herpes type 2 usually causes infections of the genitals. It is typically spread by sexual contact and is thus rare in children.

About one-third of those infected with herpes have bouts of red, painful blisters that last 5 to 10 days. Illnesses, trauma, or emotional stress may trigger these episodes.

Herpes is most contagious during and just before the time when the blisters appear. Many infected people have an itchy or tingly feeling (prodrome) a day or two before the outbreak of blisters. To lower the chance of infecting someone else, avoid sexual contact when the prodrome or blisters are present. Condoms help but don't give complete protection.

Herpes infections are associated with cancer of the cervix. Therefore, if a woman has recurrent herpes infections, she has another reason to obtain a regular Pap smear.

Home Treatment

The herpes sores heal on their own, and you can't do much for them. People with fever blisters try salves, calamine lotion, alcohol, and ether. Some people may get relief, but no remedy works well.

A hot bath for 5 to 10 minutes seems to speed healing. Over-the-counter products (e.g., Blistex) may provide some relief. Many people believe that reducing stress and anxiety is helpful.

Call the doctor if the problem lasts for more than two weeks or if you're unsure your condition is herpes.

To locate a local support program, contact:

▲ American Social Health Association
P.O. Box 13827
Research Triangle Park, NC 27709
(800) 230-6039
www.ashastd.org

What to Expect at the Doctor's Office

The doctor will take the history and do a physical examination. He or she will ask about your sexual habits and other personal information. It is important that you be complete and accurate.

If you have herpes, the doctor may take a sample for laboratory analysis. There are no drugs to cure herpes, but acyclovir (Zovirax) in oral form or in an ointment may make your first attack heal sooner: in 10 to 12 days rather than 14 to 16 days. The ointment usually doesn't work as well on repeated attacks. Oral acyclovir does decrease the number and severity of recurrences if you take the drug continuously, but its side effects can include nausea, vomiting, diarrhea, dizziness, joint pain, rash, and fever.

Genital Herpes

Is there a group of small, painful blisters on reddened skin?

No → *Consider* another problem.

Yes ↓

Is this a first episode, and do you want somewhat faster healing?

Yes → Seek Medical Care Today

No ↓

Are these severe, frequent attacks?

Yes → Seek Medical Care Today

No ↓

Use Home Treatment

AIDS and Safer Sex

AIDS (acquired immunodeficiency syndrome) is caused by the human immunodeficiency virus (HIV). This virus suppresses the immune system and leaves the body susceptible to normally rare disorders, including the type of pneumonia characterized as pneumocystis, Kaposi's sarcoma (a form of skin cancer), and other opportunistic diseases (diseases that take advantage of the body's low immune defenses).

Modes of Transmission

HIV is transmitted through sexual intercourse—oral, vaginal, or anal—or through sharing needles or syringes with an infected person.

HIV has not been shown to be spread from saliva, sweat, tears, urine, or feces. You won't get AIDS from casual contact, such as working with someone with AIDS, a kiss, a telephone, a toilet seat, or a swimming pool. However, babies of infected women may be infected during pregnancy or through breastfeeding.

Some hemophiliacs and surgical patients have become infected because of transfusions of contaminated blood. The probability of receiving infected blood is now very small. There is no risk in donating blood.

Who's at Risk?

The majority of AIDS cases in North America are concentrated among male homosexuals, bisexuals, and intravenous drug users. Approximately 4% of cases have been attributed to heterosexual contact.

The rate at which AIDS is spreading within the heterosexual community isn't clear. However, there is an increase among intravenous drug abusers. Experts believe that this may be the main means of transmission within the heterosexual population. It is important to stress that though AIDS has been predominant in certain groups (that is, gay men and intravenous drug abusers), it's not who you are, it's what you do, that increases your risk of infection. Casual sex, whether homosexual or heterosexual, is the biggest threat for most people. Having sex with many different people can be very dangerous, even when condoms are used. Therefore, reducing risky behavior is the first step to preventing and controlling the spread of AIDS.

Especially risky behaviors are:

▲ Having sex with multiple partners
▲ Sharing drug needles and syringes
▲ Anal sex with or without a condom
▲ Vaginal or oral sex with someone who shoots drugs or engages in anal sex
▲ Sex with a stranger (pickup or prostitute) or with someone who is known to have multiple sex partners
▲ Vaginal sex without a condom when there is any chance the other person is infected with HIV

AIDS Testing

Here are some ground rules for AIDS testing.

Who. Men or women who have had sex with many partners or with prostitutes, who use intravenous drugs, who have gonorrhea or syphilis, who have had sex with anyone who has engaged in these behaviors, or who received a blood transfusion or blood products between 1978 and 1985.

When. Every three to six months for as long as the behavior creating the risk continues.

Why. To detect infection with HIV. If you test positive, there are treatments that can reduce the risks of complications in some patients. Testing needs to be accompanied by counseling with respect to prevention of AIDS as well as interpretation of results. Keeping results confidential may require special strategies, but notification of sexual partners is essential when results are positive.

Preventing AIDS

Currently, a number of researchers are testing AIDS vaccines. However, a vaccine for mass inoculation isn't on the immediate horizon.

Therefore, the primary means of prevention are:

▲ Celibacy—not having sex
▲ Maintaining a monogamous relationship with an uninfected person
▲ Practicing safer sex in relationships where risk of infection is possible
▲ Not sharing needles and/or syringes, or, better yet, not shooting drugs

The risk of AIDS is somewhat decreased by using a latex condom; wear the condom for a time before and after oral, anal, and vaginal intercourse, as well as during. Safety is increased by using a water-based lubricant such as K-Y jelly, Gynol II, or Corn Huskers Lotion. Don't use petroleum jelly, cold cream, or baby oil as a lubricant. These products weaken the latex and can cause it to break.

Use of a spermicide containing nonoxynol-9 in conjunction with a condom may provide further protection from HIV infection if the condom breaks.

Treatment

There are now a number of effective drugs and drug combinations, and your doctor can advise you. Treatment can be expensive, and it can cause side effects. Treatment usually must be continued for life. Very long-term effects are not yet known. How long life can be prolonged is not clear.

Therefore, for the foreseeable future, the best way to avoid AIDS is to avoid risky behavior and practice safer sex when in doubt about your partner's status.

Prevention of Other Sexually Transmitted Diseases (STDs)

The rules for AIDS prevention also decrease the risk of developing other STDs. Again, the effectiveness of condoms as a barrier to infection is not complete but can be substantial if properly used.

Preventing Unwanted Pregnancy

Every woman must decide to abstain from sex, have babies, or use a contraceptive technique. Ideally, the male partner participates in this decision, but through a well-known quirk of nature he doesn't participate in the most direct consequences. This chapter is concerned with the medical considerations involved in making decisions about contraception and childbearing. These decisions have a major effect on your health, both directly and indirectly, whether you are male or female. Childbearing and every form of contraception have definite risks.

Few women will pursue one course of action for all their childbearing years. Not having sex is most effective but will be a reasonable choice for only a few people. For most, it is neither a practical nor a healthy suggestion. An exception: Postponing the onset of sexual activity can often assist the emotional transition to adulthood. The majority of women employ some form of contraception except for specific times when they are attempting to get pregnant or aren't engaging in sexual intercourse. Choosing a method of contraception is one of the most intensely personal decisions you will make, and the rest of us should respect your right to make up your own mind. Ideally, your choice depends on you and your partner.

Forms of Contraception

Here are brief descriptions of the most popular forms of contraception.

Surgeries. If you are sure that you don't want any more children, the safest methods for ensuring this are surgeries. Women can have their fallopian tubes tied (tubal ligation), preventing sperm from reaching their eggs. Men can have a vasectomy operation, which keeps sperm out of their semen. Neither surgery interferes with sexual performance or pleasure.

Birth Control Hormones. Birth control pills ("the pill") and Depo-Provera are the most common medications taken by women to prevent pregnancy.

Birth control pills use hormones to prevent pregnancy and must be taken on a daily basis. When used correctly, they are very effective in preventing pregnancy. However, the pill may cause blood clots, which have been fatal on occasion. It may also contribute to high blood pressure. There are less dangerous but annoying side effects such as weight gain, nausea, fluid retention, migraine headaches, vaginal bleeding, and vaginal yeast infections.

Birth control pills can also be used as emergency contraception on "the morning after." Up to 72 hours after intercourse, a woman who is worried that she may have been impregnated can take two doses of birth control pills 12 hours apart. This will reduce her chance of becoming pregnant by at least 75%. Depending on which pill is used, each dose is two or four times the usual daily dose of birth control pills. Therefore, it is helpful to ask advice from a doctor or clinic before trying this method. Since the dosages of hormone are so much higher, side effects are more common; nausea occurs for 50% to 70% of women using this method and vomiting occurs for about 20%.

Depo-Provera is a long-lasting injection of hormones that provides contraception for about three months.

Intrauterine Device (IUD). This device is inserted into the uterus by a doctor and remains there until removed or expelled. If the IUD is expelled, it may not be noticed. In such cases, some pregnancies have resulted. The IUD may also cause bleeding and cramps. In rare instances, it is associated with serious infections of the uterus, although the type of IUD most frequently associated with these uterine infections—the Dalkon Shield—has been removed from the market. Intrauterine devices, if well tolerated, are a low-cost, low-upkeep choice.

Diaphragm, Cervical Cap. A diaphragm is a rubber membrane that fits over the opening to the uterus in the vagina. It must be inserted before intercourse and kept in place for at least six hours afterward. There are no side effects or complications from diaphragms. They are best used with a spermicidal foam or jelly. Cervical caps are more sturdy variations of the diaphragm and always contain spermicide. Caps are more effective for women who have never given birth.

Foams, Jellies, and Suppositories. These ointments contain chemicals that kill or immobilize the man's sperm. In the past, they were used by themselves but now are almost always used in conjunction with a diaphragm. Side effects are unusual and consist of some irritation to the walls of the vagina. Their effect lasts only about 60 minutes, and many people

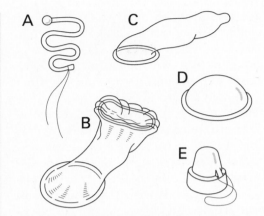

Contraceptive devices. (A) intrauterine device, or IUD (this figure shows a Lippes Loop; other types are available); (B) female condom; (C) male condom; (D) diaphragm; (E) cervical cap.

find these preparations inconvenient and just plain messy.

Condoms. Male condoms are enjoying a resurgence of popularity. If used correctly, latex condoms are 90% effective in preventing pregnancy. They have no side effects, and they are inexpensive and widely available. However, the male must remember to use a condom properly, and some designs do decrease the male's physical sensitivity. Female condoms have been used less but appear to have similar advantages and disadvantages. Condoms are the only form of birth control to give substantial protection against sexually transmitted diseases, including AIDS. They work best when used with a spermicide.

Periodic Abstinence. In this technique, the couple avoids intercourse during the time when they expect the woman to ovulate. Such techniques are often taught as "natural family planning," and are preferred by many couples with a religious or moral dislike for other forms of birth control. The "rhythm method" requires the woman to have fairly regular periods and to carefully take daily temperatures in order to predict the time of ovulation. Under the best of circumstances, it is only moderately effective. More recently developed techniques based on frequent measurement of the acidity of the cervical mucus are a slight improvement. All such methods require highly motivated people to make them work.

Finally, we will mention two methods that reduce the chance of pregnancy somewhat, but in the long run aren't reliable enough to prevent it. In withdrawal (coitus interruptus), the male removes his penis from the vagina just before ejaculation. Because there are sperm present in the secretions of the penis before ejaculation occurs and because withdrawal at just the right time is a tricky business at best, this method rather frequently fails. Douching after intercourse also decreases the number of sperm in the vagina, but it too is far from reliable.

Deciding to Give Birth

You may decide to become pregnant for the best of reasons—your own reasons. One of the most popular reasons to have sex without birth control is that you wish to raise a family. Many women have ethical or religious objections to abortion—or to other forms of contraception, for that matter. A pregnant woman who won't be able to care for her baby but can't accept an abortion has the option of allowing the newborn to be adopted.

Table 9: Effectiveness of Contraceptive Methods

Percentage of women who become pregnant during the first year of using each contraceptive method (the lower the number, the more effective the method)

Method	Typical Use	Perfect Use
No contraception	85%	85%
Spermicides only	21	6
Periodic abstinence	20	4*
Withdrawal	19	4
Cervical cap women who have never given birth	18	9
women who have given birth	36	26
Diaphragm	18	6
Female condom	21	5
Male condom	12	3
Pill	3	0.3*
IUD	1*	0.6*
Female sterilization	0.4	0.4
Depo-Provera	0.3	0.3
Male sterilization	0.2	0.1

* This number is an average of the percentages produced by different methods within this category.

Another common reason not to use contraception is simply not wanting to bother with it. Not smart. Deciding to have sex without birth control is, over the long run, the same as deciding to become pregnant.

A woman who chooses to give birth to a child deserves good medical care. This lowers the health risks of pregnancy and childbirth and provides for a healthier, happier baby. We and Dr. Robert H. Pantell discuss pregnancy and birth in detail in *Taking Care of Your Child.*

Erectile Dysfunction (ED)

Erectile dysfunction, the inability of the male to maintain an erection sufficient to complete intercourse, has now become a syndrome for both private and public discussion. Its frequency increases with age and with some diseases, such as diabetes.

First, consider the reversible causes. ED can result from smoking cigarettes, drinking alcohol, and taking any of a number of medications, especially drugs used to treat high blood pressure. Lack of aerobic physical exercise and obesity can sometimes contribute.

Second, effective medical treatment with Viagra and several similar medicines is now available. This is expensive, doesn't always work, and poses some hazards, particularly for men taking nitroglycerin. Long-term effects are not yet known. This can be a difficult choice. Talk with your doctor. Don't buy the drug over the Internet without this essential medical discussion.

PART III

Managing Your Professional Medical Care

CHAPTER 13

Working with Your Doctor and Your Health Care System

You should have one personal doctor in whom you trust and confide. This doctor should be your advocate and your guide through the complicated medical care system. You may require an additional consulting doctor from time to time, and your personal doctor should interpret and coordinate that consultant's recommendations. Good medical care usually doesn't result from having a different doctor for every organ of your body. Having too many doctors working in an uncoordinated manner often results in too many medications, too many medical procedures, too many side effects, and sometimes opposing approaches to treatment.

Your personal doctor doesn't need to be an expert in everything; he or she should readily seek advice from others when needed and guide you to other appropriate health professionals. But someone has to view the whole picture, to know everything that's going on. Someone needs to take responsibility for putting all the information together and making sure that nothing has been left out.

Finding the Right Doctor

What kind of doctor should your personal doctor be? He or she might appropriately be a:

▲ **Family practitioner:** specialist in family medicine
▲ **Internist:** specialist in internal medicine
▲ **Gynecologist:** specialist in female medicine or health
▲ **Geriatrician:** specialist in the medical care of older people

The family practitioner and the general internist are trained in dealing with the "whole patient" and in appropriate use of other consultants as required. Geriatrics is a relatively new specialty with practice limited to the senior population, and its practitioners take pride in recognizing the needs of the whole patient as well. Most internal medicine problems now occur after the age of 65, so the general internist has also become, in large part, a geriatrician.

If you have a particular major disease, such as heart disease or rheumatoid arthritis, it may be inefficient to have a general doctor who must frequently refer you to a specialist. See if it's possible for the specialist to serve as your primary doctor. As noted above, it's not a good idea to have two or more primary doctors at the same time.

The most important qualities that you want in a primary care doctor center on *communication* and *anticipation*. Communication is the human side of medicine. A good primary physician:

▲ **Takes time to listen.** You can help your doctor by explaining your problems clearly.

▲ **Takes time to talk with you.** The doctor will explain his or her suggested course of action clearly.

▲ **Plans ahead to prevent problems.** A substantial part of your conversation should be about how to prevent future illnesses. Problems will be anticipated and plans made before the problems become severe.

▲ **Reviews your total health program regularly.**

▲ **Has your trust and confidence.** If you can't communicate with your doctor, try another. Often two people just happen to operate on different frequencies. You want to keep the same doctor for a long time, so if a relationship with a particular doctor isn't working, find a new one early on. When you find the right doctor, stay with him or her unless there's a substantial change in your medical needs and you require a doctor with different skills.

▲ **Is available by telephone or email.** Simple questions can often be answered by phone or email. And you don't want to visit a doctor just to get a prescription refilled.

▲ **Uses medication conservatively.** You don't want a doctor who just gives a pill for everything.

There's a technical side of medicine too, and for some individuals, this will represent the most important part of modern medicine. Perhaps you need an operation on your blood vessels or your brain. Perhaps you need surgery inside your middle ear. Perhaps you need replacement of your hip joint, kidney dialysis, or even an organ transplant. In these situations, your standards for excellence in your consulting doctor are a little different. You're still interested in anticipation and communication, but you also want to pay a great deal of attention to the *technical skill* of the individual.

You'd like to know if a particular surgeon, for example, gets better or worse results than average. This is often a little hard to judge, but there are two key tests you can apply.

▲ Does the specialist have the complete confidence and approval of your primary doctor? Talk with your primary doctor about possible alternative physicians, and ask about the advantages and disadvantages of each.

▲ Ask how frequently the specialist performs the particular procedure. Technical results are generally better at institutions and with doctors who perform a technical procedure frequently. As a general rule, results are substantially better where the procedure is done at least 50 times each year and are not as good where the procedure is done only occasionally.

These considerations don't apply only to surgical specialists. Increasingly, the line between surgery and medicine has blurred. There are now "invasive cardiologists" who perform marvelous but sometimes hazardous tasks using long tubes manipulated through your blood vessels under X-ray control. The gastrointestinal endoscopist can now use long, flexible, lighted tubes to look at (and sometimes treat) a surprising amount of your insides from the outside. An arthroscopist can perform surgery inside a joint, needing only a small cut in the skin to admit a lighted tube with which to see the joint's interior. Arteriographers, often radiologists, use dye injected through long catheters to visualize your blood vessels on X-ray film. New imaging techniques include computed axial tomography (CT or CAT scans) and magnetic resonance imagery (MR or MRI). These techniques require skill both for performing the procedure and for interpreting the results.

Again, apply your two tests. Does the specialist who will do the procedure have the full agreement and confidence of your primary doctor? Does the specialist perform the procedure frequently?

Communicating with Your Doctor

You and your doctor must be able to listen, explain, ask questions, understand each other, and choose options wisely. Put simply, you and your doctor must be able to talk and work together as partners.

Medical History

When you visit your doctor, it's essential for you to give a concise, organized description of your illness. Tell it like it is. If you want to report a sexual problem, don't say that you're "tired and run-down." If you're afraid that you have cancer, don't say that you came "for a checkup." Patients who ramble or don't mention their real concerns are their own worst enemies. The ability to give a good medical history helps to preserve your health and your dollars.

Most people don't realize that every doctor uses a similar process to learn a patient's medical history and to organize those facts so as to be able to remember and analyze them. Knowing that process can help you give accurate information. Your primary physician may not go through your entire medical history on a repeat visit, but doctors will do so during a first visit or a comprehensive evaluation. Be prepared to give your doctor information under these five headings.

Chief Complaint. After greeting you, the doctor usually asks about your chief complaint. This question may take several forms: "What bothers you the most?" "What brings you here today?" "What's the trouble?" Your answer establishes the priorities for the rest of the visit. Be sure you express your problem clearly. Know in advance how to state your chief complaint: "I have a sore throat." "I have a pain in my lower right side." "I seem to have three problems: sore throat, skin rash, and cloudy urine." Think of the chief complaint as the title for the story you're about to tell the doctor. Any of the problems listed in Part II may be your chief complaint, and there are hundreds of less common problems.

Present Illness. Next your doctor will want to hear the story behind your chief complaint: "When did this problem begin?" "When were you last entirely well?" "How long has this been going on?" Think about these questions in advance so you can give a clear answer: "Yesterday." "On June 4." "About the middle of May." If you're uncertain about the date that the problem began, state the uncertainty and tell what you can: "I'm not sure when these problems began. I began to feel tired in the middle of February, but the pain in the joints didn't begin until April." After you define the starting point for the problem, the doctor will want to establish the sequence of events after that time. Tell the story in the order it occurred. Try not to use "flashbacks" or irrelevant details; you'll only confuse yourself and your doctor. The doctor may interrupt to ask specific questions or at the end ask questions about problems that you haven't mentioned.

Past Medical History. Your doctor may want more background information about your general health. Information that didn't appear important earlier may be relevant. The doctor will ask specific questions about your general health, childhood illnesses, hospitalizations, operative procedures, allergies, and medications. Give direct, reasonably brief answers. If you report a drug "allergy," describe the specific reaction you experienced; many reactions to drugs (such as nausea, vomiting, or ringing in the ears) are not allergies but common side effects. Be thorough when reporting medications, including birth control pills, vitamins, pain relievers, and laxatives.

Review of Systems. In a complete medical exam, your doctor will usually review symptoms related to the different body systems, asking standard questions for each system.

Social History. In a complete medical exam, your doctor may ask about your job, family, interpersonal stresses, smoking, drinking, use of drugs, sexual activity, even exposures to chemical or toxic substances. These questions are sometimes intensely personal. However, the answers can be of the utmost importance in determining your illness and how it can be best treated.

Supporting information can be extremely important. Know which medications you've taken before and during the course of your illness. Often it's helpful to bring the medication bottles to the doctor. Mention any allergic reactions that you have to drugs. If you're pregnant or could be pregnant, tell the doctor. If X-ray studies or laboratory tests have been performed during the course of the illness, try to make the results available to the doctor. If you've consulted other doctors, bring those medical records with you. Be a careful observer of your own illness. Your observations, carefully made and recounted, are more valuable than any other source of information.

Understanding Your Health Plan

The present variety of medical plans is somewhat bewildering. This section defines the major types of medical plans, but combination plans are common.

Managed care techniques may be found in all plans. This means the health plan rules on whether it will pay for particular parts of your care. The health plan's representative may have to approve your surgery beforehand, or make sure that you don't stay in the hospital too long. The purpose of managed care is to save money for the health plan. It is sometimes argued that managed care improves the quality of care through its surveillance techniques and that it prevents unnecessary surgery.

Traditional Indemnity. This is the traditional type of medical insurance. Your medical care charges are paid at a specified rate. Often there are deductibles (you must pay for a certain amount on your own before coverage begins) and copayments (you must pay a certain percentage of charges up to a specified limit) as a part of these plans. Increasingly, these plans include elements of managed care techniques.

Preferred Provider Organization (PPO). The medical plan provides a list of "preferred doctors." If you choose one of these doctors, you'll pay less than if you choose a doctor or hospital not on the list because those on the list charge the medical plan less. Sometimes the plan may be an Exclusive Provider Organization (EPO). This is similar to a PPO except that you'll pay essentially all the medical costs if you don't use a doctor or hospital on the list given by the medical plan.

Health Maintenance Organization (HMO). This is the original form of prepaid medical care. Virtually all HMOs today combine prepayment (sometimes called "capitation") with managed care techniques. Doctors who provide care for HMOs may be employed exclusively by the HMO or may contract to provide care for HMO patients while still providing care for patients in other medical plans. Usually HMOs won't pay for any care given by physicians or hospitals that aren't part of their HMO system except in emergencies or when you're traveling.

Point-of-Service Plan. Recognizing that choice is important to many people, some plans will let you choose among plans when you go for care, i.e., at the point of service. In other words, you can wait until you need care to decide whether you'll use traditional indemnity, an EPO, or your favorite physician. However, if you choose a doctor or hospital that costs the health plan more, you will pay more. You get more freedom of choice, but at a cost.

Health Savings Account (HSA). These relatively new plans most often will be the least expensive for people who take care of themselves. Your insurance premium is broken into two parts. The first goes to buy an insurance policy against catastrophic illness with a high deductible, perhaps $3,000. The remainder, perhaps $2,000, goes into your health savings account, and you use it to pay medical costs below the deductible. If you don't spend all the money in your health savings account, you get to keep it. Be sure, however, that you don't delay care that you really need just to save money. Follow the guidelines of this book.

Getting the Most Out of Your Visit to the Doctor

Asking Questions

To use your time with the doctor effectively, make a list of your questions before the visit. Write down your questions. Date the list. Leave space to jot down answers while you're talking with the doctor. If someone is accompanying you on the visit, perhaps he or she can write down the answers for you. Take the list to your doctor and ask each question. Go over the list and the answers again after you get home. Save the list as part of your own records. A written record can be very useful for you.

Table 10 suggests some questions that you may want to ask your doctor. As you make up your list for a particular visit, run through this list and see which questions you want to include. After the table has helped you get started, think of other questions that you may also find useful; don't just limit yourself to these.

The figure below shows what your list might look like if you make a visit to Dr. Johanson because of a problem with dizziness when standing. Your questions on the left will probably be handwritten in full and the answers on the right jotted down, so this example will give you a general idea of the process.

Problem List for Dr. Johanson, June 19 Appointment

Questions	Answers
1. Dizziness when standing?	• Low blood pressure. Decrease Aldomet to 2/day. Will check blood counts.
2. Wonder about aspirin or fish oil capsules for heart attacks?	• Not yet. Diet first. Will check cholesterol.
3. Leg cramps?	• Warm baths and massage.
4. Gray splotches on skin?	• Just age spots — OK.
5. Move to Arizona for joint pains?	• Probably not. Try vacation to hot, dry area first; see if it feels better.
6. Cost of blood pressure pills?	• Reducing dose anyway because of dizziness. Try AARP pharmacy services.

Table 10: Possible Questions for Your Doctor

General questions to ask:

▲ What is my problem?

▲ Is it a common problem?

▲ What does the diagnosis mean?

▲ What is likely to happen?

▲ Can you tell me what these words [any words you don't understand] mean?

▲ Could the problem be anything else?

▲ How likely is that?

▲ What are my options for the next step?

▲ What are the benefits, risks, and cost of each choice?

If the doctor suggests tests:

▲ What will we learn from these tests?

▲ Will they be uncomfortable?

▲ Do I need to make special arrangements (such as fasting before the test or planning transportation home)?

If the doctor suggests medication:

▲ How will the medication help?

▲ Does it have any side effects I should know about?

▲ Is it available in a generic form?

▲ Might it interact badly with other drugs or with foods?

▲ What can I expect in the next few weeks and also over the long term?

If the doctor suggests surgery or other medical procedures:

▲ What are the risks of the procedure?

▲ How frequently does this procedure relieve this kind of problem?

▲ Must the procedure be done right away? Why?

▲ Can this be done safely as an outpatient procedure?

▲ How frequently do you do this procedure?

▲ I would feel more comfortable with another opinion. Could you recommend someone for me to check with?

If the doctor suggests hospitalization:

▲ Can I have the tests or treatment done as an outpatient?

▲ What are the risks of being in the hospital?

▲ Which hospital do you suggest and why?

▲ Does the hospital staff perform this treatment frequently?

▲ Can I recover at home and shorten the hospital stay?

▲ What should I do at home?

▲ Is there anything I shouldn't do?

▲ When should I check back with you?

▲ Should I avoid aspirin for a week or more before the procedure?

It's not necessary to limit a valuable doctor visit to your most recent problem. You may have a lot of questions. The doctor visit is a good place to begin thinking about them, together with a knowledgeable expert. Table 11 (page 344) lists a few of the subjects you may wish to discuss.

You must understand all instructions the doctor gives you. If you're confused, ask more questions: "Could you go over that again?" "I don't understand how to use this medication." "How long should I apply the ice pack?" "Are there any risks to this?" Ask your doctor to write out the instructions, or write them down yourself. Do *not* depend on your memory.

Table 11: Possible Subjects to Discuss with Your Doctor	
▲ Exercise	▲ Drug or alcohol use
▲ Sexual problems	▲ Estrogen for women after menopause
▲ Diet	▲ Medication program
▲ Weight	▲ Mammography for women
▲ Calcium	▲ Screening tests
▲ Smoking	▲ Any immunizations needed

Understand the importance of each drug. In some instances, it doesn't matter if you take the medicine regularly because the drug gives only symptomatic relief and should be discontinued as soon as possible. Be sure that you understand whether or not it's necessary to continue the medication after you feel well.

Consider the entire prescribed program. You may already be taking medications your doctor doesn't know about. Perhaps you have trouble taking a medication at work, or you anticipate trouble with a diet the doctor prescribes. If the doctor prescribes more than one medication, you may want to take them all at once—is this okay? An upcoming trip could interfere with a treatment program, or you may worry about starting exercise in the winter. When such questions arise, ask the doctor in advance. Often if you raise these questions with your doctor, your treatment program can be modified so that you feel more comfortable. Be frank. Don't say that you'll do something that you know you won't. Express your worries. You don't have to be a "perfect" patient; it's all right to be persistent until your questions are answered.

Carrying Out Your Treatment Program

After you and your doctor have agreed on a program, follow it closely. If you notice possible side effects from the program, call the doctor and ask about them. If the side effects are serious, return for an examination.

Make a chart of the days of the week and the times when you are to take medications. Note on the chart when you take them; such charts are universally used in hospitals to ensure that medication schedules are maintained accurately. At home, you and your family are the custodians of your health. Don't view the task of taking medication more lightly than it is viewed by professionals. More important, if you find that you can't carry out the program, you and your doctor must make changes.

When you have pills left over at the end of a course of therapy, dispose of them properly. Check with your doctor's office—most have places to discard medications safely—or go to fda.gov for instructions on the proper way to dispose of medications and a list of locations that take back expired and unneeded medications. A medicine chest containing old prescription medicines presents multiple hazards. Every year, children and adults die from taking leftover drugs. Children take birth control pills, adults brush their teeth with corticosteroid creams, and people take the wrong medication because they mistake one bottle for another. If, for example, you give your leftover tetracycline to your children with their next cold, you may cause mottling (gray spotting) of their teeth. Taking outdated tetracycline may cause liver damage. When a new illness occurs and you take leftover medications, your condition may then confuse your doctor. Sometimes it will be impossible to make an accurate identification of a bacterium by culture, or the clinical picture of the disease may be changed by the medicine.

The doctor-patient encounter is your most reliable protection against serious illness. Value the opportunity for such attention, use it effectively, and follow the program that you and your doctor develop to the maximum extent possible.

Choosing the Right Medical Facility

Hospitals

The hospital is expensive. It's not a home or a hotel. Lives are saved and lost there. At times, you must use the hospital, and at other times, you must avoid it. To manage these contradictions, you and your family must carefully consider the need for hospitalization in each instance.

Don't use the hospital if services can be performed elsewhere. The acute (short-term) general hospital provides acute general medicine; it doesn't perform other functions well.

Don't use the hospital for a rest; it's not a good place to go for rest. It's busy, noisy, and populated with unfamiliar roommates. Its nights are punctuated with interruptions, and it has an unusual time schedule. It has many employees, a few of whom will be less thoughtful than others.

Don't use the hospital for the "convenience" of having a number of tests done in just a few days. It doesn't provide tests in the most efficient manner; indeed, many hospital laboratories and special X-ray facilities aren't open on the weekend, and just to schedule special procedures may require several days.

Current evidence suggests that for many conditions, treatment at home may work better than treatment in the hospital. Even home treatment for minor heart attacks in the elderly has been reported as possibly better than hospital treatment. It's apparent to most hospital visitors that the crisis atmosphere of the short-term acute hospital doesn't promote the calmest state of mind for the patient. Many therapeutic features of the home, such as familiar, comfortable surroundings, can't be duplicated in the hospital.

Emergency Rooms

The emergency room has become the "doctor" for many people. Those who can't find a doctor at night or who don't know where else to go increasingly go to emergency rooms. Thus, the typical emergency room is now filled with nonemergency cases. Various problems are all mixed together: trivial illnesses that could have been treated with the aid of this book, routine problems more easily and economically handled in a doctor's office, specialized problems that should have been dealt with at a time when the hospital facilities were fully available, and true emergencies. Although the emergency room isn't designed for the purpose it now serves, it does a surprisingly good job of delivering adequate care.

However, there are five major disadvantages to using an emergency room as your sole medical contact.

▲ Emergency rooms make little or no provision for continued care. You'll usually be seen by a different doctor each time. The emergency room doctor will attend to the chief problem you report but seldom has enough time to complete a full examination or to deal with underlying problems.

▲ Although simple X-ray facilities are available, procedures such as gall-bladder studies and upper GI (gastrointestinal) series are difficult to arrange. Thus, emergency rooms aren't the right place for evaluating complicated problems.

▲ When a true emergency occurs, patients with less urgent problems are shunted aside. You can't estimate with any certainty how long you'll have to wait for treatment in an emergency room.

▲ Emergency room fees, because they support equipment required to handle true emergencies, are higher than those for standard office visits.

▲ Emergency room services aren't always covered by medical insurance, even when the policy states that the costs of emergency care are included. With many policies, the *nature of the illness* determines whether or not it's covered. In other words, the medical plan may pay for emergency room care only in a true emergency. You may end up paying a large bill out of your own pocket if you go to the emergency room with a sore throat.

The smoothly functioning emergency room provides one of the finest and most dramatic examples of a service profession at work. Following the procedures outlined in this book, you can use this valuable resource appropriately.

Other Medical Facilities

Short-Term Surgery Centers

A number of facilities specially designed for short-term surgery (requiring only a short stay, overnight at the most) have recently appeared. Obviously, the surgery performed is relatively minor, and the patient must basically be in good health. Because such centers can avoid some of the overhead of a hospital, they often charge less. But because they don't have the capability to handle difficult cases or complications, you should use them only for minor procedures. The growing experience with these centers has been positive.

Walk-in Clinics

Similarly, some medical problems can be managed at walk-in or "drop-in" clinics. If you have a new, uncomplicated problem (for example, a sore throat or a minor injury), such clinics can be excellent. The decision charts in Part II will help you to determine if you should visit the doctor. Appointments at walk-in clinics aren't usually necessary, and service is swift and efficient. Often these clinics are open for long hours, including evenings and weekends. When available, such clinics should be used for nonemergency care in preference to emergency rooms. The problem with these clinics is with follow-up and sometimes with cost. Costs are rising and now approach those of emergency rooms. If you've had your problem for more than six weeks or if you expect that it will require multiple visits and more than six weeks to clear up, we think you should see your regular doctor.

Long-Term Care Facilities

Nursing homes and various types of rehabilitation facilities provide for the patient who doesn't require hospital care but can't be adequately managed at home. The quality of these facilities ranges from superb to horrible. In the best circumstances, with dedicated nursing and regular doctor attendance, a comfortable and home-like situation for the patient can accelerate the healing process. In other cases, uninterested personnel, inadequate facilities, and minimal care are the rule. Before choosing a nursing home facility, visit the facility or have a friend or relative visit it for you. In the long-term care setting, your comfort with the arrangements is essential.

Hospice Care

For patients with terminal diagnoses (usually a life expectancy of less than six months), the hospice movement tries to provide humane, caring, medically sound treatment without all the technological trappings of the hospital. This can occur either at home with professional personnel or in a hospice facility. The care approach emphasizes improving the patient's comfort. Hospice and home-care programs are becoming more available and are worthwhile. Check out a hospice facility in the same way you would a nursing home; most are good, but some aren't.

Reducing the Cost of Medications

Legal drugs are a multibillion-dollar industry. Your contribution to this industry is determined not only by your health, but also by your doctor, your pharmacy, and you.

Drugs are, at the same time, lifesaving and dangerous, curative and fraught with side effects, painful and pain relieving, and easy to misuse. Most drugs act to block one or more of the natural body defense mechanisms, such as pain, cough, inflammation, or diarrhea. Drugs can interact with other drugs, causing hazardous chemical reactions. They can have direct toxic reactions on the stomach lining and elsewhere in the body. They can cause allergic rashes and shock. They can have severe toxic effects when taken in excess. Some drugs can decrease the ability of the body to fight infections.

You don't want to take any medications you don't truly need. If you don't receive a prescription or a sample package of medication from your physician, consider this good news rather than rejection or lack of interest on the part of the doctor. Take the fewest possible drugs for the shortest possible time. When drugs are prescribed, take them regularly and as directed, but expect that your medication program will be thoroughly reviewed every time you see your doctor.

Most of today's drugs are "symptomatic medications"—that is, they don't cure your problem but give partial relief for the symptoms. The symptoms that may be relieved include pain, cough, inflammation, insomnia, stress, diarrhea, or constipation. If you report a different symptom every time you see your doctor and urgently request relief from that symptom, you're likely to be given additional medications. You're unlikely to feel much better as a result, and you may function at a lower level. Unless you have a serious illness, you'll seldom need to take more than one or two medications at a time. Perceptive observers have argued that our present practice of using drugs to control symptoms is only a temporary phase in the history of medicine.

Your Doctor Can Help

Use generic drugs whenever you can. They are almost always just as good as the brand-name product. Insurers often require pharmacies fill prescriptions with generics although, in some states, if your doctor prescribes a drug by its trade name the pharmacist must fill the prescription with that particular brand-name product. The brand-name product frequently costs many times more than its generic equivalent. Does your doctor know the relative cost of alternative drugs? Many doctors don't.

The drug-prescribing habits of different doctors can be divided into two types: the "additive" and the "substitutive." With each visit to an "additive" doctor, you receive a medication in addition to those you already have. With a "substitutive" doctor, a medication you were previously taking is discontinued, and a new medicine is substituted. Usually the "substitutive" practice is better for your health as well as your pocketbook. Even better is a doctor who likes to *decrease* the number of medications you take.

Most of the time, you can take medication by mouth. Sometimes a doctor gives medication by injection because of uncertainty that you'll take it as prescribed. However, as a thoughtful and reliable patient, you can assure your doctor that you will comply with an oral regimen. Taking medication by mouth is less painful, less likely to result in an allergic reaction, and usually far less expensive. There are exceptions, but whenever possible, you should take medication by mouth rather than by injection.

If it's clear that you must take a medication for a prolonged period, ask the doctor to allow refills on the prescription. With many drugs, it's not necessary to incur the expense of an additional doctor visit just to get a prescription written. However, under some circumstances, the doctor may prefer to examine you or get a lab test before deciding whether the drug can be safely continued or is still required.

The careful doctor will ensure that you fully understand the nature of each drug you're taking, the reasons you're taking it, the side effects that may arise, and the length of time that you can expect to take it. You and your doctor should arrange a daily medication schedule that's convenient as well as medically effective. If the program is confusing, ask for written instructions. It's crucial that you understand the why and how of your drug therapy. Don't leave the doctor's office for the pharmacy without understanding your medications.

Your Pharmacist Can Help

Studies indicate that the pharmacy you choose is a very important factor in drug costs. For the most part, the pharmacist no longer weighs and measures individual chemical formulations. Much of the activity in the pharmacy consists of relabeling and dispensing manufactured medication. Medication is thus usually identical at different pharmacies. You should choose the least expensive and the most convenient place that your medical plan allows.

Comparison-shop beforehand. Discount stores often sell the same medication at significantly lower prices. There are good mail-order sources. If a considerable sum of money is involved, you should compare prices by telephone before purchasing the medication. Don't buy from a pharmacy that won't give you price information over the phone.

Unfortunately, even when your doctor writes a prescription by generic name rather than brand name, the pharmacist often isn't required to give you the cheapest alternative. The pharmacy often stocks only one manufacturer's formulation of each drug. Thus, even though your doctor has been careful to permit a less expensive preparation, the pharmacist may substitute the more expensive alternative that's in stock. There's no way to detect this problem except to get direct price quotes from different pharmacies. Once you have found a pharmacy with fair prices and helpful pharmacists, stay with it.

Your pharmacist can help you understand your medications. If you forget to ask your doctor some key questions (see Table 10, page 343), the pharmacist can often help you with the answers. If you use the same pharmacy all of the time, the pharmacist can often spot problems in your overall treatment, such as taking two drugs that don't go well together.

You Can Help

Visits to the doctor all too frequently are requests for medication. If your satisfaction with the doctor depends on whether or not you're given medication, you're working against your own best interest.

If you go to a doctor because of a cold and request a "shot of penicillin," you're asking for poor medical practice. (Penicillin should only rarely be given by injection, and it shouldn't be given for uncomplicated colds.) Your doctor knows this but may give in to your request.

The most frequently prescribed medications in the United States, making up the bulk of drug costs, are tranquilizers, minor pain relievers, and sedatives. These drugs cause the greatest number of side effects, and they aren't really scientifically important medications. Our national prescription pattern arose, at least in part, because of ill-advised consumer demand. You can decrease the cost of medications by using some of the techniques discussed previously; you can eliminate them almost completely by decreasing your pressure to receive and take medications that you don't need.

Fortunately, our bodies heal most problems if we curb our impatience a little. The policy of "watchful waiting" without medication is usually the best one. Follow the guidelines of this book to identify the more serious situations. Doctors have a name for this most useful treatment of all: they call it "tincture of time."

Immunizations: A Family Record

Name: _____ _____ _____ _____ _____

Recommended Age: **Date**   **Date**   **Date**   **Date**   **Date**

Recommended Age	Date	Date	Date	Date	Date
Birth: Hepatitis B	___	___	___	___	___
1–4 months: Hepatitis B	___	___	___	___	___
2 months: DTaP #1	___	___	___	___	___
HIB #1	___	___	___	___	___
IPV #1	___	___	___	___	___
PCV #1	___	___	___	___	___
RV #1	___	___	___	___	___
4 months: DTaP #2	___	___	___	___	___
HIB #2	___	___	___	___	___
IPV #2	___	___	___	___	___
PCV #2	___	___	___	___	___
RV #2	___	___	___	___	___
6 months: DTaP #3	___	___	___	___	___
HIB #3	___	___	___	___	___
PCV #3	___	___	___	___	___
RV #3	___	___	___	___	___
6–18 months: Hepatitis B	___	___	___	___	___
IPV #3	___	___	___	___	___
12–15 months: HIB #4	___	___	___	___	___
PCV #4	___	___	___	___	___
MMR #1	___	___	___	___	___
Hepatitis A	___	___	___	___	___
12–18 months: Varicella	___	___	___	___	___
15–18 months: DTaP Booster	___	___	___	___	___
18–24 months: Hepatitis A	___	___	___	___	___
2–6 years: Meningococcus	___	___	___	___	___
2–18 years: PPSV	___	___	___	___	___
4–6 years: DTaP Booster	___	___	___	___	___
IPV Booster	___	___	___	___	___
MMR #2	___	___	___	___	___
Varicella	___	___	___	___	___
11–12 years: Tdap Booster	___	___	___	___	___
11–18 years: Meningococcus	___	___	___	___	___

11–18 years: *(Have additional tetanus booster for contaminated wounds more than 5 years after last booster.)*

	Date	Date	Date	Date	Date
T(d)	___	___	___	___	___
Over 65 or with a chronic illness					
Influenza (yearly)	___	___	___	___	___
PPV (once only)	___	___	___	___	___

DTaP: Diphtheria, tetanus, acellular pertussis; **Hepatitis A/B**: Hepatitis A/B; **HIB**: Hemophilus influenza type B; **Influenza**: Flu; **IPV**: Inactivated Polio-virus; **MMR**: Measles, Mumps, Rubella (German measles, three-day measles); **PCV**: Pneumococcal conjugate vaccine; **PPSV**: Pneumococcal polysaccharide vaccine; **Tdap**: Tetanus and adult diphtheria; **Varicella**: Chicken pox

PART IV

Appendixes

Taking Care of Yourself in an Age of Uncertain Risks

A Perspective on Disasters

You need to maintain perspective, an even and consistent approach to risks, a demeanor of confidence, and honest discussions with children; discussion should be aimed at what your child is capable of understanding. You need to have a family plan for a mass-exposure scenario. As with other problems in this book, you can have a certain level of personal control, decide on rational action, and use personal responsibility to reduce chances of illness.

It is good to know what to do. But the chance you will need the advice provided here is very small. Use your concern about threats to health to plan to avoid larger risks, such as smoking cigarettes, not exercising, poor diet, and taking risks while driving. Be consistent in how you approach risks; take care of the biggest ones first.

After the World Trade Center attacks of September 11, 2001, the subsequent mail-based anthrax attacks, and other acts of terror worldwide, many remarked that the world had changed forever and that we would, from now on, live in a climate of fear. Widespread emotional effects were reported in adults and children alike. The need for an expanded role for personal responsibility was apparent: a need for calm appraisal, wise counsel, and planning for the future.

The world has "changed forever" before. Part of parental wisdom comes from our experiences with the past. The world changed after Hiroshima with the proliferation of nuclear weapons. It changed with the epidemic of HIV/AIDS. These were bad changes, yet at some point, we stopped building bomb shelters. We adapted to these large but remote risks, and the positive aspects of life grew and flourished.

At this writing, the risk of international attacks is again upon us; urban gun violence is an ongoing plague; there are new viruses and prescribed medications that can lead to fatal addiction.

What Are the Risks of Mass Disasters?

We have trouble understanding risks, and we fear risks that seem catastrophic and uncontrollable. We fear risks that are new to us and that have a high "dread factor." We live with little fear of riding in automobiles despite the fact that 35,000 Americans die in accidents each year. We buckle seat belts, drive with care, and avoid driving impaired or riding with an impaired driver, but the risks are still there and largely not under our control. So it is clear that we can be comfortable with substantial risk. Many still smoke cigarettes, apparently without fear, although smoking kills 400,000 people in the United States each year. We fear earthquakes and tornados out of proportion to their actual risk. We fear great white sharks more than smoking in bed. Contradictory approaches to personal risks are the rule rather than the exception.

Terrorism risks have been much lower than our everyday risks, even though each of the several thousand terrorism deaths is an individual tragedy. Quite likely, if we could put all of the effort against domestic terrorism into reducing cigarette smoking, we could save hundreds of thousands of lives.

The underlying fear of terrorism is that a massive attack with an agent such as anthrax, a dirty atomic bomb, or a chemical gas could cause a large number of casualties. These scenarios are possible, but unlikely. These agents are hard to make and to deliver, and the casualties are largely preventable. The anthrax attacks in 2001 were dealt with quite efficiently even with an unprepared public health system, and future attacks will evoke a faster and better response. The basic rule is: reduce your most likely health risks first! Make your personal inventory of major health risks and cross them off one by one as you eliminate them. Take care of yourself!

The Example of Anthrax

Anthrax is the most likely bioterror agent, and a number of attempted attacks and accidental releases from facilities have documented the nature of the threat, although most attacks, including eight separate attacks in Japan, have fizzled. Some worst-case casualty estimates have projected hundreds of thousands of deaths. These assumed an airborne release of a large quantity of anthrax spores upwind of a large population area where everybody was outside and nobody had antibiotics.

Anthrax spores are very small, and when milled even smaller, they can get into the lungs. The spores can then germinate and the bacteria multiply; after a few days, they produce toxins that are usually fatal. It takes 5,000 or so spores to cause illness. Treatment is usually effective if begun before the toxins are formed. Prevention by use of antibiotics before actual infection occurs is highly effective. A vaccine is available but is cumbersome, has some side effects, and takes two weeks for early effectiveness and 18 months for full effectiveness.

The recommended public health response in a "contained casualty" anthrax situation has been to begin antibiotics after exposure if the chance of infection developing is greater than about 1 in 1,000. None of the exposed postal workers put on antibiotics in late 2001 got the disease, but it is not known how many would have developed illness without the antibiotics. The general exposure rule has been to treat if there has been (1) exposure to documented anthrax or (2) exposure to the same environment as a person who has tested positive for anthrax or developed illness from anthrax. Absent these criteria, the physician is advised to make a decision based on how credible an unproven exposure is and what the likelihood is that a given set of signs and symptoms might represent anthrax. Very few people, of course, will meet these criteria.

The keys to cure, then, are apparent: assessment of risk, preventive antibiotics if the risk is high, symptom watch if there isn't proof of exposure, and early treatment of possible active infection.

Other Terror Agents

Smallpox is usually considered the next most likely biological threat, since population immunity is low and smallpox is very contagious. However, there are many public health measures that could contain an epidemic, and risk for a given individual should be very low. Quarantine is the oldest method of controlling smallpox epidemics. Vaccination of exposed persons is effective in 4 days, and the disease's incubation period is 12 days, so you can successfully vaccinate even after exposure. In a smallpox epidemic, well-defined procedures will be explained by public health officials through the media.

Other bioterror agents, such as plague, tularemia, botulism toxin, and hemorrhagic fevers, appear much less likely to be used.

Chemical weapons are harder to deliver effectively. Nuclear irradiation weapons, especially "dirty bombs," remain as potential, but less likely, threats. It is highly likely that, at some time, terrorism attacks will occur in the United States and around the world. The same approach applies to these attacks as to bioterrorism.

Talking with Children

Children will hear about a threat or an attack and will often have inaccurate information. They pick up clues that suggest fear in their parents. You need to talk with them, for reassurance and about preparation.

Children under five often pick up bits and pieces. There may be increased clinginess or changes in sleeping or eating patterns. Ask them what they have heard. Be aware of what they are seeing on television and avoid live broadcasts.

Children aged six to eight may also show regressive behavior, emotional disturbance, and firmly held opinions: "This food may have anthrax in it." Try not to directly confront such statements but offer solid facts: "Anthrax is not catching." Keep television and Internet, including social media, to a minimum. Ask them what they can do to be safer. Make them part of the plan.

Children aged nine to eleven may become obsessed with details. They may wonder why someone would do a thing like that. They may have rigid opinions about risks that are not real. They may have nightmares. They are often receptive to reassurance. Keep television and Internet to a minimum.

Children twelve and over are likely to keep any thoughts to themselves. They may use a form of denial. You may need to introduce the subject as one for easy conversation, and you may need to do this every few days. Ask: "What is new?" "What does it mean?" "Do you think that this is a problem for us?"

The most important thing is to show control of your own fears. Parenting is experience, calmness, reassurance, and preparedness.

Family Defense Against Anthrax

Preparation

Your need for advance preparation is guided by the likelihood of a mass exposure that will overwhelm medical facilities in the area for some time. For most people who do not live in a likely target area, no preparation is needed.

Imagine the air containing aerosolized spores, an emergency room with thousands of people in line, an illness that can progress in hours, and relatively limited supplies of antibiotics in the immediate area. This mass-exposure scenario is the only situation in which you should begin antibiotic prevention by yourself at home from your emergency supply.

Authorities differ in their views on individuals having their own antibiotic supplies. Some believe that individuals cannot make informed decisions on their own, some are concerned that there could be an antibiotic shortage if everyone stocks up, and some fear an increase in the problem of antibiotic resistance. We believe that it is not unreasonable for families in metropolitan areas to consider maintaining a small antibiotic supply for use by the family unit in the initial week of an emergency.

What antibiotics do you need? Doxycycline and Ciprofloxacin (Cipro) are the preferred options. For children, Cipro is the recommended choice for initial treatment, despite some fears of possible arthritis. Doxycycline can cause mottling of teeth in children under age nine and may slow skeletal growth in infants.

The problem of indiscriminate antibiotic use, which is a real problem, is not affected by a small emergency pack. You do not need a large supply; the system will be back in order in a few days and a small supply for the family is enough.

You can certainly discuss this issue with your physician at your next regularly scheduled appointment. Be sure that you describe any drug allergies. If the decision is made to prescribe medicines, set these antibiotics aside and do not use them for anything else. Discard when outdated.

Depending on the circumstances, you are likely to get official recommendations for preventive antibiotics over the media, which you should follow. If your family's chances of significant exposure are remote, the recommendation may be not to use antibiotics. If antibiotics are not recommended over the media, do not take them. If you do not receive official recommendations, you may have to make the decision on your own.

What Else?

Reduce the amount of any possible exposure. Use the inside/outside rule. If the spores are inside, as with mailed envelopes, get outside. If the aerosol is outside, get inside. In a car, circulate the ventilation inside the car and keep windows closed. Under some circumstances, a visit to the emergency room may increase exposure, either on the trip or in the ER. Close up the house as best you can and plan to stay put for a couple of days. You can keep a supply of surgical masks around; get the kind that keep out 95% of particles. Listen to the radio for tips and advice. Washing hands and face, overall bathing, and washing of or discarding possible contaminated clothing can also reduce exposure. Remember, if you can dilute your exposure, you may not be exposed to enough spores to cause illness. The same principles apply to radiation exposure.

Additional Reading

Books

American College of Obstetrics and Gynecologists. *Planning for Pregnancy, Birth, and Beyond.* Washington, DC, 1999.

Fries, J. F. *Arthritis: A Take Care of Yourself Health Guide,* 5th ed. Cambridge, MA: Perseus Books, 1999.

Fries, J. F. *Living Well,* 3rd ed. Cambridge, MA: Perseus Books, 2004.

Fries, J. F., and L. M. Crapo. *Vitality and Aging.* San Francisco: W. H. Freeman, 1981.

Lorig, K., et al. *Living a Healthy Life with Chronic Conditions.* Palo Alto, CA: Bull Publishing, 2006.

Lorig, K., and J. F. Fries. *The Arthritis Helpbook,* 6th ed. Cambridge, MA: Perseus Books, 2006.

Pantell, R. H., J. F. Fries, and D. M. Vickery. *Taking Care of Your Child,* 6th ed. Cambridge, MA: Perseus Books, 2005.

Vickery, D. M. *Taking Part: A Consumer's Guide to the Hospital.* Reston, VA: The Center for Corporate Health Promotion, Inc., 1986.

Vickery, D. M. *Lifeplan: Your Personal Guide to Maintaining Health and Preventing Illness.* Reston, VA: Vicktor, 1990.

Articles

Allaire, S. H., et al. "Evidence for Decline in Disability and Improved Health Among Persons Aged 55 to 70 Years: The Framingham Heart Study." *American Journal Public Health* 89 (1999): 1678–1683.

Chakravarty, E. F., H. B. Hubert, V. B. Lingala, and J. F. Fries. "Reduced Disability and Mortality Among Aging Runners." *Archives of Internal Medicine* 168 (2008): 1638–1646.

Chakravarty, E. F., H. B. Hubert, V. B. Lingala, E. Zatarain, and J. F. Fries. "Long Distance Running and Knee Osteoarthritis:

A Prospective Study." *American Journal of Preventive Medicine* 35 (2008): 133–138.

Fries, J. F. "Aging, Natural Death, and the Compression of Morbidity." *New England Journal of Medicine* 303 (1980): 130–135.

Fries, J. F. "Compression of Morbidity: Near or Far?" *Milbank Quarterly* 67 (1990): 208–32.

Fries, J. F., D. A. Bloch, H. Harrington, N. Richardson, and R. Beck. "Two-Year Results of a Randomized Controlled Trial of a Health Promotion Program in a Retiree Population: The Bank of America Study." *American Journal of Medicine* 94 (1993): 455–462.

Fries, J. F., S. T. Fries, C. L. Parcell, and H. Harrington. "Health Risk Changes with a Low-Cost Individualized Health Promotion Program: Effects at Up to 30 Months." *American Journal of Health Promotion* 6 (1992): 364–371.

Fries, J. F., H. Harrington, R. Edwards, L. A. Kent, and N. Richardson. "Randomized Controlled Trial of Cost Reductions from a Health Education Program: The California Public Employees' Retirement System (PERS) Study." *American Journal of Health Promotion* 8 (1994): 216–223.

Fries, J. F., C. E. Koop, et al. "Beyond Health Promotion: Reducing Need and Demand for Medical Care." *Health Affairs* 17 (1998): 70–84.

Fries, J. F., C. E. Koop, C. E. Beadle, P. P. Cooper, M. J. England, R. F. Greaves, J. J. Sokolov, D. Wright, and The Health Project Consortium. "Reducing Health Care Costs by Reducing the Need and Demand for Medical Services." *New England Journal of Medicine* 329 (1993): 321–325.

Fries, J. F., and D. McShane. "Reducing Need and Demand for Medical Services in High Risk Persons: A Health Education Approach." *Western Journal of Medicine* 169 (1998): 201–207.

Fries, J. F., G. Singh, D. Morfeld, H. B. Hubert, N. E. Lane, and B. W. Brown. "Running and the Development of Disability with Age." *Annals of Internal Medicine* 121 (1994): 502–509.

Lorig, K., R. G. Kraines, B. W. Brown, and N. Richardson. "A Workplace Health Education Program Which Reduces Outpatient Visits." *Medical Care* 23 (1985): 1044–1054.

Swartz, A. "Faces of Public Health: James Fries, Healthy Aging Pioneer." *American Journal of Public Health* 98 (2008): 1163–1166.

Vickery, D. M. "Medical Self-Care: A Review of the Concept and Program Models." *American Journal of Health Promotion* 1 (1986): 23–28.

Vickery, D. M., and T. Golaszewski. "A Preliminary Study on the Timeliness of Ambulatory Care Utilization Following Medical Self-Care Interventions." *American Journal of Health Promotion* 3 (Winter 1989): 26–31.

Vickery, D. M., T. Golaszewski, et al. "Lifestyle and Organizational Health Insurance Costs." *Journal of Occupational Medicine* 28 (Nov. 1986): 1165–1168.

Vickery, D. M., T. Golaszewski, et al. "The Effect of Self-Care Interventions on the Use of Medical Service Within a Medicare Population." *Medical Care* (June 1988): 580–588.

Vickery, D. M., H. Kalmer, D. Lowry, M. Constantine, E. Wright, and W. Loren. "Effect of a Self-Care Education Program on Medical Visits." *Journal of the American Medical Society* 250 (1983): 2952–2956.

Vita, A. J., R. B. Terry, H. B. Hubert, and J. F. Fries. "Aging, Health Risks, and Cumulative Disability." *New England Journal of Medicine* 338 (1998): 1035–1041.

References (Chapter 1)

Chakravarty, E. F., H. B. Hubert, V. B Lingala, and J. F. Fries. "Reduced Disability and Mortality Among Aging Runners." *Archives of Internal Medicine* 168 (2008): 1638–1646.

Fries, J. F. "Aging, Natural Death, and the Compression of Morbidity." Special Article. *New England Journal of Medicine* 303 (1980): 130–135.

Fries, J. F. "The Theory and Practice of Active Aging." *Current Gerontology and Geriatric Research* (2012): 420637.

Fries, J. F. "Perspectives on the Conventional Wisdom." *Arthritis & Rheumatology* (November 2015): 2806–2812.

Fries J. F., B. Bruce, and E. Chakravarty. "Compression of Morbidity 1980–2011: A Focused Review of Paradigms and Progress." *Journal of Aging Research* (August 2011): 1–10.

Fries, J. F., P. W. Spitz, R. G. Kraines, and H. R. Holman. "Measurement of Patient Outcome in Arthritis." *Arthritis & Rheumatology* 23 (1980): 137–145.

Gompertz, B. *On the Nature of the Law of Human Mortality.* Royal Society of London, 1825.

Vita A. J., R. B. Terry, H. B. Hubert, and J. F. Fries. "Aging, Health Risks, and Cumulative Disability." Special Article. *New England Journal of Medicine* 338 (1998): 1035–1041.

Guinessworldrecords.com 76–78, 2017.

About the Authors

James F. Fries, MD

Dr. Fries is Professor Emeritus of Medicine at Stanford University and is internationally recognized as a leader in strategies to postpone the disabilities of aging, long-term outcome assessment, self-care, and longitudinal studies of human aging. He has published over 450 peer-reviewed articles having over 58,000 citations and authored eleven books.

In 1980 he developed the Compression of Morbidity hypothesis that preventive measures have a greater effect upon morbidity than upon mortality and that chronic diseases with onset later in life will be present for a shorter time. On this thesis he has twice addressed the Nobel Forum and twice the Institute of Medicine; editorialized and been profiled in the *American Journal of Public Health*; and presented a policy paper in *Health Affairs* and a Special Article in the *New England Journal of Medicine*.

Dr. Fries established the ARAMIS Chronic Disease databank system as an NIH program in 1975 and guided it through 33 years and over 1,000 scientific papers. He plays an important role in The Health Project, a private-public organization that seeks solutions to health care through reduction in medical need.

In 1976 Dr. Fries and Dr. Donald Vickery pioneered use of self-management algorithms to help patients toward better health decisions with *Take Care of Yourself,* now with 15 million copies in print. Four randomized controlled trials documented the effectiveness of *Take Care of Yourself* in reducing the need for physician visits. Dr. Fries also authored or coauthored *Living Well* for seniors, *The Arthritis Helpbook*, and *Arthritis: A Comprehensive Guide*.

For the past 25 years the James F. and Sarah T. Fries Foundation has annually awarded the Fries Prize for Improving Health (working with the CDC Foundation) and the Elizabeth Fries Health Education Award (working with the Society of Public Health Educators, SOPHE). The former goes to that individual judged to have done the most to improve health (see friesfoundation.org) and the latter for the greatest contribution to health education. The Foundation also has endowed the Fries Chair in Medicine at

Johns Hopkins for Lisa Cooper to examine disparities in cardiovascular health.

Dr. Fries lives with his wife of 58 years, Sarah, a horse, Harlequin Joker, and a Labrador Retriever, Princess, in Woodside, California. He has run the Boston Marathon and has climbed the highest mountain on all seven continents, summiting six. Sarah, despite serious disabilities from an active melanoma that confine her to a wheelchair, has been to all the latitudes and longitudes and all of the continents, and has explored in Antarctica, Patagonia, Svalbard, Greenland, Alaska, Burma, Tibet, Brazil, Cuba, Madagascar, and South Africa, among over 30 other wheelchair adventures. Sarah is a heroine to a lot of folks, including Jim.

Donald M. Vickery, MD

In Memoriam

Don Vickery died on November 22, 2008, at his home in Evergreen, Colorado, after a brief battle with a relentless cancer and is sorely missed by all of us who loved him. Don made major and legendary contributions to human health and improved millions of lives. He made a difference. He was the pioneering force behind "demand management" concepts and programs, showing that consumer-directed medical decision-making could improve health and reduce the need for medical care expenditures. He founded the Center for Consumer Health Education, now known as the Self-Care Institute, and Health Decisions International.

He concentrated on wellness rather than illness, prevention more than cure, and the power of the patient over that of the doctor. Throughout, he worked successfully to establish new concepts of prevention through lifestyle changes and wise consumer decisions on a base of solid scientific evidence. He authored and coauthored self-care books to bring wise decision-making to the public and also self-care articles for the health care professions. He was an original thinker, an extraordinary scholar, and a forceful advocate for better health for all.

Don trained at Harvard and Stanford Universities, was Board Certified in Internal Medicine, and was a Fellow of the American College of Physicians. He worked closely with Partnership for Prevention and the American College of Preventive Medicine, of which he was also a Fellow. He had an easy wit and a fine ironic sense of humor. He was easy to be with, motivating to talk with, and a pleasure to work with. This book, which he coauthored through eight editions for over 33 years and 20 million copies, remains a substantial part of his legacy.

Index

For advice on a common medical problem, look up the primary symptom in this index. Entries and numbers in **boldface** indicate where you can find the most information on each subject. These are usually the pages with decision charts and advice on home treatment and when to see a doctor.

911, calling, 78

AA (Alcoholics Anonymous), 305–306
Abdominal pain, 272–273
  nausea and vomiting, 266–267
Abdominal-thrust (Heimlich) maneuver, 82–85
Abrasions, 94–95
Abscess, in throat, 128
Absorbable antacids, 59–60
Abstinence, periodic (birth control), 331–332
Accidental injuries, 24–26
Acetaminophen, 54
  for children and adolescents, 164, 218
  dosage and side effects, 55
  liquid, 48, 55
  safety of, 55
  for sore throat, 128
Acne, 168–169, 170–171, **192–193**
Activities of Daily Living (ADLs), 35
Acyclovir, 326

Addiction. *See* Alcoholism; Drug abuse
Adhesive bandages, 50–52, 94
Adhesive tape, 48, 50–52
Adolescents
  Alateen for, 305–306
  aspirin hazard for, 54, 56, 127, 128, 130, 212, 214, 216, 220, 222, 286
  asthma in, 142
  immunizations for, 213
  Reye's syndrome, 54–56, 130, 214, 216, 220
  sore throat in, 128
  steroid use among, 308
  suicide and, 26
Adults
  choking treatments for, 83
  hoarseness, 144–145
  immunizations of (table), 32
  recommended screenings for (table), 28
  shingles, 215
Aerobic (endurance) exercise, 6, 7–12
Aging, six keys to health and, 5–34
Aging spots, 210–211
Agitation, from decongestant, 65
AIDS (acquired immunodeficiency syndrome), 324, **328–329**
Air bags, 24–25
Al-Anon/Alateen, 305–306
Alcohol
  acetaminophen and, 55

delirium tremens (DTs) and, 15, 304
driving and, 15, 25
erectile dysfunction and, 333
fetal alcohol syndrome, 304
grief and, 296
hyperventilation syndrome and, 298
lightheadedness and, 292
menopause, hot flashes, and, 322
in moderation, 14–15, 19
sleep disorders and, 288
Alcoholics Anonymous (AA), 305–306
Alcoholism, 15, **304–306**
Allergic conjunctivitis, 156
Allergic rhinitis, 123–124, 126, 136, 137. *See also* Hay fever
Allergy
  bacteria and virus vs., 123–125
  home remedies for, 48
  medications for, 62–63
  no response to antibiotics, 123
  runny nose and, 126–127
Alopecia areata, 174
Ambulance, 78
Amitriptyline, 229
Anabolic steroids, 308
Anesthetic creams and sprays, 110
Angina pectoris (heart pain), 12, 13, 260–261
Animal bites, 92–93

For quick access to your chapter, open to the appropriate tab.

For recommendations on a healthy lifestyle for you, Chapter 1

For advice on your Home Medicine Chest, Chapter 2

Common Injuries, Chapter 4

Ear, Nose, Throat, Eye, and Mouth Problems, Chapter 5

Skin Problems, Chapter 6

Childhood Diseases, Chapter 7

Bones, Muscles, and Joints, Chapter 8

Chest, Abdominal, and Urinary Problems, Chapter 9

Generalized Problems, such as fever, stress, or addiction, Chapter 10

Women's Health, Chapter 11

Sexual Problems and Questions, Chapter 12

Emergencies (Chapter 3)

Does the person show any of these emergency signs?
▲ Major injury
▲ No pulse or breath
▲ Unconsciousness
▲ Active bleeding
▲ Stupor or drowsiness
▲ Disorientation
▲ Shortness of breath while resting
▲ Cold sweats
▲ Severe pain

Yes

Emergency
Go to the emergency room or call 911 for help immediately. Turn to page 79, in the black-edged pages, for more instructions.

No

Is the person choking and unable to speak or cry out?

Yes

Emergency
Turn to page 82.

No

Has the person swallowed poison?

Yes

Emergency
Turn to page 86.

No

NONEMERGENCY
Identify the type of problem and turn to the beginning of the chapter with the corresponding blue tab on the edge of the book. Or look up the problem in the index or the table of contents.